# Plastic and Reconstructive Surgery in Personalized Medicine

# Plastic and Reconstructive Surgery in Personalized Medicine

Editors

**Andreas Arkudas**
**Raymund E. Horch**

MDPI • Basel • Beijing • Wuhan • Barcelona • Belgrade • Manchester • Tokyo • Cluj • Tianjin

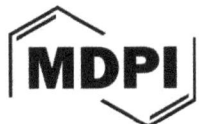

*Editors*
Andreas Arkudas
Department of Plastic and
Hand Surgery
Friedrich Alexander University
Erlangen-Nuremberg FAU
Erlangen
Germany

Raymund E. Horch
Department of Plastic and
Hand Surgery
Friedrich Alexander University
Erlangen-Nuernberg FAU
Erlangen
Germany

*Editorial Office*
MDPI
St. Alban-Anlage 66
4052 Basel, Switzerland

This is a reprint of articles from the Special Issue published online in the open access journal *Journal of Personalized Medicine* (ISSN 2075-4426) (available at: www.mdpi.com/journal/jpm/special_issues/plastic_reconstructive).

For citation purposes, cite each article independently as indicated on the article page online and as indicated below:

LastName, A.A.; LastName, B.B.; LastName, C.C. Article Title. *Journal Name* **Year**, *Volume Number*, Page Range.

**ISBN 978-3-0365-7953-5 (Hbk)**
**ISBN 978-3-0365-7952-8 (PDF)**

© 2023 by the authors. Articles in this book are Open Access and distributed under the Creative Commons Attribution (CC BY) license, which allows users to download, copy and build upon published articles, as long as the author and publisher are properly credited, which ensures maximum dissemination and a wider impact of our publications.

The book as a whole is distributed by MDPI under the terms and conditions of the Creative Commons license CC BY-NC-ND.

# Contents

**About the Editors** . . . . . . . . . . . . . . . . . . . . . . . . . . . . . . . . . . . . . . . . . . . . . . . . . . . . . . . . . . . . . . ix

**Preface to "Plastic and Reconstructive Surgery in Personalized Medicine"** . . . . . . . . . . . . xi

**Raymund E. Horch and Andreas Arkudas**
Special Issue "Plastic and Reconstructive Surgery in Personalized Medicine"
Reprinted from: *J. Pers. Med.* **2023**, *13*, 569, doi:10.3390/jpm13030569 . . . . . . . . . . . . . . . . . 1

**Jasmin S. Gruener, Raymund E. Horch, Alexander Geierlehner, Wibke Mueller-Seubert, Aijia Cai and Andreas Arkudas et al.**
Is Instillational Topical Negative Pressure Wound Therapy in Peri-Prosthetic Infections of the Breast Effective? A Pilot Study
Reprinted from: *J. Pers. Med.* **2022**, *12*, 2054, doi:10.3390/jpm12122054 . . . . . . . . . . . . . . . . 5

**Theresa Promny, Chiara-Sophia Kutz, Tina Jost, Luitpold V. Distel, Sheetal Kadam and Rafael Schmid et al.**
An In Vitro Approach for Investigating the Safety of Lipotransfer after Breast-Conserving Therapy
Reprinted from: *J. Pers. Med.* **2022**, *12*, 1284, doi:10.3390/jpm12081284 . . . . . . . . . . . . . . . . 17

**Elias Polykandriotis, Jonas Daenicke, Anil Bolat, Jasmin Grüner, Dirk W. Schubert and Raymund E. Horch**
Individualized Wound Closure—Mechanical Properties of Suture Materials
Reprinted from: *J. Pers. Med.* **2022**, *12*, 1041, doi:10.3390/jpm12071041 . . . . . . . . . . . . . . . . 33

**Hanna Luze, Sebastian Philipp Nischwitz, Paul Wurzer, Raimund Winter, Stephan Spendel and Lars-Peter Kamolz et al.**
Assessment of Mastectomy Skin Flaps for Immediate Reconstruction with Implants via Thermal Imaging—A Suitable, Personalized Approach?
Reprinted from: *J. Pers. Med.* **2022**, *12*, 740, doi:10.3390/jpm12050740 . . . . . . . . . . . . . . . . . 45

**Katharina Frank, Armin Ströbel, Ingo Ludolph, Theresa Hauck, Matthias S. May and Justus P. Beier et al.**
Improving the Safety of DIEP Flap Transplantation: Detailed Perforator Anatomy Study Using Preoperative CTA [†]
Reprinted from: *J. Pers. Med.* **2022**, *12*, 701, doi:10.3390/jpm12050701 . . . . . . . . . . . . . . . . . 55

**Chih-Kai Hsu, Rafael Denadai, Chun-Shin Chang, Chuan-Fong Yao, Ying-An Chen and Pang-Yun Chou et al.**
The Number of Surgical Interventions and Specialists Involved in the Management of Patients with Neurofibromatosis Type I: A 25-Year Analysis
Reprinted from: *J. Pers. Med.* **2022**, *12*, 558, doi:10.3390/jpm12040558 . . . . . . . . . . . . . . . . . 69

**Denis Ehrl, Nikolaus Wachtel, David Braig, Constanze Kuhlmann, Hans Roland Dürr and Christian P. Schneider et al.**
Defect Coverage after Forequarter Amputation—A Systematic Review Assessing Different Surgical Approaches
Reprinted from: *J. Pers. Med.* **2022**, *12*, 560, doi:10.3390/jpm12040560 . . . . . . . . . . . . . . . . . 79

**Alexander Geierlehner, Raymund E. Horch, Ingo Ludolph and Andreas Arkudas**
Intraoperative Blood Flow Analysis of DIEP vs. ms-TRAM Flap Breast Reconstruction Combining Transit-Time Flowmetry and Microvascular Indocyanine Green Angiography
Reprinted from: *J. Pers. Med.* **2022**, *12*, 482, doi:10.3390/jpm12030482 . . . . . . . . . . . . . . . . . 95

**Aijia Cai, Zengming Zheng, Wibke Müller-Seubert, Jonas Biggemann, Tobias Fey and Justus P. Beier et al.**
Microsurgical Transplantation of Pedicled Muscles in an Isolation Chamber—A Novel Approach to Engineering Muscle Constructs via Perfusion-Decellularization
Reprinted from: *J. Pers. Med.* **2022**, *12*, 442, doi:10.3390/jpm12030442 . . . . . . . . . . . . . . . **107**

**Amir Khosrow Bigdeli, Florian Falkner, Benjamin Thomas, Gabriel Hundeshagen, Simon Andreas Mayer and Eva-Maria Risse et al.**
The Free Myocutaneous Tensor Fasciae Latae Flap—A Workhorse Flap for Sternal Defect Reconstruction: A Single-Center Experience
Reprinted from: *J. Pers. Med.* **2022**, *12*, 427, doi:10.3390/jpm12030427 . . . . . . . . . . . . . . . **123**

**Wibke Müller-Seubert, Patrick Ostermaier, Raymund E. Horch, Luitpold Distel, Benjamin Frey and Aijia Cai et al.**
Intra- and Early Postoperative Evaluation of Malperfused Areas in an Irradiated Random Pattern Skin Flap Model Using Indocyanine Green Angiography and Near-Infrared Reflectance-Based Imaging and Infrared Thermography
Reprinted from: *J. Pers. Med.* **2022**, *12*, 237, doi:10.3390/jpm12020237 . . . . . . . . . . . . . . . **133**

**Amir K. Bigdeli, Oliver Didzun, Benjamin Thomas, Leila Harhaus, Emre Gazyakan and Raymund E. Horch et al.**
Combined versus Single Perforator Propeller Flaps for Reconstruction of Large Soft Tissue Defects: A Retrospective Clinical Study
Reprinted from: *J. Pers. Med.* **2022**, *12*, 41, doi:10.3390/jpm12010041 . . . . . . . . . . . . . . . . . **145**

**Khaled Dastagir, Doha Obed, Florian Bucher, Thurid Hofmann, Katharina I. Koyro and Peter M. Vogt**
Non-Invasive and Surgical Modalities for Scar Management: A Clinical Algorithm
Reprinted from: *J. Pers. Med.* **2021**, *11*, 1259, doi:10.3390/jpm11121259 . . . . . . . . . . . . . . . **157**

**Johannes C. Heinzel, Lucy F. Dadun, Cosima Prahm, Natalie Winter, Michael Bressler and Henrik Lauer et al.**
Beyond the Knife—Reviewing the Interplay of Psychosocial Factors and Peripheral Nerve Lesions
Reprinted from: *J. Pers. Med.* **2021**, *11*, 1200, doi:10.3390/jpm11111200 . . . . . . . . . . . . . . . **173**

**Isabel Zucal, Sebastian Geis, Lukas Prantl, Silke Haerteis and Thiha Aung**
Indocyanine Green for Leakage Control in Isolated Limb Perfusion
Reprinted from: *J. Pers. Med.* **2021**, *11*, 1152, doi:10.3390/jpm11111152 . . . . . . . . . . . . . . . **189**

**Daniel G. E. Thiem, Paul Römer, Sebastian Blatt, Bilal Al-Nawas and Peer W. Kämmerer**
New Approach to the Old Challenge of Free Flap Monitoring—Hyperspectral Imaging Outperforms Clinical Assessment by Earlier Detection of Perfusion Failure
Reprinted from: *J. Pers. Med.* **2021**, *11*, 1101, doi:10.3390/jpm11111101 . . . . . . . . . . . . . . . **199**

**Raymund E. Horch, Ingo Ludolph, Andreas Arkudas and Aijia Cai**
Personalized Reconstruction of Genital Defects in Complicated Wounds with Vertical Rectus Abdominis Myocutaneous Flaps including Urethral Neo-Orifice
Reprinted from: *J. Pers. Med.* **2021**, *11*, 1076, doi:10.3390/jpm11111076 . . . . . . . . . . . . . . . **213**

**Johannes Maximilian Wagner, Victoria Grolewski, Felix Reinkemeier, Marius Drysch, Sonja Verena Schmidt and Mehran Dadras et al.**
Posttraumatic Lymphedema after Open Fractures of the Lower Extremity—A Retrospective Cohort Analysis
Reprinted from: *J. Pers. Med.* **2021**, *11*, 1077, doi:10.3390/jpm11111077 . . . . . . . . . . . . . . . **223**

**Sebastian P. Nischwitz, Hanna Luze, Marlies Schellnegger, Simon J. Gatterer, Alexandru-Cristian Tuca and Raimund Winter et al.**
Thermal, Hyperspectral, and Laser Doppler Imaging: Non-Invasive Tools for Detection of the Deep Inferior Epigastric Artery Perforators—A Prospective Comparison Study
Reprinted from: *J. Pers. Med.* **2021**, *11*, 1005, doi:10.3390/jpm11101005 . . . . . . . . . . . . . . . . . **231**

**Alexis Combal, François Thuau, Alban Fouasson-Chailloux, Pierre-Paul Arrigoni, Marc Baud'huin and Franck Duteille et al.**
Preliminary Results of the "Capasquelet" Technique for Managing Femoral Bone Defects—Combining a Masquelet Induced Membrane and Capanna Vascularized Fibula with an Allograft
Reprinted from: *J. Pers. Med.* **2021**, *11*, 774, doi:10.3390/jpm11080774 . . . . . . . . . . . . . . . . . **245**

**Diana Heimes, Philipp Becker, Daniel G. E. Thiem, Robert Kuchen, Solomiya Kyyak and Peer W. Kämmerer**
Is Hyperspectral Imaging Suitable for Assessing Collateral Circulation Prior Radial Forearm Free Flap Harvesting? Comparison of Hyperspectral Imaging and Conventional Allen's Test
Reprinted from: *J. Pers. Med.* **2021**, *11*, 531, doi:10.3390/jpm11060531 . . . . . . . . . . . . . . . . . **255**

**Yao-Kuang Huang, Min Yi Wong, Chi-Rung Wu, Yung-Ze Cheng and Bor-Shyh Lin**
Free Myocutaneous Flap Assessment in a Rat Model: Verification of a Wireless Bioelectrical Impedance Assessment (BIA) System for Vascular Compromise Following Microsurgery
Reprinted from: *J. Pers. Med.* **2021**, *11*, 373, doi:10.3390/jpm11050373 . . . . . . . . . . . . . . . . . **271**

# About the Editors

**Andreas Arkudas**

Prof. Dr. Andreas Arkudas is a Professor of Plastic and Hand Surgery with board certifications in Plastic and Aesthetic Surgery, Hand Surgery, and General Surgery. He has published numerous scientific papers. His current Hirsch factor is 35.

**Raymund E. Horch**

Univ. Prof. Dr. med. Prof.h.c. Dr.h.c. Raymund E. Horch is a Professor of Plastic and Hand Surgery with board certifications in Plastic and Aesthetic Surgery, Hand Surgery, and General Surgery. He is the Director and Chairman of the Department of Plastic and Hand Surgery and Head of the Laboratory for Tissue Engineering and Regenerative Medicine, University Hospital Erlangen, Friedrich-Alexander University Erlangen-Nuermberg FAU in Germany, where he has been officially appointed as a tenured Professor since January 2003.

He has received numerous prestigious scientific awards and merits, including honorary doctorates and professorships, and was appointed as a honorary member of the Romanian Academy of Science, served as the President of the German Society of Plastic Reconstructive and Aesthetic Surgeons, and in the presidium of the German Society of Surgery DGCH. Since 2010, he has been a spokesman of all Surgical Departments of the University Hospital Erlangen and a vice speaker at the SFBTRR 225 Biofabrication. Clinically, he covers Plastic and Hand Surgery entirely, including Aesthetic Surgery and Microsurgery. His main research interests are tissue engineering, biofabrication, microsurgery, and wound healing. He has published numerous scientific papers, several books (currently >500 PubMed listed peer-reviewed publications and >250 non-peer-reviewed publications, book editions, and book chapters, reviews etc.). His current Hirsch factor is 43.

# Preface to "Plastic and Reconstructive Surgery in Personalized Medicine"

This Special Issue of the *Journal of Personalized Medicine* covers several trending topics, such as individualized microsurgery, flap imaging, customized perforator flaps, monitoring flap perfusion, tailored tissue engineering for reconstruction, and biofabrication applications in personalized plastic and reconstructive surgery. It also includes research into the background of what plastic surgeons do and how the science behind our operative treatments may alter or influence future developments. This Special Issue demonstrates how scientific research and clinical alertness and experience together further our ability to help aid patients with reconstructive problems.

In summary, this Special Issue shows an impressive broad spectrum of high-level clinical and basic scientific research which is currently ongoing in the field. The compilation of multiple surgical techniques, innovative imaging, and research tools is highly recommended for anybody interested in advances and updates on contemporary plastic and reconstructive surgery. It also impressively highlights that plastic surgery is definitely a trending topic, from more general to highly personalized approaches.

**Andreas Arkudas and Raymund E. Horch**
*Editors*

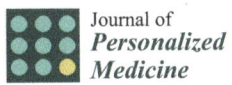 

*Editorial*

# Special Issue "Plastic and Reconstructive Surgery in Personalized Medicine"

Raymund E. Horch *  and Andreas Arkudas

Department of Plastic and Hand Surgery and Laboratory for Tissue Engineering and Regenerative Medicine, University Hospital Erlangen, Friedrich Alexander University Erlangen-Nuernberg FAU, Krankenhausstrasse 12, 91054 Erlangen, Germany
* Correspondence: raymund.horch@uk-erlangen.de

With an ever-growing knowledge in various disciplines of medicine and with rapidly evolving new techniques and operative methods in plastic surgery, it is obvious that it becomes more and more difficult to keep up with all the developments in this field at any time. Despite a plethora of scientific literature in various media, we felt that a Special Issue on the trending topics in plastic and reconstructive surgery could help to gain an overview of the recent advances in the field. We have therefore attempted to bundle the latest research and clinical data in a Special Issue on plastic and reconstructive surgery which, as such, offers a broad spectrum of different contemporary reconstructive techniques, including split skin transplantation and local as well as free flaps. Due to worldwide increasing expertise today, by means of microsurgery and perforator flaps, almost every reconstructive issue can be addressed somehow utilizing individually tailored techniques. Flaps can by their very nature comprise different tissues and can be custom designed using new imaging technologies [1–3] in order to increase the safety of the procedures and to retain the form and function of the reconstructed area in accordance with the donor site morbidity [4], as well as to reduce complications [5]. Automated devices—such as topical negative pressure application—to clean and precondition complex wounds and make them suitable for flap or skin graft coverage have found their way into daily clinical practice [2]. As with other developments of the specialty, the ingenuity of plastic surgeons leads to a continuous further evolution, and improvements of such technical tools are subject to sustained improvement and new indications. Additionally, given the modern armamentarium of surgical options today, approaches can be adjusted to increasingly personalized surgical treatment.

This issue of the Journal of Personalized Medicine covers several trending topics, such as individualized microsurgery, flap imaging, customized perforator flaps, monitoring flap perfusion, tailored tissue engineering for reconstruction, and biofabrication applications in personalized plastic and reconstructive surgery. This also includes research into the background of what plastic surgeons do and how the science behind our operative treatments may alter or influence future developments [6–9]. This Issue demonstrates how scientific research and clinical alertness and experience merge into new knowledge to further our capability to help aid patients with reconstructive problems.

In detail, Grüner et al. describe their experience with topical negative pressure therapy with instillation to cope with infected alloplastic implants in breast surgery and offer a new concept for this clinical issue [10]. Promny and coworkers discuss their findings concerning the safety of lipotransfer after breast-conserving therapy (BCT) and irradiation in breast cancer patients. They highlight that the safety of lipotransfer has still not been clarified yet due to contradictory data, and they present an innovative approach to provide more scientific data to clarify the issue [11]. Polykandriotis et al. present their research on the mechanical properties of suture materials and studies of how sutures break down under cycling loading [12]. Luze and coworkers assess the viability of skin flaps with thermal

**Citation:** Horch, R.E.; Arkudas, A. Special Issue "Plastic and Reconstructive Surgery in Personalized Medicine". *J. Pers. Med.* **2023**, *13*, 569. https://doi.org/10.3390/jpm13030569

Received: 11 March 2023
Revised: 16 March 2023
Accepted: 19 March 2023
Published: 22 March 2023

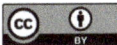

**Copyright:** © 2023 by the authors. Licensee MDPI, Basel, Switzerland. This article is an open access article distributed under the terms and conditions of the Creative Commons Attribution (CC BY) license (https:// creativecommons.org/licenses/by/ 4.0/).

imaging as a potential personalized approach [13]. Frank et al. show the improved safety of DIEP flap transplantation with a detailed perforator anatomy study [14]. Hsu et al. studied the number of surgical interventions and specialists involved in the management of patients with neurofibromatosis type I in a 25-year analysis and discuss their approach to provide comprehensive individualized care to patients with NF [15]. Geierlehner and coworkers investigated the intraoperative blood flow of DIEP vs. ms-TRAM flaps in breast reconstruction combining transit-time flowmetry and microvascular indocyanine green angiography to learn more about the various flow patterns and to establish a threshold for optimal anastomotic conditions [16]. Cai et al. successfully managed to establish a special microsurgical transplantation technique of pedicled muscles in an isolation chamber as a novel approach to engineering muscle constructs via perfusion decellularization in an animal model [17]. Bigdeli and coworkers demonstrate the value of the free myocutaneous tensor fasciae latae flap for sternal defect reconstructions in a single-center experience with a considerable number of patients [18]. In another study, they compared the use of combined versus single perforator propeller flaps for the reconstruction of large soft tissue defects in a retrospective clinical study [19]. Dastagir and coauthors describe their clinical algorithm for non-invasive and surgical modalities for scar management [20]. Müller-Seubert et al. demonstrate intra- and early postoperative evaluations of malperfused areas in an irradiated random pattern skin flap model using indocyanine green angiography and near-infrared reflectance-based imaging and infrared thermography [21]. The value of indocyanine green to control leakage in isolated limb perfusion is described as a new and effective tool by Zucal and coworkers [22]. In addition, Thiem et al. studied the value of hyperspectral imaging for the clinical assessment of free flap monitoring compared to clinical monitoring in a prospective non-randomized clinical trial [23]. Diana Heimes and coworkers also investigated hyperspectral imaging if it is suitable to assess collateral circulation prior to radial forearm free flap harvesting and compare this tool to the conventional Allen test [24]. A retrospective cohort analysis by Wagner et al. describes the detection of post-traumatic lymphedema after open fractures of the lower extremity [25].

The prospects of hyperspectral imaging are also highlighted by Nischwitz et al. who prospectively compared thermal, hyperspectral, and laser Doppler imaging as non-invasive tools to detect the deep inferior epigastric artery (DIEP) perforators [26]. On the basis of their huge experience with hundreds of pelvic reconstructions, Horch et al. described a very innovative approach using the transpelvic vertical rectus abdominis myocutaneous (VRAM) with a new modification to allow an individualized procedure, including the urethral orifice into the skin paddle of VRAM flaps (Figure 1) to circumvent urinary diversion and maintain an acceptable quality of life [27]. The use of a novel two-stage reconstruction technique for extended femoral bone defects using an allograft in accordance with the Capanna technique with an embedded vascularized fibula graft in an induced membrane according to the Masquelet technique is described by Combal and co-authors [28]. Another mode of free flap assessment is reported by Huang et al. who used a wireless bioelectrical impedance assessment system for the quantitative analysis of tissue status and potential vascular compromise following microsurgery [29]. Ehrl and co-authors address another clinically relevant problem—the challenging defect coverage after forequarter amputations—in a thorough review assessing different surgical approaches, including different flaps [30]. Adding another facete, Heinzel et al. review the interplay of psychosocial factors and peripheral nerve lesions with their carefully considered and interesting title "beyond the knife" [31].

In summary, this Special Issue shows in an impressive broad spectrum of high-level clinical and basic scientific research which is currently ongoing in the field. The present compilation of multiple surgical techniques, innovative imaging, and research tools are highly recommended for anybody interested in advances and in an update on contemporary plastic and reconstructive surgery. It also highlights in an impressive way that plastic surgery is definitely a trending topic, from more general to highly personalized approaches.

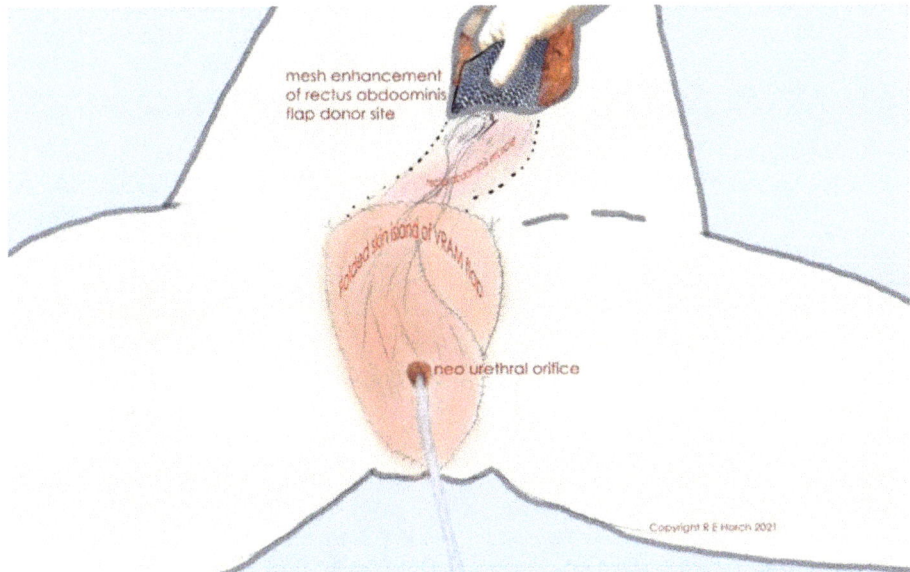

**Figure 1.** Schematic illustration of folded skin island of VRAM flap and neourethral orifice as well as of rectus abdominis muscle, tunneled subcutaneously. The flap donor site is closed with alloplastic mesh.

**Conflicts of Interest:** The authors declare no conflict of interest.

# References

1. Heiss, R.; Weber, M.A.; Balbach, E.; Schmitt, R.; Rehnitz, C.; Laqmani, A.; Sternberg, A.; Ellermann, J.J.; Nagel, A.M.; Ladd, M.E.; et al. Clinical Application of Ultrahigh-Field-Strength Wrist MRI: A Multireader 3-T and 7-T Comparison Study. *Radiology* **2023**, *2023*, 220753. [CrossRef]
2. Aslan-Horch, E.C.; Horch, R.E.; Arkudas, A.; Müller-Seubert, W.; Ludolph, I. Effects of Different Pressure Levels in Topical Negative Pressure Application-Analysis of Perfusion Parameters in a Clinical Skin Model Using Multimodal Imaging Techniques. *J. Clin. Med.* **2022**, *11*, 5133. [CrossRef]
3. Promny, D.; Grüner, J.; Hauck, T.; Horch, R.E. Paradoxical Perfusion Reaction of the contralateral Hand after Hand MRI. *Handchir. Mikrochir. Plast. Chir.* **2023**, *55*, 78–80.
4. Mulica, M.; Raymund, H.; Andreas, A.; Aijia, C.; Wibke, M.S.; Theresa, H.; Ingo, L. Corrigendum: Does indocyanine green fluorescence angiography impact the intraoperative choice of procedure in free vascularized medial femoral condyle grafting for scaphoid non-unions? *Front. Surg.* **2022**, *9*, 1101481. [CrossRef]
5. Ludolph, I.; Arkudas, A.; Müller-Seubert, W.; Cai, A.; Horch, R.E. Complications and their management following axillary, inguinal and iliac lymph node dissection. *Chirurgie* **2023**, *94*, 130–137. [CrossRef]
6. Schmitz, D.; Robering, J.W.; Weisbach, V.; Arkudas, A.; Ludolph, I.; Horch, R.E.; Boos, A.M.; Kengelbach-Weigand, A. Specific features of ex-obese patients significantly influence the functional cell properties of adipose-derived stromal cells. *J. Cell Mol. Med.* **2022**, *26*, 4463–4478. [CrossRef]
7. An, R.; Strissel, P.L.; Al-Abboodi, M.; Robering, J.W.; Supachai, R.; Eckstein, M.; Peddi, A.; Hauck, T.; Bäuerle, T.; Boccaccini, A.R.; et al. An Innovative Arteriovenous (AV) Loop Breast Cancer Model Tailored for Cancer Research. *Bioengineering* **2022**, *9*, 280. [CrossRef]
8. Vaghela, R.; Arkudas, A.; Gage, D.; Körner, C.; von Hörsten, S.; Salehi, S.; Horch, R.E.; Hessenauer, M. Microvascular development in the rat arteriovenous loop model in vivo-A step by step intravital microscopy analysis. *J. Biomed. Mater. Res. A* **2022**, *110*, 1551–1563. [CrossRef]
9. Cai, A.; Zheng, Z.M.; Himmler, M.; Schubert, D.W.; Fuchsluger, T.A.; Weisbach, V.; Horch, R.E.; Arkudas, A. Schwann Cells Promote Myogenic Differentiation of Myoblasts and Adipogenic Mesenchymal Stromal Cells on Poly-ε-Caprolactone-Collagen I-Nanofibers. *Cells* **2022**, *11*, 1436. [CrossRef]
10. Gruener, J.S.; Horch, R.E.; Geierlehner, A.; Mueller-Seubert, W.; Cai, A.; Arkudas, A.; Ludolph, I. Is Instillational Topical Negative Pressure Wound Therapy in Peri-Prosthetic Infections of the Breast Effective? A Pilot Study. *J. Pers. Med.* **2022**, *12*, 2054. [CrossRef]

11. Promny, T.; Kutz, C.S.; Jost, T.; Distel, L.V.; Kadam, S.; Schmid, R.; Arkudas, A.; Horch, R.E.; Kengelbach-Weigand, A. An In Vitro Approach for Investigating the Safety of Lipotransfer after Breast-Conserving Therapy. *J. Pers. Med.* **2022**, *12*, 1284. [CrossRef]
12. Polykandriotis, E.; Daenicke, J.; Bolat, A.; Grüner, J.; Schubert, D.W.; Horch, R.E. Individualized Wound Closure-Mechanical Properties of Suture Materials. *J. Pers. Med.* **2022**, *12*, 1041. [CrossRef]
13. Luze, H.; Nischwitz, S.P.; Wurzer, P.; Winter, R.; Spendel, S.; Kamolz, L.P.; Bjelic-Radisic, V. Assessment of Mastectomy Skin Flaps for Immediate Reconstruction with Implants via Thermal Imaging-A Suitable, Personalized Approach? *J. Pers. Med.* **2022**, *12*, 740. [CrossRef]
14. Frank, K.; Ströbel, A.; Ludolph, I.; Hauck, T.; May, M.S.; Beier, J.P.; Horch, R.E.; Arkudas, A. Improving the Safety of DIEP Flap Transplantation: Detailed Perforator Anatomy Study Using Preoperative CTA. *J. Pers. Med.* **2022**, *12*, 701. [CrossRef]
15. Hsu, C.K.; Denadai, R.; Chang, C.S.; Yao, C.F.; Chen, Y.A.; Chou, P.Y.; Lo, L.J.; Chen, Y.R. The Number of Surgical Interventions and Specialists Involved in the Management of Patients with Neurofibromatosis Type I: A 25-Year Analysis. *J. Pers. Med.* **2022**, *12*, 558. [CrossRef]
16. Geierlehner, A.; Horch, R.E.; Ludolph, I.; Arkudas, A. Intraoperative Blood Flow Analysis of DIEP vs. ms-TRAM Flap Breast Reconstruction Combining Transit-Time Flowmetry and Microvascular Indocyanine Green Angiography. *J. Pers. Med.* **2022**, *12*, 482. [CrossRef]
17. Cai, A.; Zheng, Z.; Müller-Seubert, W.; Biggemann, J.; Fey, T.; Beier, J.P.; Horch, R.E.; Frieß, B.; Arkudas, A. Microsurgical Transplantation of Pedicled Muscles in an Isolation Chamber—A Novel Approach to Engineering Muscle Constructs via Perfusion-Decellularization. *J. Pers. Med.* **2022**, *12*, 442. [CrossRef]
18. Bigdeli, A.K.; Falkner, F.; Thomas, B.; Hundeshagen, G.; Mayer, S.A.; Risse, E.M.; Harhaus, L.; Gazyakan, E.; Kneser, U.; Radu, C.A. The Free Myocutaneous Tensor Fasciae Latae Flap—A Workhorse Flap for Sternal Defect Reconstruction: A Single-Center Experience. *J. Pers. Med.* **2022**, *12*, 427. [CrossRef]
19. Bigdeli, A.K.; Didzun, O.; Thomas, B.; Harhaus, L.; Gazyakan, E.; Horch, R.E.; Kneser, U. Combined versus Single Perforator Propeller Flaps for Reconstruction of Large Soft Tissue Defects: A Retrospective Clinical Study. *J. Pers. Med.* **2022**, *12*, 41. [CrossRef]
20. Dastagir, K.; Obed, D.; Bucher, F.; Hofmann, T.; Koyro, K.I.; Vogt, P.M. Non-Invasive and Surgical Modalities for Scar Management: A Clinical Algorithm. *J. Pers. Med.* **2021**, *11*, 1259. [CrossRef]
21. Müller-Seubert, W.; Ostermaier, P.; Horch, R.E.; Distel, L.; Frey, B.; Cai, A.; Arkudas, A. Intra- and Early Postoperative Evaluation of Malperfused Areas in an Irradiated Random Pattern Skin Flap Model Using Indocyanine Green Angiography and Near-Infrared Reflectance-Based Imaging and Infrared Thermography. *J. Pers. Med.* **2022**, *12*, 237. [CrossRef]
22. Zucal, I.; Geis, S.; Prantl, L.; Haerteis, S.; Aung, T. Indocyanine Green for Leakage Control in Isolated Limb Perfusion. *J. Pers. Med.* **2021**, *11*, 1152. [CrossRef]
23. Thiem, D.G.E.; Römer, P.; Blatt, S.; Al-Nawas, B.; Kämmerer, P.W. New Approach to the Old Challenge of Free Flap Monitoring-Hyperspectral Imaging Outperforms Clinical Assessment by Earlier Detection of Perfusion Failure. *J. Pers. Med.* **2021**, *11*, 1101. [CrossRef]
24. Heimes, D.; Becker, P.; Thiem, D.G.; Kuchen, R.; Kyyak, S.; Kämmerer, P.W. Is Hyperspectral Imaging Suitable for Assessing Collateral Circulation Prior Radial Forearm Free Flap Harvesting? Comparison of Hyperspectral Imaging and Conventional Allen's Test. *J. Pers. Med.* **2021**, *11*, 531. [CrossRef]
25. Wagner, J.M.; Grolewski, V.; Reinkemeier, F.; Drysch, M.; Schmidt, S.V.; Dadras, M.; Huber, J.; Wallner, C.; Sogorski, A.; von Glinski, M.; et al. Posttraumatic Lymphedema after Open Fractures of the Lower Extremity-A Retrospective Cohort Analysis. *J. Pers. Med.* **2021**, *11*, 1077. [CrossRef]
26. Nischwitz, S.P.; Luze, H.; Schellnegger, M.; Gatterer, S.J.; Tuca, A.C.; Winter, R.; Kamolz, L.P. Thermal, Hyperspectral, and Laser Doppler Imaging: Non-Invasive Tools for Detection of The Deep Inferior Epigastric Artery Perforators-A Prospective Comparison Study. *J. Pers. Med.* **2021**, *11*, 1005. [CrossRef]
27. Horch, R.E.; Ludolph, I.; Arkudas, A.; Cai, A. Personalized Reconstruction of Genital Defects in Complicated Wounds with Vertical Rectus Abdominis Myocutaneous Flaps including Urethral Neo-Orifice. *J. Pers. Med.* **2021**, *11*, 1076. [CrossRef]
28. Combal, A.; Thuau, F.; Fouasson-Chailloux, A.; Arrigoni, P.P.; Baud'huin, M.; Duteille, F.; Crenn, V. Preliminary Results of the "Capasquelet" Technique for Managing Femoral Bone Defects-Combining a Masquelet Induced Membrane and Capanna Vascularized Fibula with an Allograft. *J. Pers. Med.* **2021**, *11*, 774. [CrossRef]
29. Huang, Y.K.; Wong, M.Y.; Wu, C.R.; Cheng, Y.Z.; Lin, B.S. Free Myocutaneous Flap Assessment in a Rat Model: Verification of a Wireless Bioelectrical Impedance Assessment (BIA) System for Vascular Compromise Following Microsurgery. *J. Pers. Med.* **2021**, *11*, 373. [CrossRef]
30. Ehrl, D.; Wachtel, N.; Braig, D.; Kuhlmann, C.; Dürr, H.R.; Schneider, C.P.; Giunta, R.E. Defect Coverage after Forequarter Amputation-A Systematic Review Assessing Different Surgical Approaches. *J. Pers. Med.* **2022**, *12*, 560. [CrossRef]
31. Heinzel, J.C.; Dadun, L.F.; Prahm, C.; Winter, N.; Bressler, M.; Lauer, H.; Ritter, J.; Daigeler, A.; Kolbenschlag, J. Beyond the Knife-Reviewing the Interplay of Psychosocial Factors and Peripheral Nerve Lesions. *J. Pers. Med.* **2021**, *11*, 1200. [CrossRef]

**Disclaimer/Publisher's Note:** The statements, opinions and data contained in all publications are solely those of the individual author(s) and contributor(s) and not of MDPI and/or the editor(s). MDPI and/or the editor(s) disclaim responsibility for any injury to people or property resulting from any ideas, methods, instructions or products referred to in the content.

## Journal of Personalized Medicine

*Article*

# Is Instillational Topical Negative Pressure Wound Therapy in Peri-Prosthetic Infections of the Breast Effective? A Pilot Study

Jasmin S. Gruener *, Raymund E. Horch, Alexander Geierlehner, Wibke Mueller-Seubert, Aijia Cai, Andreas Arkudas and Ingo Ludolph

Laboratory for Tissue Engineering and Regenerative Medicine, Department of Plastic and Hand Surgery, University Hospital Erlangen, Friedrich-Alexander-University of Erlangen-Nürnberg (FAU), 91054 Erlangen, Germany
* Correspondence: jasmin.gruener@uk-erlangen.de

**Abstract:** Peri-prosthetic breast infections pose a risk of severe complications after breast implant surgery. The need to remove the breast implant, control the infection and perform additional surgical procedures are the consequences. Reimplantation of an alloplastic implant is only appropriate after an infection-free interval. In this retrospective cohort study, we investigated the effectiveness of negative pressure wound treatment with instillation and dwell time (NPWTi-d) on peri-prosthetic breast infections in combination with implant removal and antibiotic therapy. Twelve patients treated with NPWTi-d due to breast implant infection were included in the study. The bacterial burden was analyzed using wound swabs before and after NPWTi-d. Additionally, laboratory values were determined before NPWTi-d and immediately before wound closure. A total of 13 peri-prosthetic breast infections in 12 patients were treated using implant removal and NPWTi-d. In 76.9% ($n = 10$) of the cases, the patients had undergone alloplastic breast reconstruction following cancer-related mastectomy, whereas 23.1% ($n = 3$) of the patients had undergone breast augmentation for cosmetic reasons. The bacterial burden in the breast pocket decreased statistically significant after implant removal and NPWTi-d. No shift from Gram-positive to Gram-negative bacteria was observed. Inflammatory markers rapidly decreased following treatment. NPWTi-d had a positive impact on the healing process after peri-prosthetic breast infections, leading to a decrease in bacterial burden within the wounds and contributing to uneventful healing. Therefore, secondary reimplantation of breast prostheses might be positively influenced when compared to conventional implant removal and simple secondary closure. Further studies are required to conclusively establish the beneficial long-term effects of using NPWTi-d for the treatment of peri-prosthetic breast infections.

**Keywords:** breast infection; peri-prosthetic infection; breast implant infection; silicone prostheses; negative pressure wound therapy; instillation

## 1. Introduction

According to the literature, peri-prosthetic breast infections are relatively rare events. Although autologous breast reconstruction has become a standard procedure, alloplastic breast augmentation and breast reconstruction with silicone implants continue to be popular procedures [1–5].

Peri-prosthetic breast infection (PPBI) is still a severe complication that is associated with surgical site complications and implant loss. In particular, patients undergoing tumor-associated radiation therapy of the breast before or after alloplastic breast reconstruction commonly suffer from wound-healing disorders and serious infections. Thus far, there is no consensus regarding the optimal treatment for PPBI. Standard treatment options include removal of the implant and prolonged administration of intravenous antibiotics. Subsequent issues include loss or contracture of the implant pocket, which means that the patient may need additional alloplastic or autologous breast reconstruction. Negative pressure wound therapy with instillation and dwell time (NPWTi-d) has only anecdotally been described in the context of PPBI [6].

More recent data describe the advantages of using instillational negative pressure wound therapy (NPWT) with different rinsing solutions for the treatment of acute and chronic wounds, infectious wounds and even burn injuries [7–14]. NPWTi-d with an antiseptic solution achieves a greater reduction in the number of pathogenic species within a wound compared to NPWT with no solution [15]. Furthermore, duration of hospitalization and days to wound closure in complex infected wounds can be significantly reduced with NPWTi-d compared to traditional wound care. Consequently, there can be a reduction in the cost of treating complex wounds [16,17]. However, little is known about the use of NPWT in breast infections following breast implantation. It has been demonstrated that topical negative pressure used as closed incisional NPWT on closed operation wounds improves local blood circulation and reduces edema as well [18–25].

The incidence of PPBI is between 0.1 and 2.5% [26–30]. Because the overall incidence of PPBI is low, we present this pilot study of 12 patients who underwent implant removal and NPWTi-d due to PPBI.

## 2. Materials and Methods

A retrospective analysis of 13 infected breasts in 12 female patients who underwent NPWTi-d due to peri-prosthetic breast infection was conducted. Due to the retrospective nature of this study, we did not recruit a control group of patients who received alternative treatment (PPBI without NPWTi-d). Cases were analyzed based on a complete medical record review, including regular patient follow-ups.

We used a computerized system to apply topical negative pressure with automatic instillation cycles (V.A.C. VeraFlo Therapy, Kinetic Concepts, Inc., San Antonio, TX, USA), using polyhexanide (0.4 mg/mL) (Lavasept, B. Braun Medical AG, Freiburg, Germany) as a rinsing solution. NPWTi-d was initiated immediately after removal of the implant. The first wound swab was taken directly after explantation of the implant and before irrigation of the pocket; a second wound swab was taken before wound closure. The instillation volume was adapted to the wound surface area so that the entire wound bed was covered with instillation fluid. Dwell frequency was 2-hourly. A dwell time of 20 min and pressure of −125 mmHg with continuous suction was set. Soaking time intervals were set between 2 and 3.5 h, depending on the clinical wound situation, and instillation of the wound was performed in every cycle. The foam was changed every 3–5 days with inspection of the wound bed to check for tissue granulation and signs of infection.

In all cases, a complete capsulectomy was performed. In all but one case, the patients received antibiotics perioperatively, during NPWTi-d treatment and for another 5 days after wound closure/reconstruction/reimplantation. In the other case, antibiotic treatment was only performed as a single shot preoperatively before implant removal and for another 5 days after reconstruction.

Data were analyzed for bacterial colonization of the implant pocket. Data from the first and last wound swabs before and after NPWT were collected. The wound swabs were obtained by the surgeon in a standardized manner by carefully passing the swab through the implant pocket. The number of different bacterial species (NDB) was counted, and the amount of bacteria (AB) in the culture was measured by the local Institute for Clinical Microbiology, according to recent studies [12,23]. Semiquantitative examination of the bacterial culture determined the extent of bacterial colonization of the implant pocket on an ordinal scale (1–4) for each bacteria (1: sparse, 2: moderate, 3: several, 4: plenty). Due to the heterogeneity of the bacterial colonization, the total amount of all bacteria found in the breast pocket was calculated by summing the semiquantitative ordinal scaled numbers of each bacteria. In addition, blood samples focused on inflammatory markers, including CRP and leukocyte count, were obtained before NPWTi-d and 5–6 days later during hospitalization.

Statistical analysis was performed using GraphPad Prism (Version 8.3.0 Prism 8, GraphPad Software Inc., La Jolla, CA, USA). The Wilcoxon signed-rank test was used for statistical analysis.

A $p$-value $\leq 0.05$ was defined as a statistically significant (*) difference among the treatment groups. A $p$-value $\leq 0.001$ was considered a highly significant (**) difference. Values are presented as mean $\pm$ standard deviation.

## 3. Results

### 3.1. Patient Demographics

We analyzed a total of 13 cases of PPBI in 12 female patients whose ages ranged from 24 to 94 years (median age: 52 years, mean age: 49.3 years). In 11 cases, the patients continued with regular follow-up at our outpatient clinic at 6 weeks and 6 months after the operation. In one case, follow-up ranged between 4 weeks and 5 years due to the retrospective nature of the study and the sometimes very long distance from the patient's home to the hospital. In one case, there was no further consultation in our hospital records due to the patient's advanced age of 94 years.

In 76.9% ($n$ = 10) of the cases, the patients had received a silicone gel-filled implant for reconstructive reasons following cancer-related mastectomy, while 23.1% ($n$ = 3) had received an implant for cosmetic reasons. Figure 1 shows the time range from implantation to removal of the implant due to PPBI. In one case, the time since the first implantation was unknown. The median time between implantation and explantation of the implant was 8 weeks, and the mean time in between was 36.2 weeks.

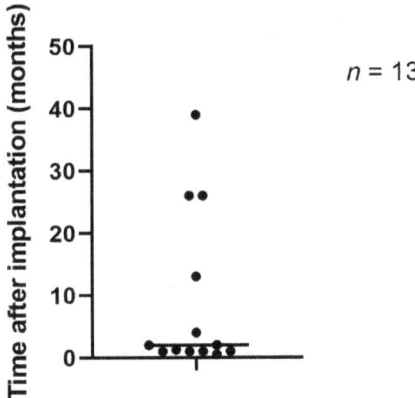

**Figure 1.** Time between implantation and explantation of the breast implant.

All patients had complete remission of their infection after NPWTi-d treatment following implant removal; the remission parameters were resolution of the clinical signs of infection (redness, swelling, pain), decreased serum CRP and serum leukocytes and absence of pus in the exudate. We performed secondary wound closures in 10 cases. One patient received a free muscle-sparing transverse rectus abdominis myocutaneous flap (ms-TRAM flap) and a free deep inferior epigastric artery perforator flap (DIEP flap) for reconstruction of both breasts in the later course, while another patient underwent repeated breast augmentation with a silicone implant. In three cases, split-thickness skin graft transplantation was necessary during the initial treatment due to the severity of the infection and related soft tissue loss. These patients received a free ms-TRAM flap or DIEP flap at a later stage.

In Table 1, patient characteristics are presented.

Table 1. Patient characteristics.

| Patient No. | Age (In Years) | Reconstructive (R)/Cosmetic (C) | Infected Side | Radiation | Relevant Concomitant Diseases |
|---|---|---|---|---|---|
| 1 | 52 | R | Both | No | Hypertension, deep vein thrombosis of the lower leg |
| 2 | 58 | R | Left | Yes | None |
| 2 | 60 | R | Right | Yes | None |
| 3 | 54 | R | Right | No | Allergy to penicillin |
| 4 | 40 | R | Both | Yes | Allergy to novaminsulfone, tramadol and clindamycin |
| 5 | 61 | R | Right | No | BRCA2 mutation, hepatic steatosis, allergy to amoxicillin, clindamycin and tramadol |
| 6 | 94 | R | Left | Yes | Urinary incontinence, hypertension |
| 7 | 24 | C | Both | No | Smoker |
| 8 | 41 | R | Both | No | None |
| 9 | 42 | C | Right | No | None |
| 10 | 55 | R | Right | No | Pulmonary embolism |
| 11 | 32 | C | Both | No | None |
| 12 | 46 | R | Both | No | None |

In Figure 2, an example of NPWTi-d in a 58-year-old patient with PPBI is shown. Figure 2a presents a severe infection of the skin with necessary excision and skin graft transplantation. In Figure 2b the topical treatment with NPWTi-d is illustrated. In Figure 2c a free ms1-TRAM flap is shown which was conducted five months later.

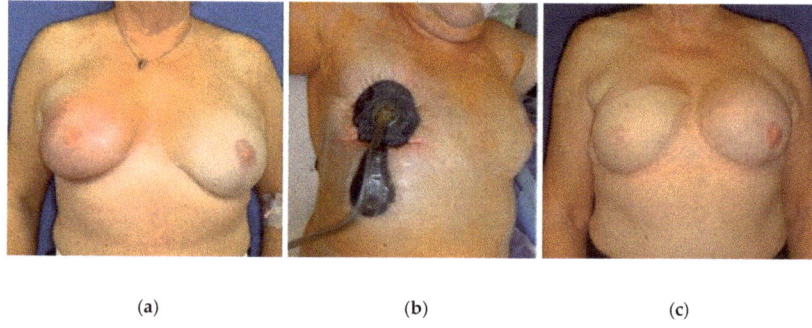

(a)       (b)       (c)

**Figure 2.** Example of NPWTi-d (**b**) in a 58-year-old patient with a history of breast cancer shown with PPBI. (**a**) Skin graft transplantation due to severe infection of the skin with necessary excision of the skin. (**c**) Five months later, the skin graft was removed, and the right breast underwent free ms1-TRAM flap reconstruction. The free ms1-TRAM flap was well perfused, and follow-up remained uneventful 6 weeks and 6 months later.

### 3.2. Bacterial Burden and Flora

In Figure 3, the bacterial burden before and after NPWTi-d is presented. Before NPWTi-d, the bacterial burden counted an average of 1.92 (1.32 SD). Before wound closure (after NPWTi-d), the bacterial burden was statistically significantly lower, with an average of 0.76 (1.47 SD, $p = 0.002$).

The average number of different types of bacteria before NPWTi-d was 0.92 (0.47 SD) and ranged from 0 to 2 different types of bacteria. In 7.7% ($n = 1$), two or more different types of bacteria were cultivated before NPWTi-d. In 76.9% ($n = 10$), there was one type of bacteria, and in 15.4% ($n = 2$), no bacteria were found. During the further course of treatment, all patients received antibiotics, including a cephalosporin and a antibiotic for anaerobic infections. Antibiotic therapy was adjusted according to the results of the wound swab cultures.

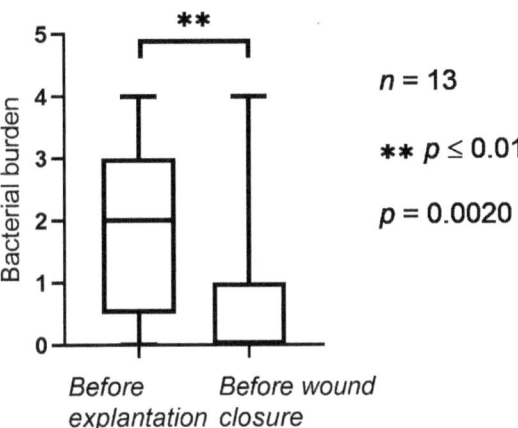

Figure 3. Bacterial burden in the implant pocket (1: sparse, 2: moderate, 3: several, 4: plenty). The horizontal lines mark the medians.

After NPWTi-d, the number of different types of bacteria decreased significantly, to an average of 0.23 (0.42 SD, $p = 0.001$). In the bacterial culture of the second wound swab, no cases showed two or more different bacteria. In 23.1% ($n = 3$) of the cases, one type of bacteria was found in the culture of the second wound swab, while in 76.9% ($n = 10$), no bacteria were found. In one case, the wound was colonized with multidrug-resistant bacteria (methicillin-resistant *Staphylococcus aureus*, MRSA) in the first wound swab. In the second wound swab (taken before wound closure), MRSA was no longer detected in the culture. The types of bacteria included MRSA, *Staphylococcus aureus*, *Staphylococcus epidermidis*, *Serratia marcescens*, *Staphylococcus warneri*, *Enterococcus faecalis*, *Proteus mirabilis* and *Bacillus* species. In 61.5% ($n = 8$) of the cases, swab analysis showed Gram-positive bacteria before NPWTi-d. No shift from Gram-positive to Gram-negative bacteria was observed.

### 3.3. Serum CRP and Number of Leukocytes

In Figures 4 and 5, CRP and the number of leukocytes in the serum are shown, respectively.

Serum CRP (Figure 4) was statistically significantly lower before wound closure (after NPWTi-d) compared to the initial values obtained before removal of the implant. The mean was 55.3 mL/L before NPWTi-d and 15.5 mL/L before wound closure ($p = 0.0002$); serum CRP ranged from 1.8 to 34.8 mL/L before wound closure.

The number of leukocytes (Figure 5) was statistically significantly lower before wound closure (after NPWTi-d) compared to the values before the first operation. The mean values were $8.16 \times 10^3/\mu L$ before NPWTi-d and $5.83 \times 10^3/\mu L$ before wound closure ($p = 0.0002$); leukocyte counts ranged from $3.13 \times 10^3/\mu L$ to $10.17 \times 10^3/\mu L$ before wound closure.

The oldest patient (94 years) had undergone alloplastic breast augmentation for cosmetic reasons more than 10 years earlier. She presented to our emergency unit in poor general condition and in extreme pain with a fever. Physical examination showed a purulent wound with central skin necrosis and a unilateral exposed implant. Inflammatory markers were very high before NPWTi-d. The other implant was removed due to capsular fibrosis (grade IV) simultaneously with the secondary wound closure of the affected side. This patient had no further consultation at our hospital due to her advanced age. At the time of discharge from the clinic, her wounds were clinically inconspicuous.

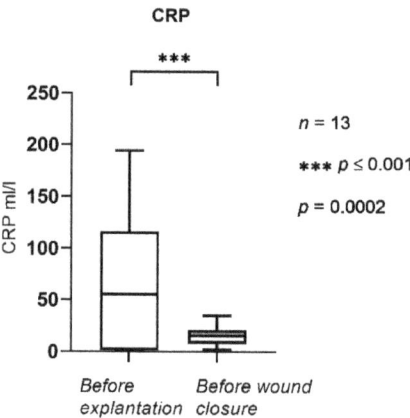

**Figure 4.** CRP levels before explantation and before wound closure. The horizontal lines mark the medians.

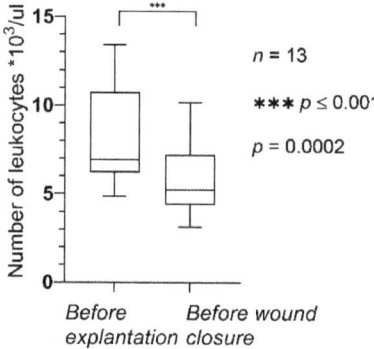

**Figure 5.** Number of leukocytes before explantation and before wound closure. The horizontal lines mark the medians.

*3.4. Additional Treatment Data*

Time to wound closure after NPWTi-d varied between 5 and 14 days, with a mean of 8.5 days (Figure 6).

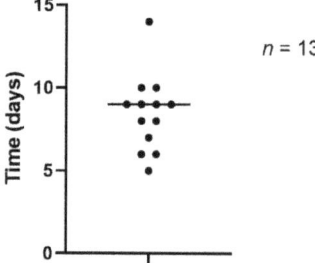

**Figure 6.** Time to wound closure after NPWTi-d.

Duration of hospitalization varied between 7 and 16 days, with a mean of 11.8 days (Figure 7).

## Duration of hospitalization

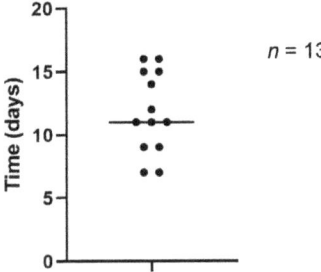

Figure 7. Duration of hospitalization.

## 4. Discussion

Peri-prosthetic breast infection is a severe complication that regularly results in multiple reoperations and risks an unsatisfactory outcome. In this context, the female breast is a unique anatomical wound location. Radiation therapy after breast cancer surgery is associated with elevated complications in terms of capsular fibrosis and surgical site infection [31,32]. Furthermore, it has been discussed that breast parenchyma is subject to bacterial colonization or contamination during breast implant procedures. Independent from the final coverage, which in irradiated breast wounds often includes a free flap to close the defect, technical advances, such as measuring the perfusion of the remaining tissue, may be necessary to ensure a successful outcome and minimize tissue loss [2,3,33,34].

Evaluating the options for PPBI treatment is difficult; data are either anecdotal or retrospectively collected because—as with other relatively infrequent surgical events—no prospective studies exist [35]. Some have called the management of severe infection or acute implant exposure following primary augmentation mammoplasty a classic surgical dilemma. According to Vasilakis et al., the inconsistency and paucity of published data preclude definitive conclusions regarding the optimal management of threatened implants [36]. However, despite insufficient published information about the effective management of these situations, Spear has recommended that device removal and delayed reinsertion is always a more conservative and predictable option, especially in seriously infected breasts or deficient soft tissue coverage when the implant does not appear to be salvageable [37]. A common treatment strategy after implant removal is reimplantation after weeks to months, but no consensus exists for standardized treatment in such cases.

Another issue is microperfusion of the skin and soft tissue in PPBI, which is essential for proper healing and hence the use of alloplastic material for reimplantation. There are currently several tools that can provide sufficient oxygenation and microperfusion to ensure adequate vascular supply to the affected tissue [2,3,18,19,33,38]. The use of noninvasive tools to validate tissue perfusion can be a helpful aid in optimizing reoperations.

In cases of PPBI, a major concern besides acute treatment is to create an ideal inflammatory-free anatomical site with maximum decontamination of the bacterial burden to facilitate reoperation and reduce the risk of further infectious sequelae.

Besides implant removal and antibiotic therapy, which was applied to all patients in this study except one, the use of NPWTi-d decreased the bacterial burden in the former implant pocket. Moreover, the inflammatory blood markers decreased markedly over a short period of time (5–6 days) after NPWTi-d was applied. Even though implant removal and intravenous antibiotics are crucial in such cases, their actual impact on the bacterial burden has not been defined exactly. Additional intermittent instillation of the breast pocket seems to positively affect the bacterial burden in the wound bed. It must be mentioned that the true extent of NPWTi-d's effect cannot be attributed exclusively to NPWTi-d without comparing its results to those of a control group. However, the reduction in bacterial load achieved through NPWTi-d reflects the results of previous studies that assessed the effects of NPWT/NPWTi-d on various types of contaminated wounds and different anatomical locations [12,35,39,40]. Especially for breast-associated interventions, such as reimplantation of an implant or autologous breast reconstruction, it is of the utmost importance to obtain clinically sterile wound conditions that are free of infection. Various complications, such as PPBI, capsular fibrosis and even breast implant-associated anaplastic large cell lymphoma, have been associated with bacterial colonization or bacterial biofilms. Within the first weeks and months after implantation, PPBI results primarily from Gram-positive bacteria, such as *Staphylococcus aureus* and *Streptococcus* [30,41]. In our study, the majority of cases (61.5%, $n$ = 8) showed Gram-positive bacterial colonization. The most common bacterial species was *Staphylococcus epidermidis*, which affirms the possible transmission of bacteria from the skin into the wound [42]. As infections of the implant pocket with multidrug-resistant bacteria (e.g., MRSA) can cause severe complications due to limited antibiotic therapy regimen options, this study focused especially on the one patient who suffered from MRSA infection of the implant pocket. After NPWTi-d and targeted antibiotic therapy, MRSA was no longer detected in the implant pocket. In all cases, the infection resolved uneventfully so that successful wound closure could be achieved.

This study demonstrated the positive effects of NPWTi-d on the healing process of peri-prosthetic wound infections and salvage of the breast implant pocket. In addition to its positive effects on bacterial burden and inflammation, NPWTi-d was able to prevent shrinkage in the former implant pocket and thereby preserve the skin envelope. Even though antibiotic use might influence bacterial analysis, it is of the utmost importance to decrease the bacterial burden in the former implant pocket, which was accomplished with NPWTi-d. The association between bacterial contamination or colonization and unfavorable sequelae following augmentation mammoplasty has been described extensively in the literature. Hence, in our opinion, NPWTi-d is a promising tool for treating PPBI, especially considering the goal of decreasing the bacterial burden as much as possible. This study presents an algorithm for problematic cases of infected and possibly exposed foreign material in the breast. Following removal of an infected breast implant, NPWTi-d using an antiseptic solution is recommended until local and systemic inflammatory markers have decreased and the local wound appears clinically clean. Between two and four changes of the NPWT dressing should be sufficient in most cases. If reimplantation with a silicone implant is planned, wound closure should be performed and reimplantation completed at the earliest 3 months after total healing of the infected breast and consecutive wounds. Planning autologous breast reconstruction offers the possibility of a direct approach following control of the local infection and treatment with NPWTi-d. This is possible because autologous breast reconstruction (e.g., using a DIEP flap) provides autologous tissue, including an independent microvascular supply. Furthermore, the patient's own tissue has the capacity to overcome any possible residual bacterial colonization. Patients should be informed about the possibility of a second stage autologous breast reconstruction after an interval of several months. Consequently, this treatment algorithm might facilitate earlier breast reconstruction after PPBI, independent of the applied technique, leading to greater patient satisfaction and lower patient burden by shortening the period the patient has to live without a reconstructed breast.

Other authors have stated that NPWTi-d, which has become a game changer in the treatment of infected wounds, is an appropriate tool for the treatment of PPBI, and we agree [43,44]. However, it should be combined with intravenous antibiotic therapy perioperatively. The prolonged use of antibiotics in addition to NPWTi-d needs to be reconsidered after trials with more cases and according to the general condition of the patient, concomitant diseases and the severity of the infection.

The findings of this study correspond to those of other publications [12,23,40,45,46]. Studies have found that, not only in PPBI but especially in chronic wounds, a significantly lower bacterial load was obtained after applying an antiseptic instillation solution as an adjunct to NPWT [12,47].

In all cases in this study, the breast implant pocket was preserved by NPWTi-d, which is consistent with the results of two studies published by Meybodi et al. in 2017 and 2021 [43,48].

Only a few previous cases have described the use of NPWT, with or without instillation, as a treatment option for peri-prosthetic infections [48–50]. Therefore, to confirm our findings, further studies with more patients are needed to develop a standardized therapy regimen or algorithm for using NPWTi-d to treat peri-prosthetic infections. As a study protocol that includes a prospective control group is not reasonable, comparing a greater number of patients with a historical patient group is recommended. Moreover, since inflammatory markers, such as CRP and leukocyte count, are not specific for any particular bacterial infection, it would be interesting to study whether indicators of systemic inflammation, such as laboratory markers, can be decreased more efficiently. This should be further investigated in the future.

An already mentioned limitation of this study is that it lacked a control group, which prevented us from comparing the NPWTi-d data with other treatments. However, these data can descriptively show relatively fast remission of clinical infection parameters and shortened time to wound closure and overall duration of hospitalization [51].

Surgical debridement and antibiotics undoubtedly influence the treatment of infected wounds. Nevertheless, the results of this study confirm those of recent studies and underline the positive effect of NPWTi-d on bacterial burden.

## 5. Conclusions

Based on an analysis of 13 breast implant-related peri-prosthetic infections, the positive effects of NPWTi-d (which were already known from applications in complex and contaminated wounds in different anatomical locations) were confirmed in the unique context of breast infections. Based on these results, the use of NPWTi-d should be considered a valuable adjunct to the treatment of peri-prosthetic breast infections in addition to implant removal and antibiotic therapy. NPWTi-d could contribute to earlier second-stage breast reconstruction following an infection-free interval. However, further investigations with more cases are necessary to establish a treatment algorithm.

**Author Contributions:** Conceptualization, J.S.G., I.L. and R.E.H.; methodology, J.S.G., I.L., R.E.H., A.G., W.M.-S., A.C. and A.A.; software, J.S.G.; validation, J.S.G. and I.L.; formal analysis, J.S.G. and I.L.; investigation, J.S.G. and I.L.; data curation, J.S.G.; writing—original draft preparation, J.S.G.; writing—review and editing, J.S.G., I.L., R.E.H., A.G., W.M.-S., A.C. and A.A.; visualization, J.S.G.; resources, R.E.H.; supervision, J.S.G., I.L. and R.E.H.; project administration, J.S.G. All authors have read and agreed to the published version of the manuscript.

**Funding:** This research received no external funding.

**Institutional Review Board Statement:** The study was conducted according to the guidelines of the Declaration of Helsinki and approved by the Ethics Committee of Friedrich-Alexander-University of Erlangen-Nuremberg, Germany (registration number: 70_20_B).

**Informed Consent Statement:** Informed consent was obtained from all subjects involved in the study.

**Conflicts of Interest:** R.E.H. has received third-party funding for scientific research on NPWT from KCI—an Acelity company—in the past and has served as a member of a Scientific Advisory Board of KCI–Acelity in the past. R.E.H. and A.A. served as speakers on the scientific symposia of KCI–Acelity in the past. The authors have no other relevant affiliations or financial involvement with any organizations or entities with a financial interest in or financial conflicts with the subject matter or materials discussed in the manuscript apart from those disclosed.

## References

1. Ludolph, I.; Bettray, D.; Beier, J.; Horch, R.; Arkudas, A. Leaving the perfusion zones? Individualized flap design in 100 free DIEP and ms-TRAM flaps for autologous breast reconstruction using indocyanine green angiography. *J. Plast. Reconstr. Aesthetic Surg.* **2021**, *75*, 52–60. [CrossRef] [PubMed]
2. Frank, K.; Ströbel, A.; Ludolph, I.; Hauck, T.; May, M.S.; Beier, J.P.; Horch, R.E.; Arkudas, A. Improving the Safety of DIEP Flap Transplantation: Detailed Perforator Anatomy Study Using Preoperative CTA. *J. Pers. Med.* **2022**, *12*, 701. [CrossRef] [PubMed]
3. Geierlehner, A.; Horch, R.E.; Ludolph, I.; Arkudas, A. Intraoperative Blood Flow Analysis of DIEP vs. ms-TRAM Flap Breast Reconstruction Combining Transit-Time Flowmetry and Microvascular Indocyanine Green Angiography. *J. Pers. Med.* **2022**, *12*, 482. [CrossRef] [PubMed]
4. Hauck, T.; Arkudas, A.; Horch, R.E.; Ströbel, A.; May, M.S.; Binder, J.; Krautz, C.; Ludolph, I. The third dimension in perforator mapping—Comparison of Cinematic Rendering and maximum intensity projection in abdominal-based autologous breast reconstruction. *J. Plast. Reconstr. Aesthetic Surg.* **2021**, *75*, 536–543. [CrossRef]
5. Bach, A.D.; Morgenstern, I.H.; Horch, R.E. Secondary "Hybrid Reconstruction" Concept with Silicone Implants After Autologous Breast Reconstruction-Is It Safe and Reasonable? *Med. Sci. Monit.* **2020**, *26*, e921329. [CrossRef]
6. Cheong, J.Y.; Goltsman, D.; Warrier, S. A New Method of Salvaging Breast Reconstruction After Breast Implant Using Negative Pressure Wound Therapy and Instillation. *Aesthetic Plast. Surg.* **2016**, *40*, 745–748. [CrossRef]
7. Siqueira, M.B.; Ramanathan, D.; Klika, A.K.; A Higuera, C.; Barsoum, W.K. Role of negative pressure wound therapy in total hip and knee arthroplasty. *World J. Orthop.* **2016**, *7*, 104825. [CrossRef]
8. Söylemez, M.S.; Erinc, S.; Kilic, B.; Ozkan, K. Intermittent negative pressure wound therapy with instillation for the treatment of persistent periprosthetic hip infections: A report of two cases. *Ther. Clin. Risk Manag.* **2016**, *12*, 161–166. [CrossRef]
9. Hodson, T.; West, J.M.; Poteet, S.J.; Lee, P.H.; Valerio, I.L. Instillation Negative Pressure Wound Therapy: A Role for Infected LVAD Salvage. *Adv. Wound Care* **2019**, *8*, 118–124. [CrossRef]
10. Hehr, J.D.; Hodson, T.S.; West, J.M.; Schulz, S.A.; Poteet, S.J.; Chandawarkar, R.Y.; Valerio, I.L. Instillation negative pressure wound therapy: An effective approach for hardware salvage. *Int. Wound J.* **2019**, *17*, 387–393. [CrossRef]
11. Lehner, B.; Bernd, L.V.A.C. V.A.C.-instill therapy in periprosthetic infection of hip and knee arthroplasty. *Zent. Chir.* **2006**, *131* (Suppl. S1), S160–S164. [CrossRef] [PubMed]
12. Ludolph, I.; Fried, F.W.; Kneppe, K.; Arkudas, A.; Schmitz, M.; E Horch, R. Negative pressure wound treatment with computer-controlled irrigation/instillation decreases bacterial load in contaminated wounds and facilitates wound closure. *Int. Wound J.* **2018**, *15*, 978–984. [CrossRef] [PubMed]
13. Beckmann, N.A.; Hanslmeier, M.G.; Omlor, G.W.; Feisst, M.; Maier, M.W.; Lehner, B. Is Negative Pressure Wound Therapy with Instillation Suitable for the Treatment of Acute Periprosthetic Hip Joint Infection? *J. Clin. Med.* **2021**, *10*, 3264. [CrossRef]
14. Altomare, M.; Benuzzi, L.; Molteni, M.; Virdis, F.; Spota, A.; Cioffi, S.P.B.; Reitano, E.; Renzi, F.; Chiara, O.; Sesana, G.; et al. Negative Pressure Wound Therapy for the Treatment of Fournier's Gangrene: A Rare Case with Rectal Fistula and Systematic Review of the Literature. *J. Pers. Med.* **2022**, *12*, 1695. [CrossRef] [PubMed]
15. Stichling, M.; Wiessner, A.; Kikhney, J.; Gatzer, R.; Müller, M.; Scheuermann-Poley, C.; Moter, A.; Willy, C. Negative pressure wound therapy with instillation and dwell time (NPWTi-d) with antiseptic solution leads to a greater reduction in the number of pathogen species detected compared to conventional NPWT despite the recontamination of the wound by eluates with high bacterial load. *Int. Wound J.* **2022**, *16*, 1740–1749. [CrossRef]
16. Gabriel, A.; Shores, J.; Heinrich, C.; Baqai, W.; Kalina, S.; Sogioka, N.; Gupta, S. Negative pressure wound therapy with instillation: A pilot study describing a new method for treating infected wounds. *Int. Wound J.* **2008**, *5*, 399–413. [CrossRef] [PubMed]
17. Kim, P.J.; Attinger, C.E.; Steinberg, J.S.; Evans, K.K.; Powers, K.A.; Hung, R.W.; Lavery, L. The impact of negative-pressure wound therapy with instillation compared with standard negative-pressure wound therapy: A retrospective, historical, cohort, controlled study. *Plast. Reconstr. Surg.* **2014**, *133*, 709–716. [CrossRef]
18. Müller-Seubert, W.; Herold, H.; Graf, S.; Ludolph, I.; Horch, R.E. Evaluation of the Influence of Short Tourniquet Ischemia on Tissue Oxygen Saturation and Skin Temperature Using Two Portable Imaging Modalities. *J. Clin. Med.* **2022**, *11*, 5240. [CrossRef]
19. Aslan-Horch, E.C.; Horch, R.E.; Arkudas, A.; Müller-Seubert, W.; Ludolph, I. Effects of Different Pressure Levels in Topical Negative Pressure Application—Analysis of Perfusion Parameters in a Clinical Skin Model Using Multimodal Imaging Techniques. *J. Clin. Med.* **2022**, *11*, 5133. [CrossRef]
20. Renno, I.; Boos, A.M.; Horch, R.E.; Ludolph, I. Changes of perfusion patterns of surgical wounds under application of closed incision negative pressure wound therapy in postbariatric patients1. *Clin. Hemorheol. Microcirc.* **2019**, *72*, 139–150. [CrossRef]
21. Horch, R.E.; Ludolph, I.; Müller-Seubert, W.; Zetzmann, K.; Hauck, T.; Arkudas, A.; Geierlehner, A. Topical negative-pressure wound therapy: Emerging devices and techniques. *Expert Rev. Med. Devices* **2020**, *17*, 139–148. [CrossRef]
22. Argenta, L.C.; Morykwas, M.J. Vacuum-assisted closure: A new method for wound control and treatment: Clinical experience. *Ann. Plast. Surg.* **1997**, *38*, 563–577. [CrossRef] [PubMed]
23. Geierlehner, A.; Horch, R.E.; Müller-Seubert, W.; Arkudas, A.; Ludolph, I. Limb salvage procedure in immunocompromised patients with therapy-resistant leg ulcers—The value of ultra-radical debridement and instillation negative-pressure wound therapy. *Int. Wound J.* **2020**, *17*, 1496–1507. [CrossRef]
24. Wang, J.; Chapman, Z.; Cole, E.; Koide, S.; Mah, E.; Overstall, S.; Trotter, D. Use of Closed Incision Negative Pressure Therapy (ciNPT) in Breast Reconstruction Abdominal Free Flap Donor Sites. *J. Clin. Med.* **2021**, *10*, 5176. [CrossRef] [PubMed]

25. Hsu, K.F.; Kao, L.T.; Chu, P.Y.; Chen, C.Y.; Chou, Y.Y.; Huang, D.W.; Tzeng, Y.S. Simple and Efficient Pressure Ulcer Reconstruction via Primary Closure Combined with Closed-Incision Negative Pressure Wound Therapy (CiNPWT)-Experience of a Single Surgeon. *J. Pers. Med.* **2022**, *12*, 182. [CrossRef] [PubMed]
26. Khan, U.D. Periprosthetic Infection in Primary and Secondary Augmentation Mammaplasty Using Round Silicone Gel Breast Implants: Comparative Analysis of 2521 Primary and 386 Secondary Mammoplasties in a Single Surgeon Practice. *Aesthetic Plast. Surg.* **2020**, *45*, 1–10. [CrossRef]
27. Araco, A.; Gravante, G.; Araco, F.; Delogu, D.; Cervelli, V.; Walgenbach, K. A Retrospective Analysis of 3,000 Primary Aesthetic Breast Augmentations: Postoperative Complications and Associated Factors. *Aesthetic Plast. Surg.* **2007**, *31*, 532–539. [CrossRef]
28. Alderman, A.K.; Collins, E.D.; Streu, R.; Grotting, J.C.; Sulkin, A.L.; Neligan, P.; Haeck, P.C.; Gutowski, K.A. Benchmarking Outcomes in Plastic Surgery: National Complication Rates for Abdominoplasty and Breast Augmentation 'Outcomes Article'. *Plast. Reconstr. Surg.* **2009**, *124*, 2127–2133. [CrossRef]
29. Kjøller, K.; Hölmich, L.R.; Jacobsen, P.H.; Friis, S.; Fryzek, J.; McLaughlin, J.K.; Lipworth, L.; Henriksen, T.F.; Jørgensen, S.; Bittmann, S.; et al. Epidemiological Investigation of Local Complications After Cosmetic Breast Implant Surgery in Denmark. *Ann. Plast. Surg.* **2002**, *48*, 229–237. [CrossRef]
30. Washer, L.L.; Gutowski, K. Breast Implant Infections. *Infect. Dis. Clin. North Am.* **2012**, *26*, 111–125. [CrossRef]
31. Sörgel, C.A.; Schmid, R.; Stadelmann, N.; Weisbach, V.; Distel, L.; Horch, R.E.; Kengelbach-Weigand, A. IGF-I and Hyaluronic Acid Mitigate the Negative Effect of Irradiation on Human Skin Keratinocytes. *Cancers* **2022**, *14*, 588. [CrossRef] [PubMed]
32. Zhou, Y.; Liu, Y.; Wang, Y.; Wu, Y. Comparison of Oncoplastic Breast-Conserving Therapy and Standard Breast-Conserving Therapy in Early-Stage Breast Cancer Patients. *J. Pharmacol. Exp. Ther.* **2020**, *26*, e927015. [CrossRef] [PubMed]
33. Müller-Seubert, W.; Ostermaier, P.; Horch, R.E.; Distel, L.; Frey, B.; Cai, A.; Arkudas, A. Intra- and Early Postoperative Evaluation of Malperfused Areas in an Irradiated Random Pattern Skin Flap Model Using Indocyanine Green Angiography and Near-Infrared Reflectance-Based Imaging and Infrared Thermography. *J. Pers. Med.* **2022**, *12*, 237. [CrossRef] [PubMed]
34. Müller-Seubert, W.; Roth, S.; Hauck, T.; Arkudas, A.; Horch, R.E.; Ludolph, I. Novel imaging methods reveal positive impact of topical negative pressure application on tissue perfusion in an in vivo skin model. *Int. Wound J.* **2021**, *18*, 932–939. [CrossRef]
35. Diehm, Y.F.; Fischer, S.; Wirth, G.A.; Haug, V.; Orgill, D.P.; Momeni, A.; Horch, R.E.; Lehner, B.; Kneser, U.; Hirche, C. Management of Acute and Traumatic Wounds With Negative-Pressure Wound Therapy With Instillation and Dwell Time. *Plast. Reconstr. Surg.* **2020**, *147*, 43S–53S. [CrossRef]
36. Vasilakis, V.; Yamin, F.; Reish, R.G. Surgeons' Dilemma: Treatment of Implant-Associated Infection in the Cosmetic Breast Augmentation Patient. *Aesthetic Plast. Surg.* **2019**, *43*, 905–909. [CrossRef]
37. Spear, S.L.; Howard, M.A.; Boehmler, J.H.; Ducic, I.; Low, M.; Abbruzzesse, M.R. The Infected or Exposed Breast Implant: Management and Treatment Strategies. *Plast. Reconstr. Surg.* **2004**, *113*, 1634–1644. [CrossRef]
38. Müller-Seubert, W.; Cai, A.; Arkudas, A.; Ludolph, I.; Fritz, N.; Horch, R.E. A Personalized Approach to Treat Advanced Stage Severely Contracted Joints in Dupuytren's Disease with a Unique Skeletal Distraction Device—Utilizing Modern Imaging Tools to Enhance Safety for the Patient. *J. Pers. Med.* **2022**, *12*, 378. [CrossRef]
39. Anchalia, M.; Upadhyay, S.; Dahiya, M. Negative Pressure Wound Therapy With Instillation and Dwell Time and Standard Negative Pressure Wound Therapy in Complex Wounds: Are They Complementary or Competitive? *Wounds* **2020**, *32*, E84–E91.
40. Schreiner, W.; Ludolph, I.; Dudek, W.; Horch, R.E.; Sirbu, H. Negative Pressure Wound Therapy Combined With Instillation for Sternoclavicular Joint Infection. *Ann. Thorac. Surg.* **2020**, *110*, 1722–1725. [CrossRef]
41. Dassoulas, K.R.; Wang, J.; Thuman, J.; Ndem, I.; Schaeffer, C.; Stovall, M.; Campbell, C.A. Reducing Infection Rates in Implant-Based Breast Reconstruction: Impact of an Evidence-based Protocol. *Ann. Plast. Surg.* **2018**, *80*, 493–499. [CrossRef] [PubMed]
42. Wixtrom, R.N.; Stutman, R.L.; Burke, R.M.; Mahoney, B.A.K.; Codner, M.A. Risk of Breast Implant Bacterial Contamination From Endogenous Breast Flora, Prevention With Nipple Shields, and Implications for Biofilm Formation. *Aesthetic Surg. J.* **2012**, *32*, 956–963. [CrossRef] [PubMed]
43. Meybodi, F.; Sedaghat, N.; Elder, E.; French, J.; Adams, K.; Hsu, J.; Kanesalingam, K.; Brennan, M. Salvaging the Unsalvageable: Negative Pressure Wound Therapy for Severe Infection of Prosthetic Breast Reconstruction. *Plast. Reconstr. Surg. Glob. Open* **2021**, *9*, e3456. [CrossRef] [PubMed]
44. Accurso, A.; Rocco, N.; Accardo, G.; Reale, P.; Salerno, C.; Mattera, E.; D'Andrea, F. Innovative Management of Implant Exposure in ADM/Implant-Based Breast Reconstruction with Negative Pressure Wound Therapy. *Aesthetic Plast. Surg.* **2016**, *41*, 36–39. [CrossRef]
45. Horch, R.E.; Braumann, C.; Dissemond, J.; Lehner, B.; Hirche, C.; Woeste, G.; Willy, C. Use of Negative Pressure Wound Therapy with Instillation and Dwell Time for Wound Treatment-Results of an Expert Consensus Conference. *Zent. Chir.* **2018**, *143*, 609–616.
46. Stumpfe, M.C.; E Horch, R.; Geierlehner, A.; Ludolph, I. Rare Pseudotumor-like Hematoma at the Latissimus Dorsi Muscle Flap Donor Site: A Treatment Strategy Utilizing Negative Pressure Wound Therapy With Instillation and Dwell Time. *Wounds* **2020**, *32*, E101–E105.
47. Stumpfe, M.C.; Horch, R.E.; Arkudas, A.; Cai, A.; Müller-Seubert, W.; Hauck, T.; Ludolph, I. The Value of Negative-Pressure Wound Therapy and Flap Surgery in Hidradenitis Suppurativa—A Single Center Analysis of Different Treatment Options. *Front. Surg.* **2022**, *9*, 867487. [CrossRef]
48. Meybodi, F.; Sedaghat, N.; French, J.; Keighley, C.; Mitchell, D.; Elder, E. Implant salvage in breast reconstruction with severe peri-prosthetic infection. *ANZ J. Surg.* **2015**, *87*, E293–E299. [CrossRef]

49. Kendrick, A.S.; Chase, C.W. Salvage of an Infected Breast Tissue Expander with an Implant Sizer and Negative Pressure Wound Management. *Plast. Reconstr. Surg.* **2008**, *121*, 138e–139e. [CrossRef]
50. Liao, E.; Breuing, K.H. Breast Mound Salvage Using Vacuum-Assisted Closure Device as Bridge to Reconstruction With Inferolateral AlloDerm Hammock. *Ann. Plast. Surg.* **2007**, *59*, 218–224. [CrossRef]
51. Albright, S.B.; Xue, A.S.; McKnight, A.; Wolfswinkel, E.M.; Hollier, L.H.; Brown, R.H.; Bullocks, J.M.; Izaddoost, S.A. One-Step Salvage of Infected Prosthetic Breast Reconstructions Using Antibiotic-Impregnated Polymethylmethacrylate Plates and Concurrent Tissue Expander Exchange. *Ann. Plast. Surg.* **2016**, *77*, 280–285. [CrossRef] [PubMed]

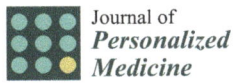

## Article

# An In Vitro Approach for Investigating the Safety of Lipotransfer after Breast-Conserving Therapy

Theresa Promny [1,*], Chiara-Sophia Kutz [1], Tina Jost [2], Luitpold V. Distel [2], Sheetal Kadam [1], Rafael Schmid [1], Andreas Arkudas [1], Raymund E. Horch [1] and Annika Kengelbach-Weigand [1]

[1] Department of Plastic and Hand Surgery, University Hospital Erlangen, Friedrich-Alexander-Universität Erlangen-Nürnberg, 91054 Erlangen, Germany
[2] Department of Radiation Oncology, University Hospital Erlangen, Friedrich-Alexander-Universität Erlangen-Nürnberg, 91054 Erlangen, Germany
* Correspondence: theresa.promny@uk-erlangen.de; Tel.: +49-9131-853327

**Abstract:** The application of lipotransfer after breast-conserving therapy (BCT) and irradiation in breast cancer patients is an already widespread procedure for reconstructing volume deficits of the diseased breast. Nevertheless, the safety of lipotransfer has still not been clarified yet due to contradictory data. The goal of this in vitro study was to further elucidate the potential effects of lipotransfer on the irradiated remaining breast tissue. The mammary epithelial cell line MCF-10A was co-cultured with the fibroblast cell line MRC-5 and irradiated with 2 and 5 Gy. Afterwards, cells were treated with conditioned medium (CM) from adipose-derived stem cells (ADSC), and the effects on the cellular functions of MCF-10A cells and on gene expression at the mRNA level in MCF-10A and MRC-5 cells were analyzed. Treatment with ADSC CM stimulated transmigration and invasion and decreased the surviving fraction of MCF-10A cells. Further, the expression of cytokines, extracellular, and mesenchymal markers was enhanced in mammary epithelial cells. Only an effect of ADSC CM on irradiated fibroblasts could be observed. The present data suggest epithelial–mesenchymal transition-like changes in the epithelial mammary breast cell line. Thus, the benefits of lipotransfer after BCT should be critically weighed against its possible risks for the affected patients.

**Keywords:** adipose-derived stem cells; ADSC; MCF-10A; mammary epithelial cells; irradiation; fibroblasts; epithelial-mesenchymal transition; mesenchymal markers

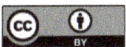

## 1. Introduction

Multimodal treatment of breast cancer consists of surgical treatment as well as systemic therapies and adjuvant radiation, depending on the underlying breast cancer subtype and breast cancer stage. Thereby, surgical therapy has become more conservative over the last decades and breast-conserving therapy (BCT), usually followed by radiation therapy, has evolved into a widespread alternative to mastectomy for patients with early breast cancer [1,2]. However, BCT might provide disfiguring results, so patients and surgeons aim to reconstruct the original anatomical contours of the breast [3–5]. This can be achieved by lipofilling or lipotransfer, a procedure in which fat is harvested via liposuction from typically used donor-sites (e.g., the abdomen, flank, thighs) and subsequently transplanted into the breast. Besides its many advantages including a natural appearance and texture, low donor-site morbidity, and easy availability, autologous fat transplants often show a low rate of graft survival [6]. The fat grafts include a minor fraction of adipose-derived stem cells (ADSC). To ameliorate graft viability, supplementation of the fat grafts with ADSC has been proposed [7,8]. ADSC have immunomodulatory and paracrine characteristics and secrete several cytokines, chemokines, and growth factors, e.g., vascular endothelial growth factor (VEGF), fibroblast growth factor 2 (FGF-2), and insulin-like growth factor 1 (IGF-1) [9–11]. These capacities are associated with regenerative effects and might contribute to higher fat engraftment, especially in irradiated tissues [12]. On the other hand, they might confer an oncological potential on the grafted fat. The issue of the oncological safety of lipotransfer, particularly to a site where malignancy was treated, has been discussed widely and controversially in the literature. Whereas predominantly clinical studies claim a safe use of lipotransfer [13–18], pre-clinical studies suggested an ADSC-induced promotion of breast cancer growth and tumor angiogenesis [9,19–22]. Among other factors, the role of vascularization in any recipient tissue for cell ingrowth or proliferation is certainly relevant [23–25]. Further, previous studies showed that ADSC can also influence healthy breast tissue and induce an epithelial-to-mesenchymal transition in mammary epithelial cells [26]. This observation should not be neglected, as many patients undergo lipotransfer after BCT with the remaining tissue consisting partially of mammary epithelial cells. In most of the cases, this tissue has also been irradiated. Radiotherapy has an outstanding role in the treatment of breast cancer to eliminate (residual) cancer cells. However, it has also an effect on the surrounding tissue. There is evidence that the microenvironment contributes to the initiation, proliferation, and metastasis of a tumor [27–29]. Thereby, fibroblasts, the predominant cellular component of the tumor microenvironment, play a decisive role. Previous investigations showed that stromal fibroblasts are involved in the control of the growth and morphogenesis of normal and tumorigenic breast epithelial cells [30,31]. Additionally, they can be activated by endogenous stimuli, such as cytokines and growth factors secreted by tumor cells, or by external stimuli, such as radiation therapy [32–34]. Those activated "cancer-associated fibroblasts" (CAF) are considered fundamental actors in tumor progression and were shown to promote tumor growth, invasion, and metastasis [35]. Further, they have been attributed a role in stroma-mediated radiotherapy resistance [36]. Thus, tumor development, growth, recurrence, and resistance to therapies is dependent on various factors. When investigating the oncological safety of lipotransfer after BCT, the interplay of different cell types and external stimuli should be considered.

The present experimental in vitro study aims to further elucidate the effect of lipotransfer on breast tissue. Therefore, we investigated the influence of ADSC on mammary epithelial cells after exposure to irradiation while taking into account an important element of the microenvironment, the fibroblasts, by using a co-cultivation model. Thereby, functional analysis was performed, and alterations in gene expression profiles were investigated.

## 2. Materials and Methods

### 2.1. Cell Lines and Cell Culture

MCF-10A (ATCC® CRL-10317™), a human mammary epithelial cell line, was a kind gift from Matthias Rübner, Department of Obstetrics and Gynaecology, University Hospital Erlangen. MCF-10A cells were cultivated in Mammary Epithelial Cell Growth Medium (MECGM; PromoCell GmbH, Heidelberg, Germany) supplemented with 5 µg/mL insulin, 0.5 µg/mL hydrocortisone, 10 ng/mL epidermal growth factor (EGF), 0.004 mL/mL bovine pituitary extract (BPE; PromoCell), 100 ng/mL cholera toxin (Sigma Aldrich, St. Louis, MO, USA), and 1% penicillin/streptomycin (Sigma Aldrich).

The human fibroblast cell line MRC-5 was purchased from ATCC (ATCC® MRC-5 CCL-171™). It was cultivated in Eagle's Minimum Essential Medium (EMEM; ATCC, Manassas, VA, USA) supplemented with 10% fetal calf serum superior (FCS superior; Sigma Aldrich). ASC/TERT1, a human-adipose-tissue-derived telomerase-immortalized mesenchymal stem cell line, was purchased from Evercyte (Evercyte GmbH, Vienna, Austria). For their cultivation we used the Endothelial Cell Growth Medium (EGM)-2 BulletKit™ (Lonza Group AG, Basel, Switzerland), a culture system containing Endothelial Cell Basal Medium-2 (EBM™-2) and EGM™-2 SingleQuots™ Supplements, enriched with 200 µg/mL Geneticin™ (Gibco® Life Technologies, Carlsbad, CA, USA) and 2% FCS superior (Sigma Aldrich). All cells were cultivated at 37 °C and 5% $CO_2$. The medium was changed every 2–3 days.

*2.2. Experimental Setup*

A total of $2 \times 10^4$ MCF-10A cells were seeded in their standard medium into the lower compartment of a 6-well transwell system (pore size 0.4 µm) and cultivated until 50–60% confluency. Subsequently, the medium was replaced by a mixed co-culture medium consisting of 2/3 MEGM and 1/3 EMEM, including their respective supplements, and $6 \times 10^5$ MRC-5 cells were placed into the transwells (6-Well ThinCert™ Cell Culture Inserts, Greiner Bio-One, Frickenhausen, Germany). For the control group, MCF-10A cells were seeded into the transwells. Irradiation with 0 (control), 2, and 5 Gy was applied after 24 h of co-cultivation. After another 24 h, co-cultures were either treated with ADSC conditioned medium (CM) for 48 h for later RNA isolation and flow cytometry or irradiated co-cultures were cultivated for a further 48 h with a mixed co-culture medium. Thereafter, MCF-10A cells were collected for later transmigration and invasion analysis with ADSC CM.

For an analysis of gene expression of MRC-5 cells, MRC-5 cells in the transwells were harvested for RNA isolation. For monoculture control, $4 \times 10^3$ MRC-5 cells were seeded in the lower compartment and cultivated until 50–60% confluency. The further procedure was analogous to the setup described above.

*2.3. Preparation of ADSC Conditioned Medium (CM)*

ASC/TERT1 were seeded in 75 cm$^2$ cell culture flasks with EBM-2 medium containing standard supplements. They were cultivated until they reached 90% confluency. After washing the cells with phosphate-buffered saline (PBS; Sigma Aldrich), ADSC were incubated in EBMTM-2 without supplements for 24 h. Filter tubes (Amicon® Ultra-15 Centrifugal Filter Devices, 3 K; Merck KGaA, Darmstadt, Germany) were used for concentrating CM. CM was centrifuged at $4000 \times g$ for 30 min, and the ultrafiltrate of 15 mL CM was diluted with 2/3 MECGM containing 5% supplement mix and 1/3 EMEM supplemented with 0.5% FCS superior (in the following described as "reduced mixed co-culture medium") up to a total volume of 5 mL to obtain 3-fold concentrated CM. The control medium (EBM-2 medium containing standard supplements without cells) was incubated under the same conditions and concentrated as above.

*2.4. Irradiation*

Irradiation was conducted with X-rays at a voltage of 120 kV and a 2 mm aluminum filter using an Isovolt Titan 160 X-ray machine (GE Sensing & Inspection Technologies, Ahrensburg, Germany). The focus-field distance was 21 cm. Irradiation doses of 2 Gy or 5 Gy were achieved at a dose rate of 2 Gy per minute. 0 Gy was utilized as control.

*2.5. Flow Cytometry for Analysis of Apoptosis and Necrosis*

After the irradiation and treatment of the cells with ADSC CM (including controls), cells including the supernatant were harvested. Cells were washed, resuspended in 200 µL of Ringer solution, and stained with 10 µL of a 1:1 mixture of Annexin V-APC (BD Biosciences, Heidelberg, Germany) and 7-amino-actinomycin D (7-AAD; BD Biosciences) for 30 min on ice. Cell suspensions were transferred to 96-well plates to investigate apoptosis and necrosis via the Cytoflex flow cytometer (Cytoflex, Beckman Coulter, Brea, CA, USA). Excitation at 660/10 nm was used to measure Annexin V-APC stained cells; excitation at 546 nm was used to measure 7-AAD stained cells. For data evaluation, FlowJo™ Analysis Software v10 (FlowJo LCC, BD Biosciences, Ashland, OR, USA) was used. Annexin V-APC-positive and 7AAD-negativ cells were defined as apoptotic cells, and Annexin V-APC-positive and 7AAD-positive cells as necrotic cells. Double-negative cells (Annexin V-APC-negative and 7AAD-negative) were defined as viable cells. Cells without any staining were used for a negative control, and cells treated with 56° C for 20 min served as positive control. Flow cytometry was performed in technical triplicate and in three independent experiments.

## 2.6. Invasion and Transmigration Assay

Invasion and transmigration assays were performed in a 24-well plate using transwell inserts with a pore size of 8 µm (ThinCert™, Greiner Bio-One GmbH, Frickenhausen, Germany), whereby transwells for invasion assays were coated with 2.4 mg/mL collagen type I from bovine skin (Sigma-Aldrich). A total of 72 h after irradiation, MCF-10A cells were harvested, and $1 \times 10^5$ cells were seeded with 300 µl reduced mixed co-culture medium into the transwells. A total of 700 µl of ADSC CM or corresponding control medium was filled into the lower chamber. The cells were incubated for 8 h at 37 °C and 5% $CO_2$. Thereafter, the transwell inserts were washed with PBS, followed by fixation with ice-cold methanol and staining with 1 µg/mL 4′,6-diamidino-2-phenylindole (DAPI) for 10 min (Life technologies). A PBS-coated cotton swab was used in twisting motions to remove the remaining cells in the inner part of the transwells. For counting transmigrated and invaded cells in the four quadrants of each transwell, an Olympus IX83 microscope (cellSens Software, Olympus Corporation, Tokio, Japan) was used for 40-fold magnification. Transmigration and invasion assays were performed in technical triplicate and in three independent experiments. Transmigrated or invaded cells, respectively, were semi-automatically measured with Fiji Is Just ImageJ (Fiji) [37].

## 2.7. Quantitative Real-Time PCR

Expression of selected cytokines, extracellular matrix (ECM) markers, and mesenchymal markers was analyzed at the mRNA level. Therefore, RNA was extracted using the RNeasy Mini Kit (Qiagen, Hilden, Germany). QuantiTect Reverse Transcription Kit with a DNase I incubation (Qiagen) was used for the reverse transcription of RNA into cDNA. Quantitative real-time PCR was conducted with a Bio-Rad CFX96 Real-Time PCR detection system (Bio-Rad Laboratories, Hercules, CA, USA) with the SsoAdvanced™ Universal SYBR® Green Supermix (Bio-Rad Laboratories). The kits were used according to the manufacturers' recommendations. Detected transcript levels were normalized to the housekeeping genes Tyrosine 3-monooxygenase/tryptophan 5-monooxygenase activation protein, zeta (*YWHAZ*), and Glyceraldehyde-3-phosphate dehydrogenase (*GAPDH*) using the $2^{-\Delta\Delta CT}$-method. Samples were tested in technical triplicate and PCR was performed in three independent experiments. Primer sequences are specified in Table 1.

**Table 1.** Primer sequences.

| Gene | Forward | Reverse |
|---|---|---|
| FGF2 | CCACCTATAATTGGTCAAAGTGGTT | TCATCAGTTACCAGCTCCCCC |
| TNF-Alpha | TGGGATCATTGCCCTGTGAG | GGTGTCTGAAGGAGGGGGTA |
| IL1B | GCTCGCCAGTGAAATGATGG | GGTGGTCGGAGATTCGTAGC |
| TGFB1 | CATGGAGGACCTGGATGCC | TCCTGAAGACTCCCCAGACC |
| COL1A1 | GCTCTTGCAACATCTCCCCT | CCTTCCTGACTCTCCTCCGA |
| MMP2 | GCCGTGTTTGCCATCTGTTT | AGCAGACACCATCACCTGTG |
| FN1 | GAGAAGTATGTGCATGGTGTCAG | AATACTTCGACAGGACCACTTGA |
| VIM | AATCCAAGTTTGCTGACCTCTC | GTCTCCGGTACTCAGTGGACTC |
| CDH2 | TCAATGACAATCCTCCAGAGTTTA | TGATCCTTATCGGTCACAGTTAGA |
| YWHAZ | ATGAGCTGGTTCAGAAGGCC | AAGATGACCTACGGGCTCCT |
| GAPDH | TCCACCCATGGCAAATTCCA | TTCCCGTTCTCAGCCTTGAC |

*FGF2*: fibroblast growth factor-2, *TNF-Alpha*: tumor necrosis factor alpha, *IL1B*: interleukin-1β, *TGFB1*: transforming growth factor-β, *COL1A1*: collagen type I alpha 1 chain, *MMP2*: matrix metallopeptidase 2, *FN1*: fibronectin 1, *VIM*: vimentin, *CDH2*: cadherin-2/N-cadherin, *YWHAZ*: tyrosine 3-monooxygenase/tryptophan 5-monooxygenase activation protein, zeta, *GAPDH*: glyceraldehyde-3-phosphate dehydrogenase.

## 2.8. Statistics

Data are presented as mean ± standard deviation. All assays were performed in three replicate experiments. Statistical analysis was performed using the Mann–Whitney U test; the asymptotic significance was used (SPSS v.21.0 Software/IBM, Armonk, NY, USA). Fig-

## 3. Results

*3.1. ADSC CM Stimulated the Transmigration, Invasion, and Decreased Survival of MCF-10A Cells after Irradiation with 5 Gy*

ADSC CM significantly stimulated the transmigration of MCF-10A in monoculture, as well as in co-culture with MRC-5 ($p = 0.037$; Figure 1A). In the 5 Gy irradiated cells, this effect decreased compared to non-irradiated samples or samples irradiated with 2 Gy. Additionally, the invasion ability of MCF-10A cells increased after treatment with ADSC CM in MCF-10A monoculture with 0 Gy irradiation and in both monoculture and co-culture after irradiation with 5 Gy ($p = 0.037$; Figure 1B). Apoptosis and necrosis analysis using flow cytometry detected lower cell survival after treatment with ADSC CM within the 5 Gy irradiation group ($p = 0.037$; Figure 1C).

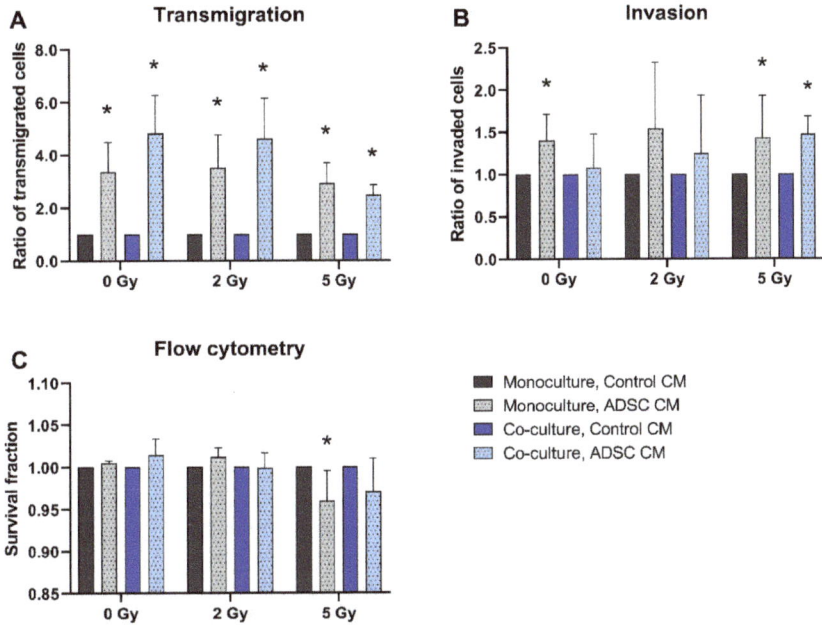

**Figure 1.** Effect of adipose-derived stem cell conditioned medium (ADSC CM) on the transmigration (**A**), invasion (**B**), and cell survival (**C**) of MCF-10A cells. MCF-10A cells were cultured as a mono- or co-culture with fibroblasts; irradiated with 0, 2, or 5 Gy; and treated with either ADSC CM or control CM. Data from the ADSC CM treatment group were normalized to the corresponding group treated with control CM (control = 1). (**A–C**) Columns show the ratio of transmigrated cells (**A**), invaded cells (**B**), and the survival fraction (**C**) compared to the control group (y-axis) in mono- and co-cultured cells in varying irradiation doses treated with ADSC CM or control CM (x-axis). $n = 3$ replicate experiments, and values are presented as mean ± SD. * $p < 0.05$, and the ADSC CM was compared to the control CM (Mann–Whitney U-test).

For analyzing the effects of ADSC CM, data of cells treated with ADSC CM were normalized to the corresponding mono- or co-culture group that were treated with control CM.

### 3.2. Co-Cultivation with Fibroblasts had a Small Effect on Transmigration and No Effect on the Invasion and Survival of MCF-10A Cells

The transmigration rate of co-cultured and 5 Gy-irradiated MCF-10A cells treated with control CM was significantly higher compared to monocultures ($p = 0.037$; Figure 2A). Co-culture with fibroblasts had no significant effect on MCF-10A invasion or cell survival (Figure 2B,C).

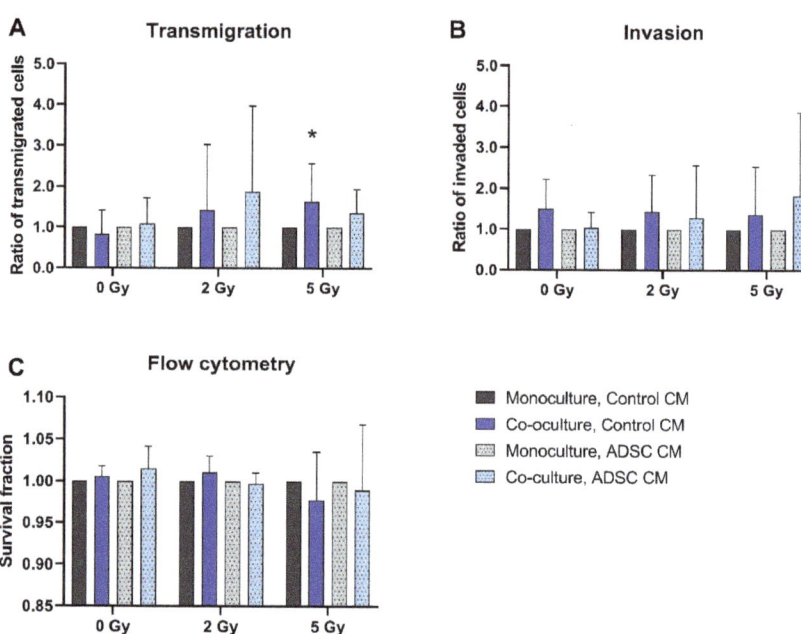

**Figure 2.** Effect of co-cultured fibroblasts on the transmigration (**A**), invasion (**B**), and cell survival (**C**) of MCF-10A cells compared to monocultured MCF-10A cells. MCF-10A cells were cultured as mono- or co-culture with fibroblasts; irradiated with 0, 2, or 5 Gy; and treated either with adipose-derived stem cell conditioned medium (ADSC CM) or control CM. Data from the co-culture group were normalized to the corresponding monoculture group (control = 1). (**A–C**) Columns show the ratio of transmigrated cells (**A**), invaded cells (**B**), and the survival fraction (**C**) compared to the control group (y-axis) in mono- and co-cultured cells in varying irradiation doses and treated with ADSC CM or control CM (x-axis). $n = 3$ replicate experiments, and values are presented as mean ± SD. * $p < 0.05$, and the co-culture was compared to the monoculture (Mann-Whitney U-Test).

### 3.3. Irradiation of Mono- and Co-Cultures Decreased Transmigration and Cell Survival and Stimulated the Invasion Rates of MCF-10A Cells

A total of 5 Gy irradiation inhibited the transmigration of MCF-10A cells in monocultures and in co-cultures treated with ADSC CM compared to non-irradiated cells ($p = 0.037$; Figure 3A). In contrast, the invasion of monocultured MCF-10A cells treated with control CM and of co-cultured MCF-10A cells treated with ADSC CM was significantly increased after irradiation with 5 Gy ($p = 0.037$; Figure 3B). Irradiation decreased the cell survival of MCF-10A cells significantly, whereby the surviving fraction was lower after irradiation with the higher irradiation dose (Figure 3C).

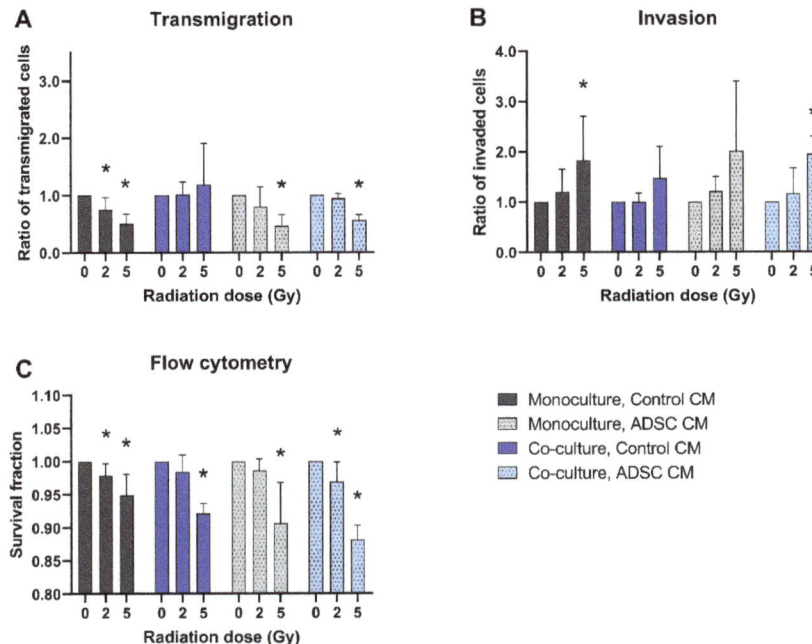

**Figure 3.** Effect of radiation on the transmigration (**A**), invasion (**B**), and cell survival (**C**) of MCF-10A cells compared to non-irradiated cells. MCF-10A cells were cultured as mono- or co-culture with fibroblasts; irradiated with 0, 2, or 5 Gy, and treated either with adipose-derived stem cell conditioned medium (ADSC CM) or control CM. Irradiation with 0 Gy was set 1 for each group. (**A–C**) Columns show the ratio of transmigrated cells (**A**), invaded cells (**B**), and the percentage of live cells (**C**; y-axis) in varying radiation doses and for mono- and co-cultured cells treated with ADSC CM or control CM (x-axis). $n = 3$ replicate experiments, and values are presented as mean ± SD. *: $p < 0.05$, and 5 Gy and 2 Gy were compared to 0 Gy (Mann–Whitney U-test).

*3.4. Treatment with ADSC CM Induced Alterations in the Gene Expression Profile in Co-cultured and Irradiated MCF-10A Cells*

For investigating changes in the gene expression of MCF-10A cells, we tested the expression of several cytokines, ECM markers, and mesenchymal markers. Thereby, alterations after treatment with ADSC CM could be mainly observed in co-cultivated and irradiated MCF-10A cells. Results are summarized in Figure 4A. Co-cultured MCF-10A cells showed an increase in the expression of tumor necrosis factor alpha (*TNF-α*), independently of the applied radiation dose ($p = 0.037$). Further, the expression of fibroblast growth factor-2 (*FGF2*) was enhanced in 2 Gy-irradiated monocultured and co-cultured MCF-10A cells after treatment with ADSC CM compared to treatment with control CM ($p = 0.037$). mRNA levels of interleukin-1β (*IL-1β*) were up-regulated significantly after treatment with ADSC CM in monocultured and co-cultured, non-irradiated MCF-10A cells ($p = 0.037$). Transforming growth factor-β (*TGF-β*) appears to play a minor role and was only enhanced in monocultured, non-irradiated MCF-10A cells after treatment with ADSC CM ($p = 0.037$). Regarding ECM markers, we observed an ADSC CM-induced upregulation of matrix metallopeptidase 2 (*MMP2*) in 2 Gy-irradiated monocultured and in 2 and 5 Gy-irradiated co-cultured MCF-10A cells. Further, ADSC CM stimulated the expression of collagen type I alpha 1 chain (*COL1A1*) in 5 Gy-irradiated co-cultured MCF-10A cells ($p = 0.037$), suggesting an influence of ADSC on ECM remodeling. Moreover, treatment with ADSC CM induced an upregulation of mesenchymal markers. Thereby, the expression of fibronectin 1 (*FN1*) was upregulated in irradiated, as well as in non-irradiated, MCF-10A cells, whereas the mRNA levels of N-cadherin (*CDH2*) and vimentin (*VIM*) were only enhanced in irradiated cells, indicating the involvement of radiation-induced pathways.

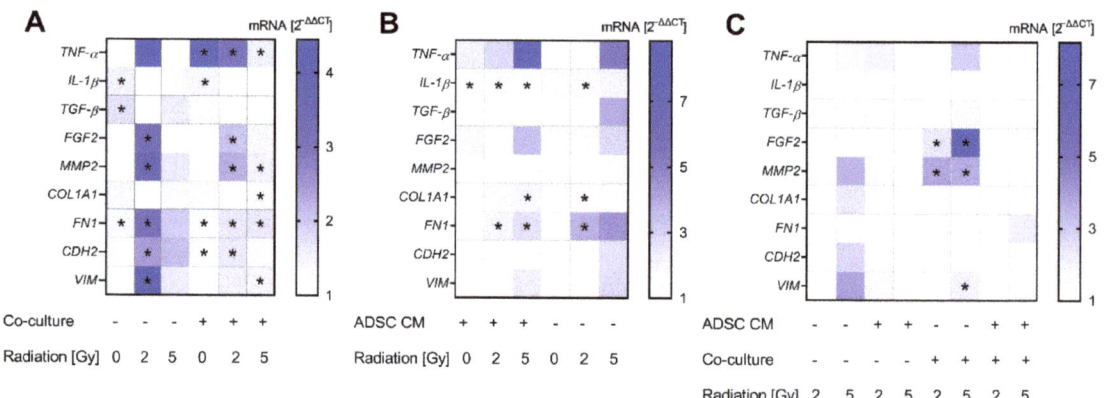

**Figure 4.** Alterations in gene expression profiles at the mRNA level in MCF-10A cells. The heatmaps show mean relative mRNA expression in MCF-10A cells compared to *GAPDH/YWHAZ* and to the corresponding control group, $n = 3$ replicate experiments. (**A**) Shows the effect of treatment with conditioned medium (CM) of adipose-derived stem cells (ADSC) normalized to treatment with control CM. (**B**) Presents the effect of co-cultivation with fibroblasts normalized to monocultures. The effect of irradiation is demonstrated in (**C**), whereby irradiation with 2 Gy and 5 Gy is normalized to 0 Gy. Values were calculated using the $2^{-\Delta\Delta CT}$ method, $2^{-\Delta\Delta CT}$ of control = 1. White fields: $2^{-\Delta\Delta CT} < 1$; * $p < 0.05$, increased compared to the corresponding control (Mann–Whitney U-test). *TNF-α*: tumor necrosis factor alpha, *IL-1β*: interleukin-1β, *TGF-β*: transforming growth factor-β, *FGF2*: fibroblast growth factor-2, *MMP2*: matrix metallopeptidase 2, *COL1A1*: collagen type I alpha 1 chain, *FN1*: fibronectin 1, *CDH2*: cadherin-2/N-cadherin, *VIM*: vimentin.

Data on co-cultures were also normalized to the corresponding conditions in monoculture to analyze the effect of co-cultivation with fibroblasts (Figure 4B). Thereby, we found a small, but significant, increase in *IL-1β* expression in co-cultured MCF-10A cells in the ADSC CM treatment group ($p = 0.037$). Moreover, *COL1A1* and *FN1* were enhanced in irradiated co-cultured MCF-10A cells.

Normalizing the data of 2 Gy- and 5 Gy-irradiated groups to the corresponding non-irradiated cells revealed a 2 and 5 Gy irradiation-induced upregulation of *FGF2* and *MMP2* in co-cultured MCF-10A cells treated with control CM ($p = 0.037$; Figure 4C). Furthermore, 5 Gy irradiation induced an enhanced expression of *VIM* in co-cultured and non-irradiated MCF-10A cells ($p = 0.037$).

*3.5. In MRC-5 Cells, Co-Cultured MRC-5 Cells Revealed an Upregulation of IL-1β, and Irradiation of Co-Cultured MRC-5 Cells Showed a Higher Expression of TGF-β*

For a gene expression analysis of MRC-5 cells, the selected cytokines and ECM marker according to recent results were examined. Altogether, we observed a minor effect from ADSC CM and irradiation on the gene expression of fibroblasts, apart from *TGF-β*. Results are summarized in Figure 5. Treatment with ADSC CM revealed an increased expression of *TGF-β* in non-irradiated and 5 Gy-irradiated and co-cultured MRC-5 cells ($p = 0.037$; Figure 5A). Further, we observed an enhanced expression of *COL1A1* in co-cultured and 5 Gy-irradiated fibroblasts after treatment with ADSC CM ($p = 0.037$; Figure 5A).

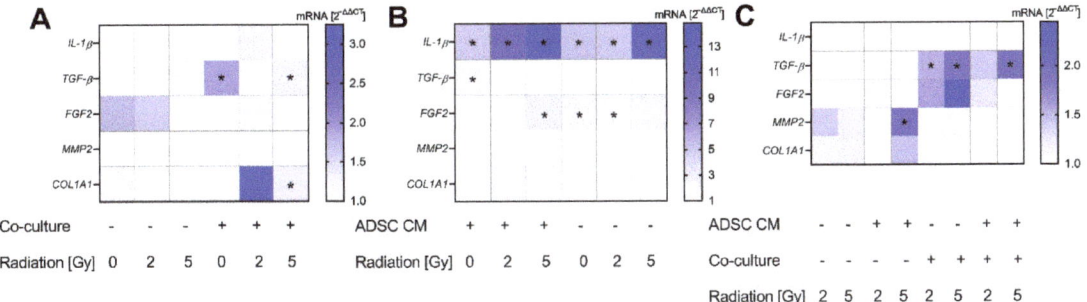

**Figure 5.** Alterations in gene expression profiles at the mRNA level in MRC-5 cells. The heatmaps show mean relative mRNA expression in MRC-5 cells compared to *GAPDH/YWHAZ* and to the corresponding control group, $n = 3$ replicate experiments. (**A**) Shows the effect of treatment with conditioned medium (CM) of adipose-derived stem cells (ADSC) normalized to treatment with control CM. (**B**) Presents the effect of co-cultivation with MCF-10A cells normalized to fibroblast monocultures. The effect of irradiation is demonstrated in (**C**), whereby irradiation with 2 Gy and 5 Gy is normalized to 0 Gy. Values were calculated using the $2^{-\Delta\Delta CT}$ method, $2^{-\Delta\Delta CT}$ of control = 1. White fields: $2^{-\Delta\Delta CT} < 1$; * $p < 0.05$, increased compared to the corresponding control (Mann–Whitney U-test). *IL-1β*: interleukin-1β, *TGF-β*: transforming growth factor-β, *FGF2*: fibroblast growth factor-2, *MMP2*: matrix metallopeptidase 2, *COL1A11*: collagen type I alpha 1 chain.

The co-cultivation of MRC-5 with MCF-10A cells showed an upregulation of *IL-1β* ($p = 0.037$) with an up-to-14-fold increase in 5 Gy-irradiated cells and independently from treatment with ADSC CM (Figure 5B). Moreover, co-cultivation stimulated the expression of *FGF2* in 5 Gy-irradiated fibroblasts treated with ADSC CM and in 0 and 2 Gy-irradiated fibroblasts treated with control CM ($p = 0.037$). *TGF-β* was only upregulated in the non-irradiated and ADSC CM group. However, irradiation evoked higher *TGF-β* mRNA levels in co-cultured fibroblasts (Figure 5C). Whereas no stimulatory effect of ADSC CM and co-culture per se could be observed in *MMP2* expression, irradiation with 5 Gy revealed higher mRNA levels of *MMP2* in monocultured and ADSC CM-treated fibroblasts compared to the non-irradiated cells ($p = 0.037$), supporting an influence of irradiation on MMP activation and ECM digestion.

## 4. Discussion

Despite contradictory data regarding the safety of lipotransfer, the application of lipotransfer after BCT in breast cancer patients is an already widespread procedure for reconstructing volume deficits of the diseased breast. Concerns particularly arise with regard to the regeneration of tissue at an anatomic region where cancer has been treated. The question whether lipotransfer induces or accelerates the development of a subclinical tumor, locoregional disease recurrence, or tumor dissemination has not yet been clarified. Further experimental and standardized clinical studies are urgently needed to answer this question from different perspectives and to draw reliable conclusions. As irradiation of the residual breast tissue is an integral part after BCT in most of the cases, the effect of irradiation should not be neglected. Further, the tumor microenvironment was described as an essential part of malignant transformation. Thus, investigations on the influence of lipotransfer should include the tumor microenvironment. In this study, we analyzed the effects of lipotransfer on irradiated and non-irradiated MCF-10 cells in monoculture or in co-culture with fibroblasts as the main cellular component of the tumor microenvironment. Moreover, alterations in gene expression in fibroblasts were examined.

In the present study we observed a strong stimulatory effect of ADSC CM on the transmigration of mammary epithelial cells. Further, the invasion of MCF-10A cells was stimulated by ADSC CM, though to a lesser extent compared to transmigration capability.

Additionally, the mesenchymal cell markers *FN1*, *CDH2*, and *VIM* were upregulated in irradiated MCF-10A cells after treatment with ADSC CM compared to control CM. *FN1* participates in cell growth, migration, and wound healing under homeostatic conditions. In mammary epithelium, the targeted deletion of *FN* leads to the growth restriction of branching ducts and deficient alveologenesis [38]. However, it has also been found to be increased in several types of cancers and to play a central role in tumorigenesis [39]. *CDH2* was correlated with upregulated motility and invasion in human breast epithelial and breast carcinoma cell lines [40,41]. Similarly, the enhanced expression of *VIM* was associated with the increased migration and invasion of cancer cells [42]. Moreover, the upregulation of *FN1*, *CDH2*, and *VIM* is commonly associated with the epithelial–mesenchymal transition (EMT) in breast cancer and also in mammary epithelial cells [43]. The gain of mesenchymal cell markers and the increased migratory and invasive capabilities of MCF-10A cells observed in the present study represent features of EMT [44]. MCF-10A represents a breast cell line with intrinsic plasticity sharing stem-cell-like characteristics and was shown to be able to undergo EMT or EMT-like phenotypic changes [45]. EMT is evident for epithelial plasticity during embryogenesis, tissue homeostasis, and tissue repair or wound healing, respectively [46]. On the other hand, previous data suggested the involvement of EMT in early or later phases of breast cancer development [47]. It is still equivocal whether EMT in mammary epithelial cells leads to the production of stems cells [46].

We further observed an increase in the expression of cytokines in MCF10A cells after treatment with ADSC CM. Thereby, the ADSC CM treatment of MCF-10A cells in co-culture with fibroblasts lead to an enhanced expression of *TNF-α* in MCF-10A cells. Previous studies reported a potential cytotoxic and anti-tumor effect, as well as an important role in breast cancer progression and the local recurrence of *TNF-α* [48,49]. Thereby, *TNF-α* was suggested to be able to induce EMT in healthy breast epithelial cells like MCF-10A cells and malignant breast cells [50,51]. Further, treatment with ADSC CM led to a higher expression of *FGF2* in irradiated MCF-10A cells. *FGF2* plays an important role in fibroblast ECM synthesis and remodeling. In organotypic 3D co-cultures, FGF2 signaling was shown to increase the fibroblast-induced branching of mammary epithelium [52]. Reduced activity in FGF signaling under physiological conditions inhibits epithelial branching. However, the upregulation of *FGF* was shown to disrupt cell polarity and to induce cell proliferation, migration, and invasion capability, resembling molecular processes during breast cancer development [53]. Thus, the enhanced expression of cytokines might promote tumor development in healthy breast tissue. Moreover, an upregulation of cytokines in mammary epithelial cells by ADSC in the course of breast reconstruction might be relevant in case of residual adjacent malignant cells persisting after BCT that might be activated by those cytokines.

Treatment with ADSC CM had only a minor effect on the expression of *IL-1β* of MCF-10A cells. However, the co-cultivation of mammary epithelial cells with fibroblasts treated with ADSC CM revealed a higher expression of *IL-1β* compared to cells cultivated in monocultures. Previous findings demonstrated a correlation of upregulated *IL-1β* with neoplasm initiation and development. Thereby, an overexpression of *IL-1β* was found in both epithelial cells and in fibroblasts [54]. In the present study, we also found an upregulation of *IL-1β* in mammary epithelial cells and in fibroblasts in co-cultures compared to their monocultures, whereby the effect was more pronounced in fibroblasts, especially after 5 Gy irradiation. These findings suggest an interplay of mammary epithelial cells and fibroblasts that stimulates *IL-1β* expression mainly in fibroblasts under "physiological" conditions without ADSC and without irradiation as well as after 2 and 5 Gy-irradiation. However, the stimulatory effect on *IL-1β* expression of fibroblasts was enhanced by irradiation, indicating the involvement of radiation-induced pathways. Moreover, whereas treatment with ADSC CM and co-cultivation with fibroblasts had only a slight effect on the expression of *TGF-β* in MCF-10A cells, the irradiation of co-cultivated fibroblasts showed an upregulation of *TGF-β* in those cells. TGF-β was shown to induce a more aggressive cancer phenotype in breast cancer cells. Additionally, it is considered a potent EMT-promoting cytokine and was suggested to stimulate the neoplastic progression of transformed epithelial cells [55].

However, it was recently reported that TGF-β alone scarcely induces EMT [56]. Interestingly, a previous study could show that radiation-induced signaling pathways provoke heritable phenotypes that might be involved in carcinogenesis and that a single exposure to irradiation can sensitize mammary epithelial cells to undergo TGF-β-mediated EMT [57]. These findings support the relevance of irradiation in the pathophysiology of breast cancer development and progression. A further observation induced by irradiation in the present study is the enhanced invasion capability of MCF-10A. Whereas transmigration rates were inhibited after irradiation, MCF-10A cells showed increased invasion rates after irradiation with 5 Gy. No significant stimulation was observed after 2 Gy irradiation, which is in concordance with previous findings [58], indicating that higher irradiation doses are necessary to evoke this effect. As already expected and reported in earlier studies, irradiation decreased the survival rates of MCF-10A cells [58]. Although a regenerative effect is ascribed to ADSC, the ADSC CM decreased the surviving fraction of MCF-10A cells after irradiation with 5 Gy.

The ECM has been attributed not only a role in normal breast development and differentiation but has also been attributed an evident function in breast cancer tumorigenesis due to imbalances in the ECM remodeling processes [59]. MMPs are involved in the reorganization of the tumor stroma and are supposed to have a decisive role in breast cancer invasion and metastasis [60]. Thereby, MMP2 and MMP9 can stimulate cell proliferation and angiogenesis and have been attributed a role in early-stage tumorigenesis and cancer progression [61,62]. COL1A1, as a further essential component of the ECM, was also correlated with breast cancer progression and metastasis [63]. In breast cancer stroma, *COL1A1* was identified as one of the most promising genes for tumor detection and treatment [64]. In the present study, treatment with ADSC CM enhanced the expression of *MMP2* and *COL1A1* in irradiated MCF-10A cells. Moreover, in fibroblasts, treatment with ADSC CM promoted the mRNA levels of *COL1A1* in irradiated cells, and irradiation enhanced the mRNA levels of *MMP2*. Interestingly, we could not observe any effect on *MMP2* or *COL1A1* in non-irradiated groups, suggesting an essential role of irradiation in inducing those upregulations of ECM markers. An upregulation of collagen genes might also contribute to a radiation-associated secondary breast cancer [65].

We also want to discuss several limitations of this study. Firstly, breast tissue consists of many additional components with a heterogeneous cell population, including i.a. endothelial cells, adipocytes, or immune-competent cells that were not addressed in this study. Therefore, the study is only of limited significance and only partially transferable into clinical practice. Nevertheless, the inclusion of further cell types would lead to more complex data in which the detected effects would be more difficult to assign to the respective subgroup. Additionally, the interval between irradiation and lipotransfer is much longer in patients so that the effect of irradiation in vitro might not depict the clinical reality. Another limitation is that direct cell–cell interactions between ADSC, mammary epithelial cells and fibroblasts were not taken into account. However, the data of the present study indicate that the use of lipotransfer should still be evaluated critically. Our data suggest EMT-like changes in the epithelial mammary breast cell line that might contribute to improved tissue regeneration. On the other hand, those changes might also induce the neoplastic transformation of the breast. Further, residual adjacent malignant cells persisting after BCT might be activated by ADSC. Thus, the benefits of lipotransfer after BCT should be critically weighed against its possible risks for the affected patients. Subgroup analyses in the past showed that some conditions are associated with higher recurrence rates after lipotransfer [66]. Thereby, e.g., breast cancer subtype, high-grade histology, age, Ki-67 expression, and the number of positive axillary nodes seem to play an important role [67,68]. Therefore, it is of special importance to identify high-risk patients and to discuss lipotransfer in a personalized approach for each patient.

More standardized and prospective clinical studies that include a considerable number of patients who underwent BCT are needed to further elucidate that issue on the clinical side. Moreover, there is a need of further in vitro and in vivo studies to provide a better understanding of the underlying cellular mechanisms. Thereby, translating experimental studies to clinical reality is difficult. Future experimental studies should include the surrounding microenvironment, e.g., within the context of 3D experiments. In addition, the effect of lipotransfer on the remaining breast cancer cells, including different breast cancer subtypes, surrounded by cancer-associated fibroblasts should be examined more closely.

## 5. Conclusions

Treatment with ADSC CM promoted the transmigration and invasion of MCF-10A cells and stimulated the expression of mesenchymal markers, suggesting EMT-like changes in mammary epithelial cells. Further, ADSC CM, in combination with irradiation, revealed increased mRNA levels of ECM markers in mammary epithelial cells and fibroblasts. We further observed the enhanced expression of tumor-promoting cytokines, which might play an important role in the presence of microscopic residual tumor foci after BCT. The data of the present study suggest a careful consideration of the need for lipotransfer after BCT of the individual patient.

**Author Contributions:** Conceptualization: T.P., A.K.-W.; methodology: T.P., A.K.-W., C.-S.K., T.J., S.K., R.S.; validation: C.-S.K., T.P., A.K.-W.; formal analysis: C.-S.K., T.P., A.K.-W., T.J.; investigation: C.-S.K., T.J.; data curation: C.-S.K.; writing—original draft preparation: T.P., A.K.-W.; writing—review and editing: C.-S.K., T.J., L.V.D., S.K., R.S., A.A., R.E.H.; visualization: T.P., C.-S.K.; supervision: T.P., A.K.-W., L.V.D., R.E.H., A.A.; project administration: A.K.-W., T.P.; funding acquisition: T.P., A.K.-W. All authors have read and agreed to the published version of the manuscript.

**Funding:** This research was funded by Manfred Roth Foundation, the Forschungsstiftung Medizin University Hospital Erlangen, and ELAN FAU (grant number 18-12-19-1). We further want to acknowledge support by Boya Marshall. C.-S.K. was supported by the interdisciplinary center for clinical research (IZKF) at Friedrich-Alexander-Universität Erlangen-Nürnberg, Erlangen, Germany. We acknowledge financial support by Deutsche Forschungsgemeinschaft and Friedrich-Alexander-Universität Erlangen-Nürnberg within the funding programme "Open Access Publication Funding".

**Institutional Review Board Statement:** Not applicable.

**Informed Consent Statement:** Not applicable.

**Data Availability Statement:** The datasets generated during and/or analyzed during the current study are available from the corresponding author on reasonable request.

**Acknowledgments:** We would like to thank Matthias Rübner, Department of Obstetrics and Gynaecology, for providing us with the MCF10A cell line and Stefan Fleischer and Ilse Arnold-Herberth for their excellent technical support. The present work was performed in (partial) fulfilment of the requirements for obtaining the degree "Dr. med." for Chiara-Sophia Kutz.

**Conflicts of Interest:** The authors declare no conflict of interest.

## References

1. Veronesi, U.; Cascinelli, N.; Mariani, L.; Greco, M.; Saccozzi, R.; Luini, A.; Aguilar, M.; Marubini, E. Twenty-year follow-up of a randomized study comparing breast-conserving surgery with radical mastectomy for early breast cancer. *N. Engl. J. Med.* **2002**, *347*, 1227–1232. [CrossRef] [PubMed]
2. Chen, K.; Zhang, J.; Beeraka, N.M.; Tang, C.; Babayeva, Y.V.; Sinelnikov, M.Y.; Zhang, X.; Zhang, J.; Liu, J.; Reshetov, I.V.; et al. Advances in the Prevention and Treatment of Obesity-Driven Effects in Breast Cancers. *Front. Oncol.* **2022**, *12*, 820968. [CrossRef] [PubMed]
3. Bajaj, A.K.; Kon, P.S.; Oberg, K.C.; Miles, D.A. Aesthetic outcomes in patients undergoing breast conservation therapy for the treatment of localized breast cancer. *Plast. Reconstr. Surg.* **2004**, *114*, 1442–1449. [CrossRef]
4. Kelly, D.A.; Wood, B.C.; Knoll, G.M.; Chang, S.C.; Cranford, J.C.; Bharti, G.D.; Levine, E.A.; Thompson, J.T. Outcome analysis of 541 women undergoing breast conservation therapy. *Ann. Plast. Surg.* **2012**, *68*, 435–437. [CrossRef]
5. Chen, K.; Beeraka, N.M.; Sinelnikov, M.Y.; Zhang, J.; Song, D.; Gu, Y.; Li, J.; Reshetov, I.V.; Startseva, O.I.; Liu, J.; et al. Patient Management Strategies in Perioperative, Intraoperative, and Postoperative Period in Breast Reconstruction with DIEP-Flap: Clinical Recommendations. *Front. Surg.* **2022**, *9*, 729181. [CrossRef]

6. Herly, M.; Ørholt, M.; Glovinski, P.V.; Pipper, C.B.; Broholm, H.; Poulsgaard, L.; Fugleholm, K.; Thomsen, C.; Drzewiecki, K.T. Quantifying Long-Term Retention of Excised Fat Grafts: A Longitudinal, Retrospective Cohort Study of 108 Patients Followed for up to 8.4 Years. *Plast. Reconstr. Surg.* **2017**, *139*, 1223–1232. [CrossRef]
7. Kølle, S.F.; Fischer-Nielsen, A.; Mathiasen, A.B.; Elberg, J.J.; Oliveri, R.S.; Glovinski, P.V.; Kastrup, J.; Kirchhoff, M.; Rasmussen, B.S.; Talman, M.L.; et al. Enrichment of autologous fat grafts with ex-vivo expanded adipose tissue-derived stem cells for graft survival: A randomised placebo-controlled trial. *Lancet* **2013**, *382*, 1113–1120. [CrossRef]
8. Yoshimura, K.; Sato, K.; Aoi, N.; Kurita, M.; Hirohi, T.; Harii, K. Cell-assisted lipotransfer for cosmetic breast augmentation: Supportive use of adipose-derived stem/stromal cells. *Aesthet. Plast. Surg.* **2008**, *32*, 48–57. [CrossRef]
9. Fajka-Boja, R.; Szebeni, G.J.; Hunyadi-Gulyás, É.; Puskás, L.G.; Katona, R.L. Polyploid Adipose Stem Cells Shift the Balance of IGF1/IGFBP2 to Promote the Growth of Breast Cancer. *Front. Oncol.* **2020**, *10*, 157. [CrossRef]
10. Schweizer, R.; Tsuji, W.; Gorantla, V.S.; Marra, K.G.; Rubin, J.P.; Plock, J.A. The role of adipose-derived stem cells in breast cancer progression and metastasis. *Stem Cells Int.* **2015**, *2015*, 120949. [CrossRef]
11. Kucerova, L.; Kovacovicova, M.; Polak, M.; Bohac, M.; Fedeles, J.; Palencar, D.; Matuskova, M. Interaction of human adipose tissue-derived mesenchymal stromal cells with breast cancer cells. *Neoplasma* **2011**, *58*, 361–370. [CrossRef] [PubMed]
12. Rigotti, G.; Marchi, A.; Galiè, M.; Baroni, G.; Benati, D.; Krampera, M.; Pasini, A.; Sbarbati, A. Clinical treatment of radiotherapy tissue damage by lipoaspirate transplant: A healing process mediated by adipose-derived adult stem cells. *Plast. Reconstr. Surg.* **2007**, *119*, 1409–1422. [CrossRef] [PubMed]
13. Goncalves, R.; Mota, B.S.; Sobreira-Lima, B.; Ricci, M.D.; Soares, J.M., Jr.; Munhoz, A.M.; Baracat, E.C.; Filassi, J.R. The oncological safety of autologous fat grafting: A systematic review and meta-analysis. *BMC Cancer* **2022**, *22*, 391. [CrossRef]
14. Cohen, O.; Lam, G.; Karp, N.; Choi, M. Determining the Oncologic Safety of Autologous Fat Grafting as a Reconstructive Modality: An Institutional Review of Breast Cancer Recurrence Rates and Surgical Outcomes. *Plast. Reconstr. Surg.* **2017**, *140*, 382e–392e. [CrossRef] [PubMed]
15. Largo, R.D.; Tchang, L.A.; Mele, V.; Scherberich, A.; Harder, Y.; Wettstein, R.; Schaefer, D.J. Efficacy, safety and complications of autologous fat grafting to healthy breast tissue: A systematic review. *J. Plast. Reconstr. Aesthet. Surg.* **2014**, *67*, 437–448. [CrossRef]
16. Mestak, O.; Hromadkova, V.; Fajfrova, M.; Molitor, M.; Mestak, J. Evaluation of Oncological Safety of Fat Grafting After Breast-Conserving Therapy: A Prospective Study. *Ann Surg Oncol* **2016**, *23*, 776–781. [CrossRef]
17. Silva-Vergara, C.; Fontdevila, J.; Descarrega, J.; Burdio, F.; Yoon, T.S.; Grande, L. Oncological outcomes of lipofilling breast reconstruction: 195 consecutive cases and literature review. *J. Plast. Reconstr. Aesthet. Surg.* **2016**, *69*, 475–481. [CrossRef]
18. Krastev, T.; van Turnhout, A.; Vriens, E.; Smits, L.; van der Hulst, R. Long-term Follow-up of Autologous Fat Transfer vs Conventional Breast Reconstruction and Association with Cancer Relapse in Patients With Breast Cancer. *JAMA Surg.* **2019**, *154*, 56–63. [CrossRef]
19. Massa, M.; Gasparini, S.; Baldelli, I.; Scarabelli, L.; Santi, P.; Quarto, R.; Repaci, E. Interaction Between Breast Cancer Cells and Adipose Tissue Cells Derived from Fat Grafting. *Aesthet. Surg. J.* **2016**, *36*, 358–363. [CrossRef]
20. Wang, Y.; Liu, J.; Jiang, Q.; Deng, J.; Xu, F.; Chen, X.; Cheng, F.; Zhang, Y.; Yao, Y.; Xia, Z.; et al. Human Adipose-Derived Mesenchymal Stem Cell-Secreted CXCL1 and CXCL8 Facilitate Breast Tumor Growth by Promoting Angiogenesis. *Stem Cells* **2017**, *35*, 2060–2070. [CrossRef]
21. Mandel, K.; Yang, Y.; Schambach, A.; Glage, S.; Otte, A.; Hass, R. Mesenchymal stem cells directly interact with breast cancer cells and promote tumor cell growth in vitro and in vivo. *Stem Cells Dev.* **2013**, *22*, 3114–3127. [CrossRef] [PubMed]
22. Trivanović, D.; Nikolić, S.; Krstić, J.; Jauković, A.; Mojsilović, S.; Ilić, V.; Okić-Djordjević, I.; Santibanez, J.F.; Jovčić, G.; Bugarski, D. Characteristics of human adipose mesenchymal stem cells isolated from healthy and cancer affected people and their interactions with human breast cancer cell line MCF-7 in vitro. *Cell Biol. Int.* **2014**, *38*, 254–265. [CrossRef] [PubMed]
23. Müller-Seubert, W.; Ostermaier, P.; Horch, R.E.; Distel, L.; Frey, B.; Cai, A.; Arkudas, A. Intra- and Early Postoperative Evaluation of Malperfused Areas in an Irradiated Random Pattern Skin Flap Model Using Indocyanine Green Angiography and Near-Infrared Reflectance-Based Imaging and Infrared Thermography. *J. Pers. Med.* **2022**, *12*, 237. [CrossRef] [PubMed]
24. Vaghela, R.; Arkudas, A.; Gage, D.; Körner, C.; von Hörsten, S.; Salehi, S.; Horch, R.E.; Hessenauer, M. Microvascular development in the rat arteriovenous loop model in vivo-A step by step intravital microscopy analysis. *J. Biomed. Mater. Res. A* **2022**, *110*, 1551–1563. [CrossRef]
25. Steiner, D.; Mutschall, H.; Winkler, S.; Horch, R.E.; Arkudas, A. The Adipose-Derived Stem Cell and Endothelial Cell Coculture System-Role of Growth Factors? *Cells* **2021**, *10*, 2074. [CrossRef]
26. Kengelbach-Weigand, A.; Tasbihi, K.; Strissel, P.L.; Schmid, R.; Marques, J.M.; Beier, J.P.; Beckmann, M.W.; Strick, R.; Horch, R.E.; Boos, A.M. Plasticity of patient-matched normal mammary epithelial cells is dependent on autologous adipose-derived stem cells. *Sci. Rep.* **2019**, *9*, 10722. [CrossRef]
27. Quail, D.F.; Joyce, J.A. Microenvironmental regulation of tumor progression and metastasis. *Nat. Med.* **2013**, *19*, 1423–1437. [CrossRef]
28. Taghizadeh-Hesary, F.; Behnam, B.; Akbari, H.; Bahadori, M. Targeted Anti-mitochondrial Therapy: The Future of Oncology. **2022**; *in press.* [CrossRef]
29. Chen, K.; Lu, P.; Beeraka, N.M.; Sukocheva, O.A.; Madhunapantula, S.V.; Liu, J.; Sinelnikov, M.Y.; Nikolenko, V.N.; Bulygin, K.V.; Mikhaleva, L.M.; et al. Mitochondrial mutations and mitoepigenetics: Focus on regulation of oxidative stress-induced responses in breast cancers. *Semin. Cancer Biol.* **2022**, *83*, 556–569. [CrossRef]

30. Lühr, I.; Friedl, A.; Overath, T.; Tholey, A.; Kunze, T.; Hilpert, F.; Sebens, S.; Arnold, N.; Rösel, F.; Oberg, H.-H.; et al. Mammary fibroblasts regulate morphogenesis of normal and tumorigenic breast epithelial cells by mechanical and paracrine signals. *Cancer Lett.* **2012**, *325*, 175–188. [CrossRef]
31. Krause, S.; Maffini, M.V.; Soto, A.M.; Sonnenschein, C. A novel 3D in vitro culture model to study stromal-epithelial interactions in the mammary gland. *Tissue Eng. Part C Methods* **2008**, *14*, 261–271. [CrossRef]
32. Steer, A.; Cordes, N.; Jendrossek, V.; Klein, D. Impact of Cancer-Associated Fibroblast on the Radiation-Response of Solid Xenograft Tumors. *Front. Mol. Biosci.* **2019**, *6*, 70. [CrossRef] [PubMed]
33. Piper, M.; Mueller, A.C.; Karam, S.D. The interplay between cancer associated fibroblasts and immune cells in the context of radiation therapy. *Mol. Carcinog.* **2020**, *59*, 754–765. [CrossRef] [PubMed]
34. Wang, Z.; Tang, Y.; Tan, Y.; Wei, Q.; Yu, W. Cancer-associated fibroblasts in radiotherapy: Challenges and new opportunities. *Cell Commun. Signal.* **2019**, *17*, 47. [CrossRef] [PubMed]
35. Eiro, N.; González, L.; Martínez-Ordoñez, A.; Fernandez-Garcia, B.; González, L.O.; Cid, S.; Dominguez, F.; Perez-Fernandez, R.; Vizoso, F.J. Cancer-associated fibroblasts affect breast cancer cell gene expression, invasion and angiogenesis. *Cell. Oncol.* **2018**, *41*, 369–378. [CrossRef]
36. Ji, X.; Zhu, X.; Lu, X. Effect of cancer-associated fibroblasts on radiosensitivity of cancer cells. *Future Oncol.* **2017**, *13*, 1537–1550. [CrossRef]
37. Schindelin, J.; Arganda-Carreras, I.; Frise, E.; Kaynig, V.; Longair, M.; Pietzsch, T.; Preibisch, S.; Rueden, C.; Saalfeld, S.; Schmid, B.; et al. Fiji: An open-source platform for biological-image analysis. *Nat. Methods* **2012**, *9*, 676–682. [CrossRef]
38. Liu, K.; Cheng, L.; Flesken-Nikitin, A.; Huang, L.; Nikitin, A.Y.; Pauli, B.U. Conditional knockout of fibronectin abrogates mouse mammary gland lobuloalveolar differentiation. *Dev. Biol.* **2010**, *346*, 11–24. [CrossRef]
39. Wang, J.P.; Hielscher, A. Fibronectin: How Its Aberrant Expression in Tumors May Improve Therapeutic Targeting. *J. Cancer* **2017**, *8*, 674–682. [CrossRef]
40. Nieman, M.T.; Prudoff, R.S.; Johnson, K.R.; Wheelock, M.J. N-Cadherin Promotes Motility in Human Breast Cancer Cells Regardless of Their E-Cadherin Expression. *J. Cell Biol.* **1999**, *147*, 631–644. [CrossRef]
41. Hazan, R.B.; Phillips, G.R.; Qiao, R.F.; Norton, L.; Aaronson, S.A. Exogenous Expression of N-Cadherin in Breast Cancer Cells Induces Cell Migration, Invasion, and Metastasis. *J. Cell Biol.* **2000**, *148*, 779–790. [CrossRef]
42. Gilles, C.; Polette, M.; Mestdagt, M.; Nawrocki-Raby, B.; Ruggeri, P.; Birembaut, P.; Foidart, J.M. Transactivation of vimentin by beta-catenin in human breast cancer cells. *Cancer Res.* **2003**, *63*, 2658–2664. [CrossRef] [PubMed]
43. Li, C.W.; Xia, W.; Huo, L.; Lim, S.O.; Wu, Y.; Hsu, J.L.; Chao, C.H.; Yamaguchi, H.; Yang, N.K.; Ding, Q.; et al. Epithelial-mesenchymal transition induced by TNF-α requires NF-κB-mediated transcriptional upregulation of Twist1. *Cancer Res.* **2012**, *72*, 1290–1300. [CrossRef] [PubMed]
44. Huber, M.A.; Kraut, N.; Beug, H. Molecular requirements for epithelial-mesenchymal transition during tumor progression. *Curr. Opin. Cell Biol.* **2005**, *17*, 548–558. [CrossRef] [PubMed]
45. Sarrió, D.; Rodriguez-Pinilla, S.M.a.; Hardisson, D.; Cano, A.; Moreno-Bueno, G.; Palacios, J. Epithelial-Mesenchymal Transition in Breast Cancer Relates to the Basal-like Phenotype. *Cancer Res.* **2008**, *68*, 989–997. [CrossRef] [PubMed]
46. Thiery, J.P.; Acloque, H.; Huang, R.Y.J.; Nieto, M.A. Epithelial-Mesenchymal Transitions in Development and Disease. *Cell* **2009**, *139*, 871–890. [CrossRef] [PubMed]
47. Haslam, S.Z.; Woodward, T.L. Host microenvironment in breast cancer development: Epithelial-cell-stromal-cell interactions and steroid hormone action in normal and cancerous mammary gland. *Breast Cancer Res.* **2003**, *5*, 208–215. [CrossRef]
48. Cruceriu, D.; Baldasici, O.; Balacescu, O.; Berindan-Neagoe, I. The dual role of tumor necrosis factor-alpha (TNF-α) in breast cancer: Molecular insights and therapeutic approaches. *Cell. Oncol.* **2020**, *43*, 1–18. [CrossRef]
49. Soria, G.; Ofri-Shahak, M.; Haas, I.; Yaal-Hahoshen, N.; Leider-Trejo, L.; Leibovich-Rivkin, T.; Weitzenfeld, P.; Meshel, T.; Shabtai, E.; Gutman, M.; et al. Inflammatory mediators in breast cancer: Coordinated expression of TNFα & IL-1β with CCL2 & CCL5 and effects on epithelial-to-mesenchymal transition. *BMC Cancer* **2011**, *11*, 130. [CrossRef]
50. Bhat-Nakshatri, P.; Appaiah, H.; Ballas, C.; Pick-Franke, P.; Goulet, R., Jr.; Badve, S.; Srour, E.F.; Nakshatri, H. SLUG/SNAI2 and tumor necrosis factor generate breast cells with CD44+/CD24- phenotype. *BMC Cancer* **2010**, *10*, 411. [CrossRef]
51. Asiedu, M.K.; Ingle, J.N.; Behrens, M.D.; Radisky, D.C.; Knutson, K.L. TGFbeta/TNF(alpha)-mediated epithelial-mesenchymal transition generates breast cancer stem cells with a claudin-low phenotype. *Cancer Res.* **2011**, *71*, 4707–4719. [CrossRef]
52. Sumbal, J.; Koledova, Z. FGF signaling in mammary gland fibroblasts regulates multiple fibroblast functions and mammary epithelial morphogenesis. *Development* **2019**, *146*, dev185306. [CrossRef] [PubMed]
53. Avagliano, A.; Fiume, G.; Ruocco, M.R.; Martucci, N.; Vecchio, E.; Insabato, L.; Russo, D.; Accurso, A.; Masone, S.; Montagnani, S.; et al. Influence of Fibroblasts on Mammary Gland Development, Breast Cancer Microenvironment Remodeling, and Cancer Cell Dissemination. *Cancers* **2020**, *12*, 1697. [CrossRef]
54. Wu, T.; Hong, Y.; Jia, L.; Wu, J.; Xia, J.; Wang, J.; Hu, Q.; Cheng, B. Modulation of IL-1β reprogrammes the tumor microenvironment to interrupt oral carcinogenesis. *Sci. Rep.* **2016**, *6*, 20208. [CrossRef] [PubMed]
55. Lindley, L.E.; Briegel, K.J. Molecular characterization of TGFβ-induced epithelial-mesenchymal transition in normal finite lifespan human mammary epithelial cells. *Biochem. Biophys. Res. Commun.* **2010**, *399*, 659–664. [CrossRef] [PubMed]
56. Brown, K.A.; Aakre, M.E.; Gorska, A.E.; Price, J.O.; Eltom, S.E.; Pietenpol, J.A.; Moses, H.L. Induction by transforming growth factor-β1 of epithelial to mesenchymal transition is a rare event in vitro. *Breast Cancer Res.* **2004**, *6*, R215. [CrossRef]

57. Andarawewa, K.L.; Erickson, A.C.; Chou, W.S.; Costes, S.V.; Gascard, P.; Mott, J.D.; Bissell, M.J.; Barcellos-Hoff, M.H. Ionizing radiation predisposes nonmalignant human mammary epithelial cells to undergo transforming growth factor beta induced epithelial to mesenchymal transition. *Cancer Res.* **2007**, *67*, 8662–8670. [CrossRef]
58. Pereira, L.; Lima, A.G.F.; Ferreira, M.T.; Salata, C.; Ferreira-Machado, S.C.; Morandi, V.; Magalhães, L.A.G. Evaluation of Biological Effect in Breast Cell Irradiated with Dose 2 Gy in Radiotherapy. 2021. Available online: https://europepmc.org/article/ppr/ppr433264 (accessed on 4 July 2022).
59. Kaushik, S.; Pickup, M.W.; Weaver, V.M. From transformation to metastasis: Deconstructing the extracellular matrix in breast cancer. *Cancer Metastasis Rev.* **2016**, *35*, 655–667. [CrossRef]
60. Davies, K.J. The Complex Interaction of Matrix Metalloproteinases in the Migration of Cancer Cells through Breast Tissue Stroma. *Int. J. Breast Cancer* **2014**, *2014*, 839094. [CrossRef]
61. Gialeli, C.; Theocharis, A.D.; Karamanos, N.K. Roles of matrix metalloproteinases in cancer progression and their pharmacological targeting. *FEBS J.* **2011**, *278*, 16–27. [CrossRef]
62. Hojilla, C.V.; Mohammed, F.F.; Khokha, R. Matrix metalloproteinases and their tissue inhibitors direct cell fate during cancer development. *Br. J. Cancer* **2003**, *89*, 1817–1821. [CrossRef]
63. Liu, J.; Shen, J.X.; Wu, H.T.; Li, X.L.; Wen, X.F.; Du, C.W.; Zhang, G.J. Collagen 1A1 (COL1A1) promotes metastasis of breast cancer and is a potential therapeutic target. *Discov. Med.* **2018**, *25*, 211–223. [PubMed]
64. Wang, Y.; Xu, H.; Zhu, B.; Qiu, Z.; Lin, Z. Systematic identification of the key candidate genes in breast cancer stroma. *Cell. Mol. Biol. Lett.* **2018**, *23*, 44. [CrossRef] [PubMed]
65. Yao, G.; Zhao, K.; Bao, K.; Li, J. Radiation increases COL1A1, COL3A1, and COL1A2 expression in breast cancer. *Open Med. (Wars)* **2022**, *17*, 329–340. [CrossRef] [PubMed]
66. Cohen, S.; Sekigami, Y.; Schwartz, T.; Losken, A.; Margenthaler, J.; Chatterjee, A. Lipofilling after breast conserving surgery: A comprehensive literature review investigating its oncologic safety. *Gland Surg.* **2019**, *8*, 569–580. [CrossRef] [PubMed]
67. Biazus, J.V.; Stumpf, C.C.; Melo, M.P.; Zucatto, A.E.; Cericatto, R.; Cavalheiro, J.A.; Damin, A.P. Breast-Conserving Surgery with Immediate Autologous Fat Grafting Reconstruction: Oncologic Outcomes. *Aesthet. Plast. Surg.* **2018**, *42*, 1195–1201. [CrossRef]
68. Petit, J.Y.; Rietjens, M.; Botteri, E.; Rotmensz, N.; Bertolini, F.; Curigliano, G.; Rey, P.; Garusi, C.; De Lorenzi, F.; Martella, S.; et al. Evaluation of fat grafting safety in patients with intraepithelial neoplasia: A matched-cohort study. *Ann. Oncol.* **2013**, *24*, 1479–1484. [CrossRef]

Article

# Individualized Wound Closure—Mechanical Properties of Suture Materials

Elias Polykandriotis [1,2,*], Jonas Daenicke [3], Anil Bolat [4], Jasmin Grüner [2], Dirk W. Schubert [3] and Raymund E. Horch [2]

1. Department of Plastic, Hand and Microsurgery, Sana Hospital Hof, 95032 Hof, Germany
2. Department of Plastic and Hand Surgery, University of Erlangen Medical Center, 91054 Erlangen, Germany; jasmin.gruener@uk-erlangen.de (J.G.); raymund.horch@uk-erlangen.de (R.E.H.)
3. Department of Materials Science and Engineering, Friedrich-Alexander-University Erlangen-Nürnberg, 91054 Erlangen, Germany; jonas.daenicke@fau.de (J.D.); dirk.schubert@fau.de (D.W.S.)
4. Department of Orthopedics, Theresien Hospital, 90491 Nürnberg, Germany; anil.bolat@icloud.com
* Correspondence: elias.polykandriotis@gmail.com; Tel.: +49-15161-068069

**Abstract:** Wound closure is a key element of any procedure, especially aesthetic and reconstructive plastic surgery. Therefore, over the last decades, several devices have been developed in order to assist surgeons in achieving better results while saving valuable time. In this work, we give a concise review of the literature and present a biomechanical study of different suturing materials under mechanical load mimicking handling in the operating theatre. Nine different suture products, all of the same USP size (4-0), were subjected to a standardized crushing load by means of a needle holder. All materials were subjected to 0, 1, 3 and 5 crushing load cycles, respectively. The linear tensile strength was measured by means of a universal testing device. Attenuation of tensile strength was evaluated between materials and between crush cycles. In the pooled analysis, the linear tensile strength of the suture materials deteriorated significantly with every cycle ($p < 0.0001$). The suture materials displayed different initial tensile strengths (in descending order: polyglecaprone, polyglactin, polydioxanone, polyamid, polypropylene). In comparison, materials performed variably in terms of resistance to crush loading. The findings were statistically significant. The reconstructive surgeon has to be flexible and tailor wound closure techniques and materials to the individual patient, procedure and tissue demands; therefore, profound knowledge of the physical properties of the suture strands used is of paramount importance. The crushing load on suture materials during surgery can be detrimental for initial and long-term wound repair strength. As well as the standard wound closure methods (sutures, staples and adhesive strips), there are promising novel devices.

**Keywords:** suture materials; crush load; mechanical properties; wound closure

## 1. Introduction

Most surgical fields are defined by an anatomical system. Visceral surgery, for instance, is the surgery of the bowel and neurosurgery is deployed in the central or peripheral nervous system. However, in the epicenter of aesthetic and reconstructive surgery lies a concept, rather than an anatomical system. It is all about reconstitution of tissue defects and functional deficits. In this task, the reconstructive surgeon is challenged by the fact that many tissue elements and suture materials have to be used in many different ways. Profound knowledge of these materials and their biomechanical properties is invaluable. There are numerous reports on surgical suturing techniques and patterns, as well as on different suture materials. Although each suture material must undergo excessive testing procedures before it is officially approved as a medical device, there are few data concerning changes in the strength and behavior of sutures during surgical handling and mechanical suture trauma. In open surgery, it is standard that only the end of the suture—that will be discarded—should be mechanically grasped to avoid weakening of the suture. However, when repeated instrument handling is necessary, such as in laparoscopic or robotic surgery, mostly resorbable sutures may well lead to a breakdown of the material, which, according to Bariol et al. [1], has not been well investigated so far [2]. It is obvious that repeated instrument handling of sutures with a needle holder might damage the surface or texture of any suture. Additional care should be taken.

Abhari et al. performed an excellent overview of the current developments in suture materials, postulating that there are still limitations in their use [3]. Until recently, there has been low academic interest in the evolution of suturing devices. Advancements were mainly industry-driven, promoting low cost and strict compliance to the regulatory setting. Polymer optimizations and antimicrobial coating were the main advances. However, suture failure is still a problem, with challenges such as knot slippage, cheese wiring, tearing of the suture through tissue when under tension remaining unsolved. Maybe the suture–tissue interface presents the single weakest link in soft tissue repair. In the near future, bioactive products will probably shift the role of suture materials from mechanical and biologically inert threads to healing-promoting devices [3].

In this work, we give a concise review of the literature and present a biomechanical study of different suturing materials under mechanical load mimicking during surgery.

## 2. Materials and Methods

### 2.1. Suture Materials

For this study, nine products were compared to each other in respect to their linear tensile strength after a standardized crushing load by a needle holder. For the sake of comparability, only threads of the size 4-0 USP (United States Pharmakopeia (UPS)) were used. A summary of the different materials used is provided in Table 1. The effect of crushing load is displayed in Figure 1. Similar study designs for comparison of suture materials have been used in the past [4].

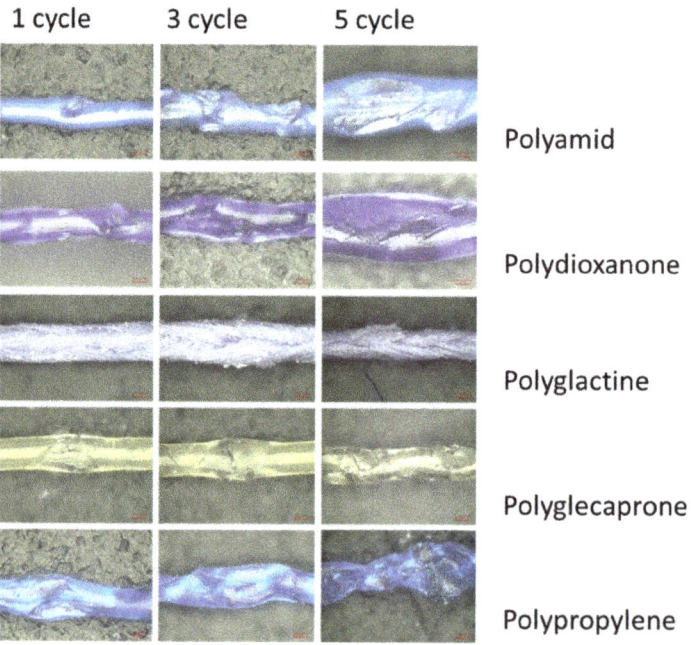

**Figure 1.** Mechanical distortion after 1, 3 and 5 crushes.

**Table 1.** A list of the used suture threads. All threads were 4-0 USP.

| Product | Manufacturer | Material | Type | Absorbable | Coating |
|---|---|---|---|---|---|
| Vicryl® Plus | Ethicon | Polyglactine 910 | Braided | + | + |
| Vicryl® | Ethicon | Polyglactine 910 | Braided | + | − |
| Monocryl® Plus | Ethicon | Polyglecaprone 25 | Braided | + | + |
| PDS® Plus | Ethicon | Polydioxanone | Monofil. | + | + |
| PDS® II | Ethicon | Polydioxanone | Monofil. | + | − |
| Prolene® | Ethicon | Polypropylene | Monofil. | − | − |
| Surgipro® | Covidien | Polypropylene-Polyethylene | Monofil. | − | − |
| Seratan® | Serag-Wiessner | Polyamide | Monofil. | − | + |
| Resolon® | Resorba | Polyamide | Monofil. | − | − |

Coating for Vicryl plus, Monocryl plus and PDS plus is a broad spectrum antibiotic (Triclosan), coating for Seratan is Titanium. Monofil. = monofilamentous. + = with, − = without.

### 2.2. Group Allocation

Nine different suture products were used for this line of experiments. Forty threads from every product were used for the study. In groups of 10, they were subjected to 0, 1, 3 or 5 cycles of crush loading by means of a standard needle holder (4U Medikal, Ankara, Turkey). Every one of these threads was measured and described in an experimental array later. There were 360 measurements altogether.

### 2.3. Experimental Array

A standard needle holder (4U Medikal, Ankara, Turkey) was used for all experiments. With this instrument, a crushing load was applied on the threads. The threads were crushed 0, 1, 3 or 5 times prior to measurement of the linear tensile strength. The clamp mechanism of the needle holder was used for locking the jaws on the thread. The force needed to lock the jaws of the needle holder was determined in a separate experiment, as follows.

To perform this particular measurement, the needle holder was mounted on a compression dynamometer (ZwickRoell GmbH & Co. KG, Ulm, Germany) (Figure 1). The force required to lock the instrument by compressing the clamping mechanism to its maximum (3 notches) with a 0.2 mm spacer between the jaws was found to be approximately 35 N. A thread diameter of 0.15–0.2 corresponds to USP 4-0 (Figure 2).

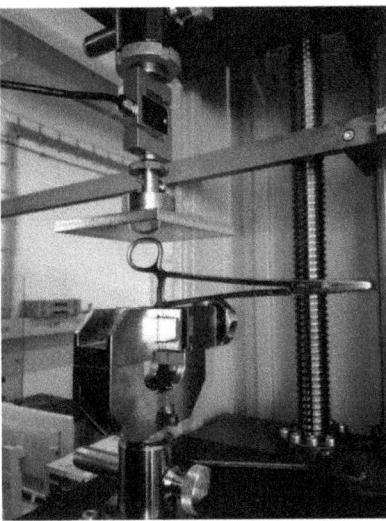

**Figure 2.** Experimental array for determination of the force (N) required to lock the jaws of the needle holder using the clamp mechanism. It was found to be 35 N.

Subsequently, for the measurements of the tensile strength of the threads, a Zwick Z050 universal dynamometer (ZwickRoell GmbH & Co. KG, Ulm, Germany) was used. For the measurement, a 100 N measuring component was mounted with a velocity setting of 300 mm/min. This method has been validated before [5,6]. The force required to evoke tear of the material was recorded. For evaluation of the results, the testXpert software (ZwickRoell GmbH & Co. KG, Ulm, Germany) was used (Figure 3).

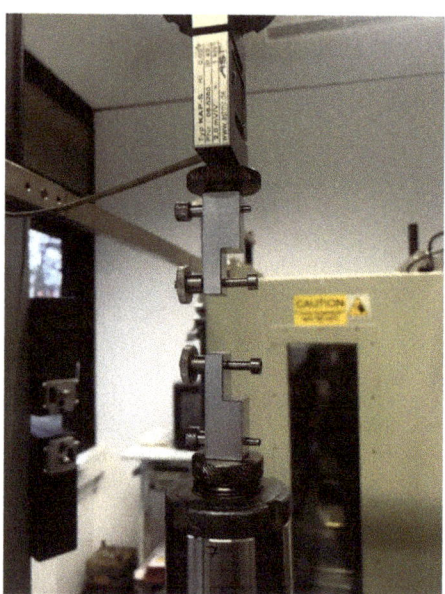

**Figure 3.** Experimental array for determination of the linear tensile strength of the suture materials.

*2.4. Statistical Analysis*

Two-way ANOVA was used for comparison between the groups using the Bonferroni correction for multiple comparisons. Parameters are generally displayed as mean values with standard deviation (±) and range.

### 3. Results

The pooled mean tensile strength in the group with zero crush load was 19.21 N (±6.371, 11.66–30.72). It deteriorated to 12.70 (±5.13, 7.62–21.33) after one crush, to 9.75 (±4.63, 4.48–18.24) after three crushes and down to 7.36 (±3.45, 3.49–15.18) after five crush cycles. All comparisons were highly significant ($p < 0.0001$). These results are demonstrated in Table 2 and Figure 4.

**Table 2.** Crush cycles, pooled data over all suture materials. All comparisons displayed high statistical significance.

| Crushing Load (Cycles) | Mean Tensile Strength (N) | Tensile Strength Remaining (%) |
|---|---|---|
| 0 | 19.21 (±6.371, 11.66–30.72) | 100.0 |
| 1 | 12.70 (±5.13, 7.62–21.33) | 66.1 |
| 3 | 9.75 (±4.63, 4.48–18.24) | 50.0 |
| 5 | 7.36 (±3.45, 3.49–15.18) | 38.3 |

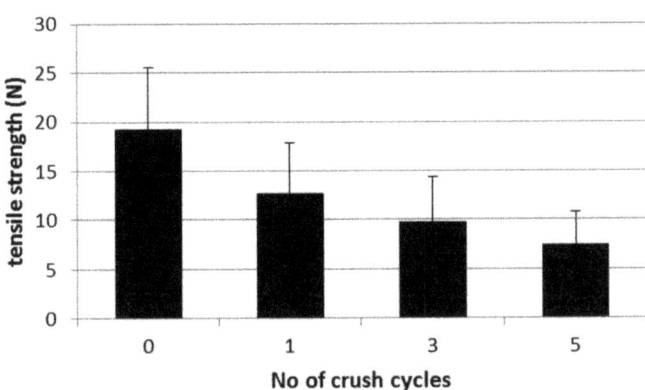

**Figure 4.** Deterioration of tensile strength of the suture materials with increasing cycles of crush load. All comparisons between the groups were highly significant ($p < 0.0001$).

After one crush cycle, all the products displayed a significant deterioration in tensile strength, except Vicryl® ($p = 0.077$) and Surgipro® ($p = 0.496$). In the comparison between zero and three crush cycles, all the products showed a significant deterioration in tensile strength. The detailed results listed by product description are displayed in Table 3 and Figure 5.

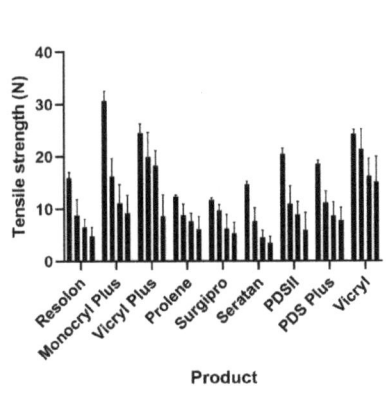
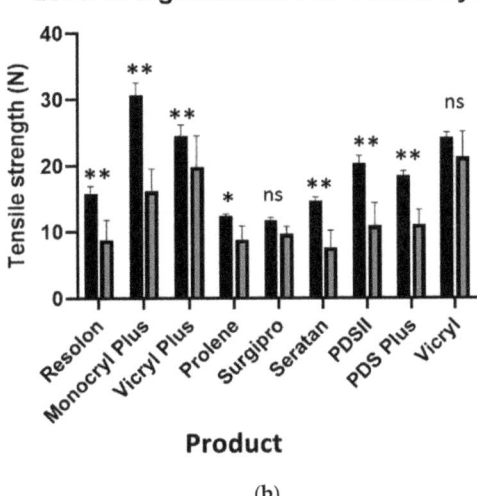

(a) (b)

**Figure 5.** (a) Attenuation of tensile strength for all suture products. (b) Attenuation of tensile strength for all suture products between 0 and 1 crush cycles. ** = highly significant, * = significant, ns = non significant, black color: tensile strength prior to crushing load, grey color: tensile strength after one crushing load with needle-holder.

Table 3. Tensile strength deterioration detailed for all suture products.

| Product | 0 Crushing Load | | 1× Crushing Load | | 3× Crushing Load | | 5× Crushing Load | |
|---|---|---|---|---|---|---|---|---|
| | Mean | (SD) | Mean | (SD) | Mean | (SD) | Mean | (SD) |
| Resolon | 15.87 | (1.13) | 8.78 | (3.03) | 6.50 | (1.55) | 4.86 | (1.63) |
| Monocryl Plus | 30.72 | (1.82) | 16.24 | (3.37) | 11.06 | (3.60) | 9.19 | (3.43) |
| Vicryl Plus | 24.52 | (1.69) | 19.91 | (4.66) | 18.24 | (2.88) | 8.55 | (4.15) |
| Prolene | 12.30 | (0.35) | 8.80 | (2.09) | 7.60 | (1.59) | 6.10 | (2.43) |
| Surgipro | 11.66 | (0.44) | 9.65 | (1.14) | 6.28 | (2.67) | 5.33 | (2.12) |
| Seratan | 14.62 | (0.59) | 7.62 | (2.56) | 4.48 | (1.35) | 3.49 | (1.23) |
| PDSII | 20.43 | (1.16) | 10.85 | (3.49) | 8.86 | (2.51) | 5.87 | (3.37) |
| PDS Plus | 18.53 | (0.72) | 11.08 | (2.25) | 8.64 | (2.61) | 7.74 | (2.49) |
| Vicryl | 24.22 | (0.78) | 21.33 | (3.85) | 16.17 | (3.33) | 15.18 | (4.75) |

When analyzed by material, all the comparisons after one or three crush cycles were significant. The corresponding results are summarized in Table 4 (descriptive), Table 5 (inferential statistics) and Figures 6 and 7.

Table 4. Tensile strength deterioration detailed for all suture materials.

| Material | 0 Crushing Load | | 1× Crushing Load | | 3× Crushing Load | | 5× Crushing Load | |
|---|---|---|---|---|---|---|---|---|
| | Mean (SD) | Remaining Linear Strength | Mean (SD) | Remaining Linear Strength | Mean (SD) | Remaining Linear Strength | Mean (SD) | Remaining Linear Strength |
| Polyamid | 15.25 (1.09) | 100% | 8.20 (2.80) | 53.79% | 5.49 (1.75) | 36.01% | 5.10 (1.85) | 33.42% |
| Polydioxanone | 19.48 (1.35) | 100% | 10.97 (2.86) | 56.29% | 8.75 (2.49) | 44.92% | 6.81 (3.04) | 34.93% |
| Polyglactine | 24.37 (1.29) | 100% | 20.62 (4.22) | 84.61% | 17.21 (3.21) | 70.60% | 11.87 (5.51) | 48.69% |
| Polyglecaprone | 30.72 (1.82) | 100% | 16.24 (3.37) | 52.86% | 11.06 (3.60) | 36.00% | 9.19 (3.43) | 29.92% |
| Polypropylene | 11.98 (0.51) | 100% | 9.23 (1.70) | 77.00% | 6.94 (2.24) | 57.93% | 5.72 (2.25) | 47.70% |

Table 5. Analysis of the effect of 0 to 5 crush loading cycles on the linear tensile strength of different suture materials (two-way ANOVA with Bonferroni correction for multiple comparisons.

| Material | 0× vs. 1× Crushing Load | 1× vs. 3× Crushing Load | 3× vs. 5× Crushing Load |
|---|---|---|---|
| | Level of Significance | Level of Significance | Level of Significance |
| Polyamid | $p < 0.0001$ (**) | $p = 0.0110$ (*) | $p > 0.9999$ (ns) |
| Polydioxanone | $p < 0.0001$ (**) | $p = 0.0639$ (ns) | $p = 0.1486$ (ns) |
| Polyglactine | $p = 0.0001$ (**) | $p = 0.0005$ (**) | $p < 0.0001$ (**) |
| Polyglecaprone | $p < 0,0001$ (**) | $p = 0.0002$ (**) | $p = 0.7571$ (ns) |
| Polypropylene | $p = 0.0092$ (**) | $p = 0.0507$ (ns) | $p = 0.9387$ (ns) |

** = highly significant, * = significant, ns = non significant.

**Tensile strength attenuation with no of crushing loads**

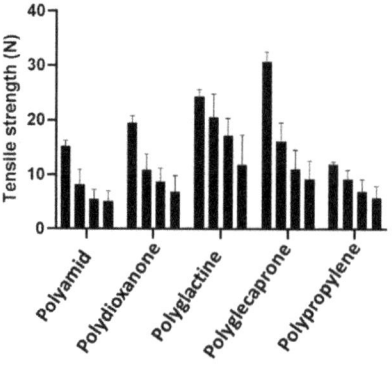

Figure 6. Graphical presentation of the findings in Table 4.

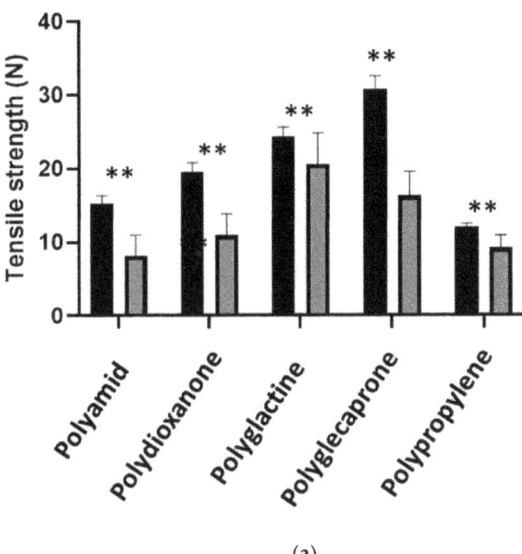

(a)

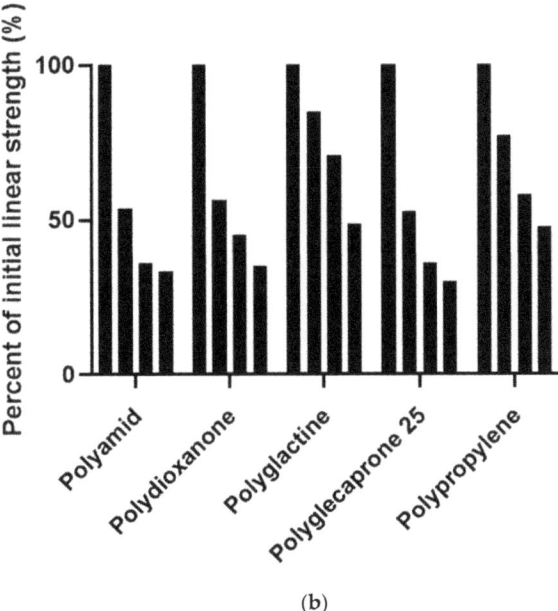

(b)

**Figure 7.** (a) A graphical presentation of the findings in Table 4 (partial results), black color: tensile strength prior to crushing load, grey color: tensile strength after one crushing load with needle-holder. (b) Attenuation of tensile strength in percent of initial linear strength. Relative values. ** = highly significant.

## 4. Discussion

Sutures are the mainstay of any surgical procedure, either as an interrupted or continuously applied closure method. Generally, the physical properties of sutures, such as the suture diameter, tensile strength, elongation, surface roughness, coefficient of friction, bending stiffness and tissue drag, and the knot characteristics are well characterized and have been studied extensively [1]. Such tests are, in fact, an integral part of the regulatory procedures before a suture is officially approved as a medical device [7]. However, only a few studies investigated the mechanical damage to sutures by repeated instrument handling during surgery [8]. According to Naleway et al., most published reports on the tensile behavior of various sutures only focus on breaking force, and detailed reports comparing other important tensile properties, such as failure elongation, failure stress, failure strain, modulus, and full stress–strain curves across suture materials, are quite limited [9]. Most researchers agree that simple knotting alone influences materials that may differ significantly in their tensile strengths and elastic/plastic deformation characteristics, but can still display comparable elongations at failure [6]. Von Fraunhofer et al. [10] described that all sutures in their study showed decreased tensile strength and elongation at failure when knotted. Most of their investigated materials showed increased tensile strength and decreased elongation at failure for smaller suture gauges (thicker strands), and this behavior is thought to be related to their internal molecular organization [11].

Clamp fixation for preventing the unfolding of a suture knot has been described to weaken the tensile strength of polypropylene sutures by Türker et al. [12]. Studies on the grip forces regarding hand and finger movements or force control reflected by individual grip force data may help to gain further data on dominant and nondominant hand influences, but do not apply in this context as the needle holder used here offered a distinct and reliable predetermined force when operated [13]. In laparoscopic and robotic surgery, it has been noted that the lack of haptic feedback has become a growing issue due to the application of excessive force that may lead to clinical problems, such as intraoperative and postoperative suture breakage [11]. Latest sensing technology and haptic feedback systems that can reduce instances of suture failure without negatively impacting performance outcomes, including knot quality, are, therefore, under investigation [11,14,15].

In these studies [11,14], it was also pointed out that the loop created in any suture is most prone to failure due to suture elongation, knot slip and suture breakage. It was found that monofilament sutures offered higher bending stiffness, but also a higher tendency to untie, compared to monofilament sutures. Interestingly, the ultimate failure load of monofilament nonabsorbable polypropylene sutures (Prolene) was significantly reduced when compared to the ultimate failure load achieved by other monofilament sutures, such as polyglyconate and nylon, as well as braided absorbable polyglactin, which were not affected by correcting the first throw of the loop, in their experimental array [12]. Mechanical grip of sutures with a clamp or needle holder is often applied when sutures have to be tied under tension to temporarily secure a knot after the first throw, to minimize unwanted gap formation until further throws are performed and fix the whole knots. Bisson et al. found that ForceFiber suture loops tied with serrated clamps were reduced by approximately 21% compared to those tied with no clamp (227 N vs. 289 N, $p = 0.003$), and approximately 18% compared to those tied with a smooth clamp [16].

In open surgery, it is a rule that only the end of the suture—that will be discarded —should be mechanically grasped to avoid weakening of the suture. However, since laparoscopic and robotic surgery has become a frequent and standard approach for many indications, the problem of suture trauma by instrument handling becomes an important issue. It has been shown that sutures in robot-assisted vascular surgery showed a significant loss of strength. Surgeons have, therefore, begun to search for materials that are most resistant against robotic mechanical handling. The properties of different sutures have been investigated to find out which materials are least susceptible to robotic manipulations and, therefore, could best be considered as materials of first choice [17].

Laparoscopic surgery necessitates the mechanical manipulation of sutures due to the limited access to the operative field. According to Bariol et al., absorbable sutures are especially bound to suffer material break-down upon repeated instrument handling. This effect has not been well investigated so far [1]. In continuous sutures, a broken suture can result in loss of achieved tissue approximation and lead to significant clinical problems. It is obvious that repeated instrument handling of sutures with a needle holder might alter the surface or texture of any suture. Until now—apart from anecdotal and rare experimental reports—it remained unclear how precisely sutures are damaged by doing so and how many grips it takes to ruin a suture. The recommendation of Bisson and coworkers, which was that temporarily clamping a knot to keep it from slipping during the tying process when securing sutures can be performed without any concern for weakening the suture or without imposing the danger of suture trauma [16], cannot be confirmed by our findings. Our experimental set up mimicked the clinical situation in a standardized way and clearly revealed the increasing damage to the various sutures with the increasing number of clamping procedures. Here, we could show, for the first time, exactly how repeated clamping with a needle holder alters the surface and texture of various suture materials and reduces their breaking strength.

Other studies that intended to define the breaking strength by repeated elongation of sutures are not directly comparable to our experiments. Dobrin and Mrkvicka found that chronic loading of polypropylene sutures increased their "acute" breaking force. They suggested that this may have resulted from increased orientation of crystals in the core of the filaments [8,18]. Dobrin et al. briefly applied stress to suture materials by disturbing the outer surface of the filament by placing a stray knot or pinching with forceps, which both resulted in a decreased "acute" breaking strength [19].

In this study, we did not tackle the challenges posed by the use of different suture–needle configurations and handling of the needle itself. Here, surgical skills are of paramount importance for adequate tissue repair [20]. One should be aware of the different indications of tapered, round, cutting and reversed cutting needle designs. Apart from that, some of the alloys (S45500) [21] used to manufacture the needles contain a substantial proportion of nickel, rendering them unsuitable for patients with a nickel allergy. Finally, grasping the needle at the "eye" weakens the link to the suture material.

As expected, our experiment confirmed that a single crush with the needle holder can significantly reduce the tensile strength of a suture strand by approximately 30%. However, when investigated separately, not all the products displayed the same effect. In particular, Vicryl® (polyglactine) and Surgipro® (polypropylene) suffered non-significant material damage in terms of linear strength. In fact, braided polyglactine (Vicryl®) showed resistance to crush load and lost the least linear tensile strength upon deformation. Polypropylene possessed the least initial linear tensile strength, but strength deterioration was relatively low. When the strands were investigated by material (and not as a separate product), a single cycle of crush load in all cases produced significant attenuation of linear tensile strength. There was no marked or significant difference between resorbable and non-resorbable materials, although the study design was inappropriate for this question.

Other newer technologies, such as staples, various skin adhesives, zipper-like devices, and polyester meshes, have gained popularity in the operating theatre [22]. Although adverse reactions to the adhesives [23] or to nickel alloys in metallic staplers have been reported, these new devices definitely have a place in orthopedic [24] and cardiovascular surgery [25], but are yet to acquire wide acceptance in plastic surgery. This might change with the development of novel degradable polyurethane-based tissue sealants [26]. Numerous reports on wound closure after knee surgery showed that zipper-like devices can produce equal or better results than staples [27]. Finally, the use in ointments and gels loaded with biomodulatory molecules [28] is yet to be fully evaluated, but seems to be an option in burns and diabetic foot ulcers. Products containing basic and acidic fibroblastic growth factor (bFGF and aFGF), granulocyte macrophage colony-stimulating growth factor (GM-CSF), platelet-derived growth factor (PDGF) as well as epidermal growth factor (EGF) are available. However, some concerns arose following reports of malignancies emerging in combination with the use of recombinant PDGF gels (becaplermin-Regranex®) [29,30].

## 5. Conclusions

Repeated instrumental handling of various suture materials inevitably leads to mechanical damage of sutures and premature break down, even with perfectly knotted sutures. Especially in continuous sutures, this can have severe clinical consequences. Our data clearly reveal the deleterious effect on sutures when they are repeatedly grasped with an instrument during knotting. It, therefore, seems advisable to take meticulous care without unnecessary grasping of the material. Reconstructive surgeons have to be flexible and tailor their wound closure techniques and materials to individual patients, as well as to the procedure and tissue demands; therefore, profound knowledge of the physical properties of the suture materials used is of paramount importance.

**Author Contributions:** Conceptualization, R.E.H.; methodology, J.D. and E.P.; software, E.P.; validation, R.E.H. and J.G.; formal analysis, E.P.; investigation, J.D. and A.B.; resources, R.E.H. and D.W.S.; data curation, E.P. and J.D.; writing—original draft preparation, R.E.H. and E.P.; writing—review and editing, E.P.; visualization, E.P. and A.B.; supervision, R.E.H. and D.W.S.; project administration, R.E.H.; funding acquisition, R.E.H. All authors have read and agreed to the published version of the manuscript.

**Funding:** This research received no external funding.

**Institutional Review Board Statement:** Not applicable.

**Informed Consent Statement:** Not applicable.

**Data Availability Statement:** Detailed data supporting the results are available with the authors.

**Conflicts of Interest:** The authors declare no conflict of interest.

## References

1. Bariol, S.V.; Stewart, G.D.; Tolley, D.A. Laparoscopic Suturing: Effect of Instrument Handling on Suture Strength. *J. Endourol.* **2005**, *19*, 1127–1133. [CrossRef] [PubMed]
2. Hong, T.; King, M.W.; Michielsen, S.; Cheung, L.W.; Mary, C.; Guzman, R.; Guidoin, R. Development of in Vitro Performance Tests and Evaluation of Nonabsorbable Monofilament Sutures for Cardiovascular Surgery. *ASAIO J.* **1998**, *44*, 776–785. [CrossRef] [PubMed]
3. Abhari, R.E.; Martins, J.A.; Morris, H.L.; Mouthuy, P.A.; Carr, A. Synthetic Sutures: Clinical Evaluation and Future Developments. *J. Biomater. Appl.* **2017**, *32*, 410–421. [CrossRef] [PubMed]
4. Abellan, D.; Nart, J.; Pascual, A.; Cohen, R.E.; Sanz-Moliner, J.D. Physical and Mechanical Evaluation of Five Suture Materials on Three Knot Configurations: An in Vitro Study. *Polymers* **2016**, *8*, 147. [CrossRef] [PubMed]
5. Polykandriotis, E.; Besrour, F.; Arkudas, A.; Ruppe, F.; Zetzmann, K.; Braeuer, L.; Horch, R.E. Flexor Tendon Repair with a Polytetrafluoroethylene (Ptfe) Suture Material. *Arch. Orthop. Trauma Surg.* **2019**, *139*, 429–434. [CrossRef]
6. Polykandriotis, E.; Ruppe, F.; Niederkorn, M.; Polykandriotis, E.; Brauer, L.; Horch, R.E.; Arkudas, A.; Gruener, J.S. Polytetrafluoroethylene (Ptfe) Suture Vs Fiberwire and Polypropylene in Flexor Tendon Repair. *Arch. Orthop. Trauma Surg.* **2021**, *141*, 1609–1614. [CrossRef]
7. Nonabsorbable Surgical Suture. In *United States Pharmacopeia and National Formulary*, Usp 29-Nf 24th ed.; United States Pharmacopeial Convention: Rockville, MD, USA, 2006; p. 2776.
8. Dobrin, P.B. Surgical Manipulation and the Tensile Strength of Polypropylene Sutures. *Arch. Surg.* **1989**, *124*, 665–668. [CrossRef]
9. Naleway, S.E.; Lear, W.; Kruzic, J.J.; Maughan, C.B. Mechanical Properties of Suture Materials in General and Cutaneous Surgery. *J. Biomed. Mater. Res. Part B Appl. Biomater.* **2015**, *103*, 735–742. [CrossRef]
10. von Fraunhofer, J.A.; Storey, R.S.; Stone, I.K.; Masterson, B.J. Tensile Strength of Suture Materials. *J. Biomed. Mater. Res.* **1985**, *19*, 595–600. [CrossRef]
11. Abiri, A.; Paydar, O.; Tao, A.; LaRocca, M.; Liu, K.; Genovese, B.; Candler, R.; Grundfest, W.S.; Dutson, E.P. Tensile Strength and Failure Load of Sutures for Robotic Surgery. *Surg. Endosc.* **2017**, *31*, 3258–3270. [CrossRef]
12. Turker, M.; Yalcinozan, M.; Cirpar, M.; Cetik, O.; Kalaycioglu, B. Clamp Fixation to Prevent Unfolding of a Suture Knot Decreases Tensile Strength of Polypropylene Sutures. *Knee Surg. Sports Traumatol. Arthrosc.* **2012**, *20*, 2602–2605. [CrossRef] [PubMed]
13. Cai, A.; Pingel, I.; Lorz, D.; Beier, J.P.; Horch, R.E.; Arkudas, A. Force Distribution of a Cylindrical Grip Differs between Dominant and Nondominant Hand in Healthy Subjects. *Arch. Orthop. Trauma. Surg.* **2018**, *138*, 1323–1331. [CrossRef] [PubMed]

14. Abiri, A.; Askari, S.J.; Tao, A.; Juo, Y.Y.; Dai, Y.; Pensa, J.; Candler, R.; Dutson, E.P.; Grundfest, W.S. Suture Breakage Warning System for Robotic Surgery. *IEEE Trans. Biomed. Eng.* **2019**, *66*, 1165–1171. [CrossRef] [PubMed]
15. Dai, Y.; Abiri, A.; Pensa, J.; Liu, S.; Paydar, O.; Sohn, H.; Sun, S.; Pellionisz, P.A.; Pensa, C.; Dutson, E.P.; et al. Biaxial Sensing Suture Breakage Warning System for Robotic Surgery. *Biomed. Microdevices* **2019**, *21*, 10. [CrossRef]
16. Bisson, L.J.; Sobel, A.D.; Godfrey, D. Effects of Using a Surgical Clamp to Hold Tension While Tying Knots with Commonly Used Orthopedic Sutures. *Knee Surg. Sports Traumatol. Arthrosc.* **2012**, *20*, 1673–1680. [CrossRef] [PubMed]
17. Diks, J.; Nio, D.; Linsen, M.A.; Rauwerda, J.A.; Wisselink, W. Suture Damage During Robot-Assisted Vascular Surgery: Is It an Issue? *Surg. Laparosc. Endosc. Percutaneous Tech.* **2007**, *17*, 524–527. [CrossRef]
18. Dobrin, P.B. Chronic Loading of Polypropylene Sutures: Implications for Breakage after Carotid Endarterectomy. *J. Surg. Res.* **1996**, *61*, 4–10. [CrossRef]
19. Dobrin, P.B.; Mrkvicka, R. Chronic Loading and Extension Increases the Acute Breaking Strength of Polypropylene Sutures. *Ann. Vasc. Surg.* **1998**, *12*, 424–429. [CrossRef]
20. Lekic, N.; Dodds, S.D. Suture Materials, Needles, and Methods of Skin Closure: What Every Hand Surgeon Should Know. *J. Hand Surg. Am.* **2022**, *47*, 160–171.e1. [CrossRef]
21. Lear, W. Instruments and Materials. In *Surgery of the Skin*, 3rd ed.; Robinson, J.K., Hanke, C.W., Siegel, D., Fratila, A., Bhatia, A., Rohrer, T., Eds.; Saunders: Philadelphia, PA, USA, 2014; pp. 64–72. ISBN 9780323260282.
22. Kim, K.Y.; Anoushiravani, A.A.; Long, W.J.; Vigdorchik, J.M.; Fernandez-Madrid, I.; Schwarzkopf, R.A. Meta-Analysis and Systematic Review Evaluating Skin Closure after Total Knee Arthroplasty-What Is the Best Method? *J. Arthroplast.* **2017**, *32*, 2920–2927. [CrossRef]
23. Knackstedt, R.W.; Dixon, J.A.; O'Neill, P.J.; Herrera, F.A. Rash with Dermabond Prineo Skin Closure System Use in Bilateral Reduction Mammoplasty: A Case Series. *Case Rep. Med.* **2015**, *2015*, 642595. [CrossRef] [PubMed]
24. Ko, J.H.; Yang, I.H.; Ko, M.S.; Kamolhuja, E.; Park, K.K. Do Zip-Type Skin-Closing Devices Show Better Wound Status Compared to Conventional Staple Devices in Total Knee Arthroplasty? *Int. Wound J.* **2017**, *14*, 250–254. [CrossRef] [PubMed]
25. Tanaka, Y.; Miyamoto, T.; Naito, Y.; Yoshitake, S.; Sasahara, A.; Miyaji, K. Randomized Study of a New Noninvasive Skin Closure Device for Use after Congenital Heart Operations. *Ann. Thorac. Surg.* **2016**, *102*, 1368–1374. [CrossRef] [PubMed]
26. Zou, F.; Wang, Y.; Zheng, Y.; Xie, Y.; Zhang, H.; Chen, J.; Hussain, M.I.; Meng, H.; Peng, J. A Novel Bioactive Polyurethane with Controlled Degradation and L-Arg Release Used as Strong Adhesive Tissue Patch for Hemostasis and Promoting Wound Healing. *Bioact. Mater.* **2022**, *17*, 471–487. [CrossRef]
27. Tian, P.; Li, Y.M.; Li, Z.J.; Xu, G.J.; Ma, X.L. Comparison between Zip-Type Skin Closure Device and Staple for Total Knee Arthroplasty: A Meta-Analysis. *BioMed Res. Int.* **2021**, *2021*, 6670064. [CrossRef]
28. Han, C.M.; Cheng, B.; Wu, P. Writing group of growth factor guideline on behalf of Chinese Burn, Association. Clinical Guideline on Topical Growth Factors for Skin Wounds. *Burn. Trauma* **2020**, *8*, tkaa035. [CrossRef]
29. Calhoun, C.C.; Cardenes, O.; Ducksworth, J.; Le, A.D. Off-Label Use of Becaplermin Gel (Recombinant Platelet-Derived Growth Factor-Bb) for Treatment of Mucosal Defects after Corticocancellous Bone Graft: Report of 2 Cases with Review of the Literature. *J. Oral Maxillofac. Surg.* **2009**, *67*, 2516–2520. [CrossRef]
30. Papanas, N.; Maltezos, E. Benefit-Risk Assessment of Becaplermin in the Treatment of Diabetic Foot Ulcers. *Drug Saf.* **2010**, *33*, 455–461. [CrossRef]

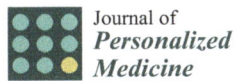

Article

# Assessment of Mastectomy Skin Flaps for Immediate Reconstruction with Implants via Thermal Imaging—A Suitable, Personalized Approach?

Hanna Luze [1,*], Sebastian Philipp Nischwitz [1], Paul Wurzer [1,2], Raimund Winter [1], Stephan Spendel [1], Lars-Peter Kamolz [1,3,4] and Vesna Bjelic-Radisic [5,6]

1. Division of Plastic, Aesthetic and Reconstructive Surgery, Department of Surgery, Medical University of Graz, 8036 Graz, Austria; sebastian.nischwitz@medunigraz.at (S.P.N.); office@wurzer-medical.at (P.W.); r.winter@medunigraz.at (R.W.); stephan.spendel@medunigraz.at (S.S.); lars.kamolz@medunigraz.at (L.-P.K.)
2. Burgenländische Krankenanstalten-Ges.m.b.H., 7000 Eisenstadt, Austria
3. COREMED–Cooperative Centre for Regenerative Medicine, JOANNEUM RESEARCH Forschungsgesellschaft mbH, 8010 Graz, Austria
4. Research Unit for Safety and Sustainability in Healthcare, Division of Plastic, Aesthetic and Reconstructive Surgery, Department of Surgery, Medical University of Graz, 8036 Graz, Austria
5. Breast Unit, Helios University Hospital, University of Witten Herdecke, 42283 Wuppertal, Germany; vesna.bjelic-radisic@helios-gesundheit.de
6. Division of General Gynaecology, Department of Obstetrics and Gynaecology, Medical University of Graz, 8010 Graz, Austria
* Correspondence: hanna.luze@medunigraz.at; Tel.: +43-316-385-30445; Fax: +43-316-385-59514690

**Abstract:** Background: Impaired perfusion of the remaining skin flap after subcutaneous mastectomy can cause wound-healing disorders and consecutive necrosis. Personalized intraoperative imaging, possibly performed via the FLIR ONE thermal-imaging device, may assist in flap assessment and detect areas at risk for postoperative complications. Methods: Fifteen female patients undergoing elective subcutaneous mastectomy and immediate breast reconstruction with implants were enrolled. Pre-, intra- and postoperative thermal imaging was performed via FLIR ONE. Potential patient-, surgery- and environment-related risk factors were acquired and correlated with the occurrence of postoperative complications. Results: Wound-healing disorders and mastectomy-skin-flap necrosis occurred in 26.7%, whereby areas expressing intraoperative temperatures less than 26 °C were mainly affected. These complications were associated with a statistically significantly higher BMI, longer surgery duration, lower body and room temperature and a trend towards larger implant sizes. Conclusion: Impaired skin-flap perfusion may be multifactorially conditioned. Preoperative screening for risk factors and intraoperative skin-perfusion assessment via FLIR ONE thermal-imaging device is recommendable to reduce postoperative complications. Intraoperatively detectable areas with a temperature of lower than 26 °C are highly likely to develop mastectomy-skin-flap necrosis and early detection allows individual treatment concept adaption, ultimately improving the patient's outcome.

**Keywords:** personalized medicine; thermal imaging; reconstructive breast surgery; mastectomy-skin-flap perfusion; mastectomy-skin-flap necrosis

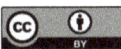

## 1. Introduction

Breast cancer (BC) ranks top in malignancies among females worldwide and represents the most common reason for death by cancer as well [1]. About two-thirds of patients with BC undergo breast-conserving surgery [2,3]. Thirty to forty per cent require a mastectomy and about 25% of these patients decide to undergo an immediate breast reconstruction (IBR) [2,3]. Besides autologous tissue reconstruction, IBR with implants is a commonly used technique and considered safe from an oncological point of view [2]. Larger varieties of sizes and shapes of implants and the use of different meshes creating a more natural appearing lower pole, may have contributed to an increased use of implants [4,5].

Due to the combination of oncoplastic and plastic surgical techniques, aesthetically pleasing reconstructive results can be achieved without compromising the oncological safety [6]. A modified radical mastectomy was replaced, e.g., by nipple-sparing mastectomy (NSM) and/or skin-sparing mastectomy (SSM), offering good aesthetic results [4].

Besides hematoma and infection listed as the most common early complications in IBR with implants, wound-healing disorders (WHD) and mastectomy-skin-flap necrosis (MSFN) occur more commonly than appreciated, with reports ranging from 5% to 41.2% [7–11]. The main reason for WHD and especially for skin-flap necrosis is attributed to an impaired perfusion of the remaining skin flap after mastectomy [11]. Subsequently, numerous challenging sequelae including wound-management problems, follow-up interventions, implant loss, delays to adjuvant therapy, aesthetic compromise and patient dissatisfaction can occur [11].

Several studies have investigated patient-related (e.g., smoking, diabetes, obesity etc.) and surgery-related risk factors (e.g., incision type, mastectomy weight, thickness of the skin flap, etc.) for WHD and MSFN to date [11,12]. Apart from screening and monitoring possible risk factors, intraoperative assessment of the individual skin-flap perfusion is considered of the utmost importance to detect areas at risk of WHD and MSFN [12]. A number of assessment methods have evolved so far, including clinical evaluation, handheld Doppler devices, laser Doppler, fluorescein angiography and indocyanine green techniques [12]. As an indicator of tissue perfusion, skin (surface) temperature can also readily and accurately be measured via thermal imaging [13,14]. The present study evaluated the feasibility of assessing the individual mastectomy-skin-flap perfusion via the thermal-imaging device FLIR ONE in patients undergoing NSM or SSM and following IBR with implants. Furthermore, possible patient-, surgery- and environment-related risk factors for postoperative complications were determined and the overall complication rate was assessed.

## 2. Methods

This prospective analysis was conducted the Medical University of Graz, Austria, Division of General Gynaecology, Department of Obstetrics and Gynaecology and Division of Plastic, Aesthetic and Reconstructive Surgery, Department of Surgery in cooperation with the Department of Surgery, LKH Graz II, Standort West, Graz, Austria between 2016 and 2018 and has been approved by the responsible ethics' committee. The surgeries were performed by two different surgeons (one female and one male) who were experienced in this field for 28 and 31 years, respectively.

*2.1. Study Population*

Fifteen female (age range 18–80 years) healthy, non-pregnant study participants were enrolled. Inclusion criteria were defined as follows: history of BC, carcinoma in situ on one or both breasts and/or known genetic BRCA I or BRCA II mutation and planned NSM or SSM, and following IBR with definite implants. Exclusion criteria were defined as follows: BC diagnosis with the contraindication for NSM or SSM (e.g., inflammatory carcinoma), use of tissue expanders; diabetes mellitus type 1 and 2, nicotine abuse, inability to fully comprehend study procedures or to provide written informed consent. The reconstruction was performed in dual plane technique using anatomical silicone implants (Mentor Deutschland GmbH, Munich, Germany), placed subpectorally. The acellular dermal matrix Strattice™ (Allergan, Dublin, Ireland) was used for implant stabilization and affixed to the musculus pectoralis major as well as in the inframammary fold. Postoperative follow-up visits were uniformly scheduled at 1, 2 and 6 weeks postoperative.

Additional patient-related, (age, Body-Mass-Index (BMI), body temperature), surgery-related (incision type and position, implant size, surgery duration) and environment-related data (room temperature) were acquired.

## 2.2. FLIR ONE

Surface temperature was acquired using measurements obtained with a FLIR ONE thermal-imaging camera (FLIR Systems, Wilsonville, OR, USA). FLIR ONE is a lightweight, pocket-sized, smartphone attachment thermal-imaging camera with a measurable temperature range from $-20\ °C$ to $120\ °C$ and a measurement accuracy of $0.10\ °C$ [15]. A Multi-Spectral Dynamic imaging technology allows for enhanced thermal imaging by embossing details from the camera onto the thermal image [15].

Four timepoints for thermal imaging with FLIR ONE were determined:

- Preoperative: immediately after anesthesia induction before disinfection
- Intraoperative 1: immediately after NSM/SSM
- Intraoperative 2: immediately after implant placement and wound closure
- Postoperative: 24 h postoperative

The distance between the FLIR ONE and patients' skin was set at 30 cm in every measuring. At recording, surgical lights were turned off and body and room temperature were assessed. Thermal images were transferred to FLIR Tools software, where highest, lowest and average temperature of each image was determined within a specialized region of interest (ROI). (See Figure 1) The ROI was manually plotted, matching the region, where the NSM/SSM was performed.

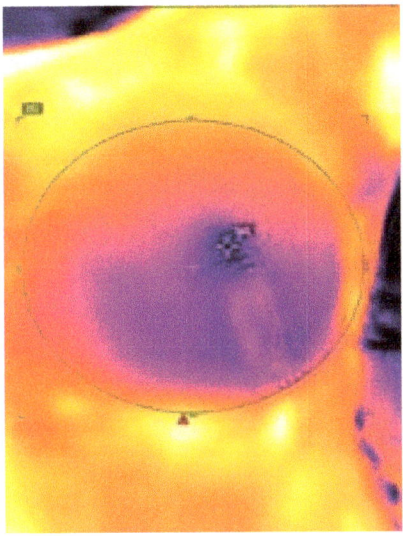

**Figure 1.** Intraoperative thermal imaging via FLIR ONE. The ROI (black circle) displays the subcutaneous mastectomy area, within the temperature was measured. Darker colors (purple, blue) indicate lower surface temperature while brighter colors (orange, yellow) indicate higher temperature.

## 2.3. Statistical Analysis

Since this study was designed as an explorative study with a small sample size, a formal sample size calculation was waived. The rationale for conducting a study with females exclusively was based on the fact that NSM/SSM with IBR with implants is primarily used in female BC patients. Data were analyzed with GraphPad Prism software (version 9.0.2; GraphPad Software, Inc., San Diego, CA, USA). Mean, median and standard deviation (SD) of numerous data were calculated and correlated to the occurrence of postoperative complications (WHD, MSFN) performing a Spearman correlation test. All statistical tests were two-tailed and differences were considered statistically significant when $p < 0.05$.

## 3. Results

Overall, 15 patients with a mean age of 44.1 years (SD ± 9.2 years) and a mean BMI of 25.9 kg/m$^2$ (SD ± 2.46 kg/m$^2$) were included in this investigation. All patients enrolled underwent neoadjuvant chemotherapy; no patient underwent radiotherapy prior to surgery. Risk-reduction mastectomy was performed in one, NSM in six and SSM in seven patients. In the patient undergoing risk-reduction mastectomy, skin-flap perfusion was assessed exclusively on the left side, since a minimally prefilled tissue expander was used on the right side. The mean surgery duration was 2 h 32 min (SD ± 108 min). 8 (53.33%) periareolar and 7 (46.67%) inframammary incisions were performed.

### 3.1. Surface Temperature of the Mastectomy Skin Flap

The preoperative mean surface temperature was 36.3 °C (SD ± 3.6 °C). The first mean intraoperative surface temperature after subcutaneous mastectomy (intraoperative 1, I1), was 33.3 °C (SD ± 4.0 °C) decreasing to 32.0 °C (SD ± 2.7 °C) and at the second timepoint after implant placement (intraoperative 2, I2). Twenty-four hours postoperative, the mean surface temperature was 36.0 °C (SD ± 1.4 °C). The preoperative mean temperature was statistically significantly higher than intraoperative 1 and intraoperative 2 ($p$ = < 0.001). Intraoperative measured mean temperatures were statistically significantly lower than postoperative (I1: $p$ = 0.024, I2: $p$ = 0.017).

The highest mean preoperative temperature was 37.5 °C (SD ± 1.1 °C). intraoperative measured mean highest temperature statistically significantly decreased to 35.5 °C (SD ± 1.3 °C) at the first timepoint and 34.6 °C (SD ± 1.9 °C) at the second (p= 0.001 and $p$ = 0.048). Twenty-four hours postoperative, the mean highest temperature was 37.4 °C (SD ± 1.2 °C), which was statistically significantly higher than both values measured intraoperatively ($p \leq 0.001$ and $p$ = 0.002).

The lowest preoperative temperature was 35.5 °C (SD ± 3.0 °C). The intraoperative measured lowest temperature statistically significantly decreased to 28.3 °C (SD ± 4.4 °C) after subcutaneous mastectomy and to 27.7 °C (SD ± 4.6 °C) after implant placement ($p \leq 0.001$ and $p$ = 0.036) in the same patients. 24 h postoperative, mean lowest temperature was 33.7 °C (SD ± 3.0 °C), which was statistically significantly higher than both values measured intraoperatively ($p$ = 0.012). An overview of surface temperatures is depicted in Table 1 and Figure 2.

**Table 1.** Surface temperatures at different measurement points. Data are presented as average values [°C] and standard deviations. An asterisk indicates statistical significance.

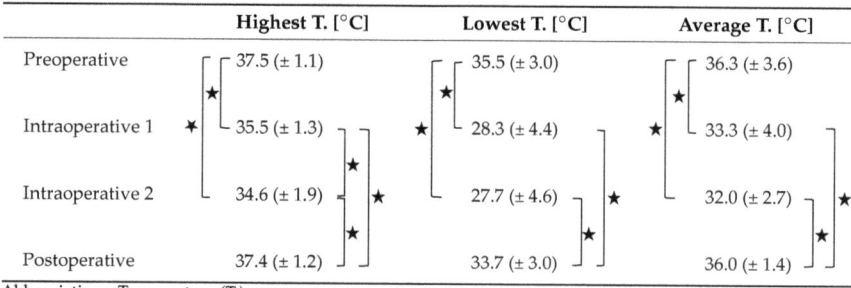

|  | Highest T. [°C] | Lowest T. [°C] | Average T. [°C] |
|---|---|---|---|
| Preoperative | 37.5 (± 1.1) | 35.5 (± 3.0) | 36.3 (± 3.6) |
| Intraoperative 1 | 35.5 (± 1.3) | 28.3 (± 4.4) | 33.3 (± 4.0) |
| Intraoperative 2 | 34.6 (± 1.9) | 27.7 (± 4.6) | 32.0 (± 2.7) |
| Postoperative | 37.4 (± 1.2) | 33.7 (± 3.0) | 36.0 (± 1.4) |

Abbreviations: Temperature (T.).

### 3.2. Wound-Healing Disorders and Necrosis

Patients were divided into a "no-complication group" and a "complication group" including WHD and MSFN for further comparisons. 4 of 15 patients (26.7%) developed WHD, which were initially treated without surgical interaction but prolonged dressing changes and administration of antibiotics. In the further course, 3 (20%) WHD converted into superficial MSFN requiring follow up interventions under local anesthesia. No implant loss was noted. In all patients of the complication group, WHD and MSFN occurred within areas with an intraoperative measured temperature lower than 26 °C.

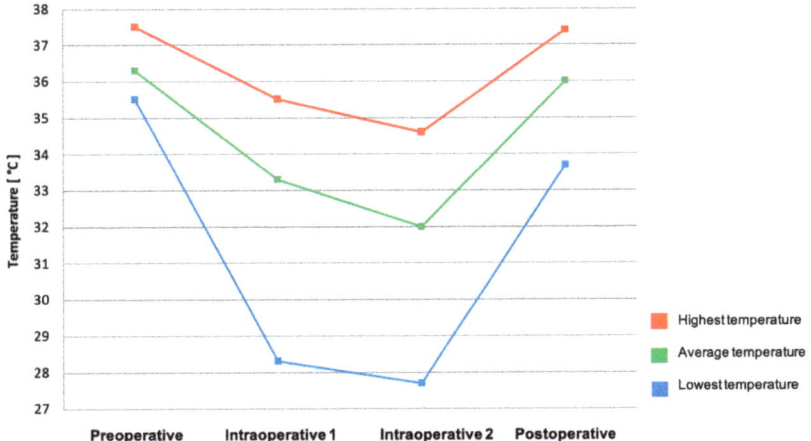

**Figure 2.** Surface temperature changes during the procedure of NSM/SSM and immediate reconstruction with implants. Data are presented as mean values [°C].

The main statistically significant difference between the no-complication and the complication group was found regarding the surface temperatures of the mastectomy skin flap. The complication group showed a statistically significantly lower mean temperature in preoperative ($p \leq 0.001$), intraoperative 1 ($p = 0.029$) and postoperative ($p \leq 0.001$) measurements. The mean lowest temperatures were statistically significantly lower during the entire procedure ($p \leq 0.001$) in the complication group, as well as the mean highest temperatures pre- and postoperative ($p = 0.021$ and $p \leq 0.001$). An overview of surface temperatures within the no-complication and complication groups is depicted in Table 2.

**Table 2.** Surface temperatures in the no-complication and the complication groups. Data are presented as average values and standard deviations. An asterisk indicates statistical significance ($p < 0.05$).

|  | Highest T. [°C] | | Lowest T. [°C] | | Average T. [°C] | |
| --- | --- | --- | --- | --- | --- | --- |
|  | No Complication | Complication | No Complication | Complication | No Complication | Complication |
| Preoperative | 37.8 (± 1.1) —★— | 36.8 (± 0.6) | 35.8 (± 1.2) —★— | 33.1 (± 4.6) | 37.0 (± 1.1) —★— | 34.3 (± 3.7) |
| Intraoperative 1 | 35.4 (± 1.3) | 35.6 (± 0.8) | 29.1 (± 3.1) —★— | 25.7 (± 3.9) | 33.9 (± 4.1) —★— | 31.6 (± 0.6) |
| Intraoperative 2 | 34.8 (± 1.7) | 34.2 (± 2.1) | 28.2 (± 3.9) —★— | 25.4 (± 2.4) | 32.1 (± 2.6) | 32.0 (± 2.5) |
| Postoperative | 37.7 (± 1.2) —★— | 36.8 (± 0.9) | 34.7 (± 2.4) —★— | 31.3 (± 2.8) | 36.4 (± 1.0) —★— | 34.7 (± 1.3) |

Abbreviations: Temperature (T.).

### 3.2.1. Surgery-Related Risk Factors

WHD rate with periareolar incisions was 37.5% vs. 14.3% with inframammary incisions. MSFN rate, requiring follow-up interventions under local anesthesia in all patients, was 25% with periareolar incisions and 14.3% with inframammary incisions. No statistically significant difference between incision type ($p = 0.36$) and NSM or SSM technique ($p = 0.29$)

was observed. An overview of incision types and postoperative complications is depicted in Figure 3.

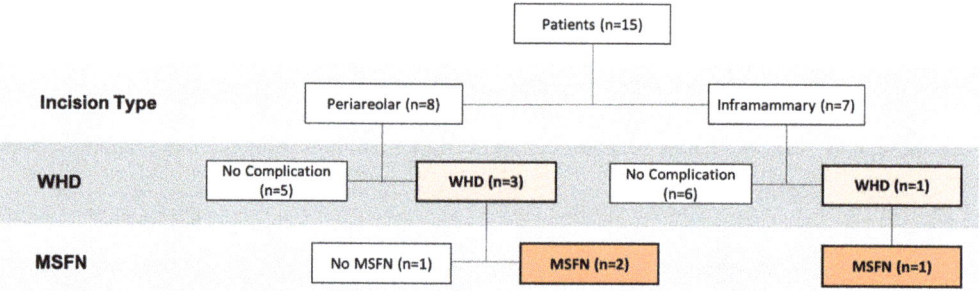

**Figure 3.** Incision types and postoperative complications. Abbreviations: Mastectomy-skin-flap necrosis (MSFN); wound-healing disorder (WHD).

A comparison of both groups showed a statistically higher average surgery duration in the complication group (2 h 58 min) compared to the no-complication group (2 h 22 min) ($p = 0.027$). Furthermore, statistically significantly lower average room temperatures (21.2 °C (SD $\pm$ 0.2 °C), $p \leq 0.001$) were observed in the complication group in comparison to the no-complication group (23.0 °C (SD $\pm$ 1.2 °C)). In all patients, mastectomy weight approximately correlated to the implant size. A trend towards larger implants was noted in the complication group (370 cm$^3$ (SD $\pm$ 43.3 cm$^3$)) compared to the no-complication group (320.5 cm$^3$ ($\pm$42.5 cm$^3$), $p = 0.223$).

### 3.2.2. Patient-Related Risk Factors

Statistically significantly lower mean body temperatures during the entire procedure (35.6 °C (SD $\pm$ 0.4 °C), $p = 0.012$) were found in the complication group when compared to the no-complication group (36.0 °C (SD $\pm$ 0.1 °C). Patients developing WHD and MSFN also had a significantly higher BMI (28.1 kg/m$^2$ (SD $\pm$ 0.6 kg/m$^2$)) than patients without complications (25.3 kg/m$^2$ (SD $\pm$ 3.0 kg/m$^2$), $p = 0.002$). No age-related significances were found ($p = 0.46$). Demographic and clinical data of the complication and no-complication groups are listed in Table 3.

**Table 3.** Patient-, surgery- and environmental-related factors. Data are presented as average values and standard deviations. An asterisk indicates statistical significance between the groups.

|  |  | No Complication | Complication |
|---|---|---|---|
| Patients ($n = 15$) |  | 11 (73.3%) | 4 (26.7%) |
| Age [years] |  | 47.6 ($\pm$10.6) | 46.3 ($\pm$1.5) |
| BMI [kg/m$^2$] |  | 25.3 ($\pm$3.0) | 28.1 ($\pm$0.6) |
| Body temperature [°C] | ★ | 36.0 ($\pm$0.1) | 35.6 ($\pm$0.4) |
| Surgery duration [min] | ★ | 142 ($\pm$0.43) | 178 ($\pm$42) |
| Implant size [cm$^3$] | ★ | 320.5 ($\pm$42.5) | 370 ($\pm$43.3) |
| Room temperature [°C] | ★ | 23.0 ($\pm$0.2) | 21.2 ($\pm$1.2) |

Abbreviations: Body mass index (BMI).

## 4. Discussion

Wound-healing disorders and mastectomy-skin-flap necrosis of the remaining skin flap after mastectomy due to hypoperfusion are highly relevant and underappreciated complications that may result in considerable challenges for the patient and health-care system. Potential consequences range from aesthetic compromise and patient dissatisfaction to limited options of reconstruction and delays in adjuvant therapies [10]. Existing evidence highlights the difficulty in assessing individual mastectomy-skin-flap perfusion despite various techniques available to date [16].

### 4.1. Examination of Skin-Flap Perfusion via Thermal Imaging

The present study demonstrated thermal imaging via FLIR ONE to be a suitable approach for the measurement of individual skin/surface temperature as a proxy indicator of tissue perfusion. The FLIR ONE particularly excels in the domains of usability, time to image acquisition, and reliably accurate results requiring minimal to no training, resulting in high-resolution images. In our opinion, these features contribute to the fact that the FLIR ONE can be considered a valuable support tool in clinics in a wider range of applications. Personalized thermal imaging may be of particular value in establishing individual treatment concepts. To date, thermal imaging via FLIR ONE has widely been clinically employed, for instance, in the individual assessment of burn wounds [13,17–19], diagnosis of complex regional pain syndrome [20], detection of perforator vessels in reconstructive surgery [14,21,22] and many other settings where thermal distribution patterns can yield proxy data. Within the field of breast oncology in particular, thermal imaging has recently been investigated as an emerging modality in breast-cancer screening [23,24] and has been considered a helpful tool in the treatment of breast-cancer-related lymphedema [25]. Apart from the low initial costs and ease of use of the FLIR ONE device, the non-invasive, no-touch character and absence of radiation are among the many advantages of this technique [22,23].

### 4.2. Detection of Hypoperfused Areas at Risk for WHD and MSFN

The procedure of mastectomy interrupts the axial perfusion of the over-lying breast dermis, leaving the relatively hypovascular skin flaps dependent on random-pattern perfusion and drainage through the subdermal plexus [26]. Studies report mastectomy flaps with a higher amount of subcutaneous fat and, therefore, better preserved blood supply, to be associated with a reduced risk of MSFN [26,27].

Evidence indicates a direct relationship between changes in tissue perfusion and temperature, therefore suggesting non-invasive surface-temperature measurement a valuable proxy marker for the analysis of (skin) perfusion [28]. In the present project, the temperature profile assessed via thermal imaging demonstrated a statistically significant drop during, and a rise after the procedure, nearly reaching initial values 24 h postoperative. The temperature drop is mainly induced due to the procedure of mastectomy and keeps increasing with increasing surgery duration, verifying the interruption the axial perfusion during the procedure. The subsequent postoperative increase may be attributed to a compensatory increase in random pattern perfusion and drainage through the subdermal plexus as well as room temperature compared to the operating room.

A comparison between patients without complications and those developing WHD and MSFN revealed significant differences in the surface temperature. We encountered significantly lower average temperatures in three out of four measuring time points, ($p \leq 0.001$, 0.029 and <0.001); and lower maximum temperatures prior to and following the procedure ($p \leq 0.001$) in the complication group. The lowest temperatures were statistically significantly lower during the entire procedure, suggesting lower tissue perfusion.

The present study revealed that areas with intraoperative temperatures lower than 26 °C are highly likely to develop WHD and MSFN, since their occurrence was exclusively noted within these areas. We derive that consideration of the proxy parameter of intraoperative temperature distribution to assess for clinically relevant hypoperfusion may lead to opportunities for early intervention in selected cases to avoid or reduce some of the possible adverse consequences. Early intervention is particularly important in IBR with implants and may comprise different strategies. The importance of the excision of non-viable skin edges to prevent WHD has often been determined in acute and chronic wound management [29]. According to our findings, excision of wound edges with a temperature of lower than 26 °C may be considered even when clinical signs of hypoperfusion are absent. If larger areas manifest with impaired skin-flap perfusion as indicated on thermal imaging with areas <26 °C, the risk of extended MSFN may be increased and the reconstruction strategy should be reconsidered; however, to our knowledge, no studies addressing this challenge exist to date.

### 4.3. Detection of Patient- and Surgery-Related Risk Factors for WHD and MSFN

In the present study, a significantly higher BMI and a trend towards larger implants matching the mastectomy weight were identified to be associated with flap morbidity. The majority of the existing literature investigating risk factors related to WHD and MSFN is limited to retrospective series [12]. Smoking, diabetes, radiotherapy, previous scars and severe medical comorbidity have been revealed as patient-related risk factors so far [12]. Similar to our results, there is also evidence that obesity and increased breast volumes may cause or contribute to impaired skin-flap perfusion [30,31].

Preoperative screening for known risk factors and incorporation into operative planning, especially if immediate breast reconstruction is performed, is of utmost importance. Unfortunately, the majority of patient-related risk factors are not modifiable prior to surgery; therefore, surgical risk factors need to be minimized. Among surgical factors, longer surgery duration is considered a risk factor for postoperative complications [12]. Our results not only revealed a statistically significant correlation to surgery duration, but also to body and room temperature. Measurements obtained during the procedure demonstrated statistically significantly lower values in both body and room temperature, in patients developing WHD and MSFN. Therefore, intraoperative temperature monitoring and management, if necessary, may be another approach to reduce postoperative complications, especially when other risk factors are present. No differences were identified between inframammary and periareolar incisions; however, other authors attribute flap morbidity to wise pattern mastectomy incisions [31].

In our setting, patients developing MSFN only required one follow-up intervention under local anesthesia and no implant loss was noted. However, extended MSFN resulting from hypoperfused areas may consequently lead to a higher chance for subsequent implant loss. Woerdeman et al. further reported an increased risk of implant loss in patients with larger-than-average-sized breasts and obese smokers [30]. In these patients, placement of breast implants may particularly need to be refrained from. As an alternative, tissue expanders may be placed first in order to minimize pressure on the skin flap and prevent subsequent implant loss.

A combination of careful preoperative planning and intraoperative monitoring may contribute to a reduced incidence of WHD resulting in MSFN. Early intervention in selected cases and deviation from the planned reconstructive procedure may reduce the overall morbidity of MSFN.

### 4.4. Limitations

This study is limited due to the small sample size, hence results and patient-related factors in particular may not be fully representative and transferable. Despite some significances that were statistically demonstrated, the small sample size might be accountable for the lack of further significances; however, we believe that tendencies were established to guide further investigation. While the study setup was designed to reduce possible bias caused by different surgeons, the thickness of the mastectomy skin flap linked to the skin-flap perfusion may not be directly comparable in all patients.

Furthermore, previous breast surgeries were not evaluated. Consequently, a bias by individual factors—such as scars potentially impairing the remaining skin flap perfusion—must be considered as a limiting factor. However, evaluation of a possible influence of previous medical interventions on skin-flap perfusion and postoperative complications may be an interesting approach for future studies. Ultimately, there is a great demand for strategies to detect risk factors contributing to WHD and MSFN. Further studies are necessary to reach the full potential of thermal imaging in the detection of areas at particular risk for developing WHD and MSFN.

## 5. Conclusions

WHD and MSFN due to compromised perfusion patterns of the remaining skin flap occur more commonly than appreciated, leading to numerous challenges. Hypoperfusion of the remaining mastectomy skin flap as a major factor contributing to WHD and MSFN is readily and accurately examined via the novel and personalized approach of thermal imaging with the FLIR device. Skin areas with a temperature lower than 26 °C are highly likely to develop subsequent WHD and MSFN and may require early intervention to avoid or reduce the incidence of MSFN. Ultimately, careful and diligent individual preoperative planning and intraoperative monitoring may contribute to a reduced incidence of WHD converting to MSFN.

**Author Contributions:** Conceptualization, H.L., S.S. and V.B.-R.; methodology, H.L. and S.P.N.; software, P.W.; validation, P.W. and R.W.; formal analysis, H.L. and S.P.N.; investigation, H.L. and V.B.-R.; resources, L.-P.K. and V.B.-R.; data curation, R.W.; writing—original draft preparation, H.L.; writing—review and editing, S.P.N., P.W., R.W., V.B.-R. and L.-P.K.; visualization, H.L.; supervision V.B.-R. and L.-P.K.; project administration, H.L.; funding acquisition, L.-P.K. and H.L. All authors have read and agreed to the published version of the manuscript.

**Funding:** This research received no specific grant from any funding agency in the public, commercial or not-for-profit sectors.

**Institutional Review Board Statement:** The study was conducted according to the guidelines of the Declaration of Helsinki, and approved by the Ethics Committee of Medical University Graz, Austria (protocol code 29-059 ex 16/17).

**Informed Consent Statement:** Informed consent was obtained from all subjects involved in the study.

**Data Availability Statement:** The authors confirm that the data supporting the findings of this study are available within the article.

**Conflicts of Interest:** The authors declare no conflict of interest.

## References

1. Bray, F.; Ferlay, J.; Soerjomataram, I.; Siegel, R.L.; Torre, L.A.; Jemal, A. Global cancer statistics 2018: GLOBOCAN estimates of incidence and mortality worldwide for 36 cancers in 185 countries. *CA Cancer J. Clin.* **2018**, *68*, 394–424. [CrossRef] [PubMed]
2. Jahkola, T.; Asko-Seljavaara, S.; von Smitten, K. Immediate Breast Reconstruction. *Scand. J. Surg.* **2003**, *92*, 249–256. [CrossRef] [PubMed]
3. Albornoz, C.R.; Cordeiro, P.G.; Pusic, A.L.; McCarthy, C.M.; Mehrara, B.J.; Disa, J.J.; Matros, E. Diminishing relative contraindications for immediate breast reconstruction: A multicenter study. *J. Am. Coll. Surg.* **2014**, *219*, 788–795. [CrossRef] [PubMed]
4. Panchal, H.; Matros, E. Current Trends in Postmastectomy Breast Reconstruction. *Plast. Reconstr. Surg.* **2017**, *140*, 7S–13S. [CrossRef] [PubMed]
5. Zenn, M.; Venturi, M.; Pittman, T.; Spear, S.; Gurtner, G.; Robb, G.; Mesbahi, A.; Dayan, J. Optimizing Outcomes of Postmastectomy Breast Reconstruction With Acellular Dermal Matrix: A Review of Recent Clinical Data. *Eplasty* **2017**, *17*, e18. [PubMed]
6. Chiappa, C.; Fachinetti, A.; Boeri, C.; Arlant, V.; Rausei, S.; Dionigi, G.; Rovera, F. Wound healing and postsurgical complications in breast cancer surgery: A comparison between PEAK PlasmaBlade and conventional electrosurgery—A preliminary report of a case series. *Ann. Surg. Treat. Res.* **2018**, *95*, 129. [CrossRef] [PubMed]
7. Antony, A.K.; Mehrara, B.M.; McCarthy, C.M.; Zhong, T.; Kropf, N.; Disa, J.J.; Pusic, A.; Cordeiro, P.G. Salvage of tissue expander in the setting of mastectomy flap necrosis: A 13-year experience using timed excision with continued expansion. *Plast. Reconstr. Surg.* **2009**, *124*, 356–363. [CrossRef]
8. Patel, K.M.; Hill, L.M.; Gatti, M.E.; Nahabedian, M.Y. Management of Massive Mastectomy Skin Flap Necrosis Following Autologous Breast Reconstruction. *Ann. Plast. Surg.* **2012**, *69*, 139–144. [CrossRef]
9. Margulies, A.G.; Hochberg, J.; Kepple, J.; Henry-Tillman, R.S.; Westbrook, K.; Klimberg, V.S. Total skin-sparing mastectomy without preservation of the nipple-areola complex. *Am. J. Surg.* **2005**, *190*, 920–926. [CrossRef]
10. Matsen, C.B.; Mehrara, B.; Eaton, A.; Capko, D.; Berg, A.; Stempel, M.; Van Zee, K.J.; Pusic, A.; King, T.A.; Cody, H.S.; et al. Skin Flap Necrosis After Mastectomy With Reconstruction: A Prospective Study. *Ann. Surg. Oncol.* **2016**, *23*, 257–264. [CrossRef]

11. Lee, K.-T.; Mun, G.-H. Necrotic Complications in Nipple-Sparing Mastectomy Followed by Immediate Breast Reconstruction: Systematic Review with Pooled Analysis. *J. Korean Soc. Microsurg.* **2014**, *23*, 51–64. [CrossRef]
12. Robertson, S.; Jeevaratnam, J.; Agrawal, A.; Cutress, R. Mastectomy skin flap necrosis: Challenges and solutions. *Breast Cancer Targets Ther.* **2017**, *9*, 141–152. [CrossRef]
13. Jaspers, M.E.H.; Carrière, M.E.; Meij-de Vries, A.; Klaessens, J.H.G.M.; van Zuijlen, P.P.M. The FLIR ONE thermal imager for the assessment of burn wounds: Reliability and validity study. *Burns* **2017**, *43*, 1516–1523. [CrossRef] [PubMed]
14. Hallock, G.G. Smartphone Thermal Imaging Can Enable the Safer Use of Propeller Flaps. *Semin. Plast. Surg.* **2020**, *34*, 161–164. [CrossRef] [PubMed]
15. FLIR ONE. Available online: https://www.flir.com/products/flir-one-gen-3/ (accessed on 19 September 2021).
16. Phillips, B.T.; Lanier, S.T.; Conkling, N.; Wang, E.; Dagum, A.B.; Ganz, J.C.; Khan, S.U.; Bui, D.T. Intraoperative Perfusion Techniques Can Accurately Predict Mastectomy Skin Flap Necrosis in Breast Reconstruction. *Plast. Reconstr. Surg.* **2012**, *129*, 778e–788e. [CrossRef]
17. Xue, E.Y.; Chandler, L.K.; Viviano, S.L.; Keith, J.D. Use of FLIR ONE Smartphone Thermography in Burn Wound Assessment. *Ann. Plast. Surg.* **2018**, *80*, S236–S238. [CrossRef] [PubMed]
18. Goel, J.; Nizamoglu, M.; Tan, A.; Gerrish, H.; Cranmer, K.; El-Muttardi, N.; Barnes, D.; Dziewulski, P. A prospective study comparing the FLIR ONE with laser Doppler imaging in the assessment of burn depth by a tertiary burns unit in the United Kingdom. *Scars Burn. Heal.* **2020**, *6*, 205951312097426. [CrossRef]
19. Nischwitz, S.P.; Luze, H.; Kamolz, L.-P. Thermal imaging via FLIR One—A promising tool in clinical burn care and research. *Burns* **2020**, *46*, 988–989. [CrossRef]
20. Dhatt, S.; Krauss, E.M.; Winston, P. The Role of FLIR ONE Thermography in Complex Regional Pain Syndrome. *Am. J. Phys. Med. Rehabil.* **2021**, *100*, e48–e51. [CrossRef]
21. Rabbani, M.J.; Ilyas, A.; Rabbani, A.; Abidin, Z.U.; Tarar, M.N. Accuracy of Thermal Imaging Camera in Identification of Perforators. *J. Coll. Physicians Surg. Pak.* **2020**, *30*, 512–515. [CrossRef]
22. Nischwitz, S.P.; Luze, H.; Schellnegger, M.; Gatterer, S.J.; Tuca, A.-C.; Winter, R.; Kamolz, L.-P. Thermal, Hyperspectral, and Laser Doppler Imaging: Non-Invasive Tools for Detection of The Deep Inferior Epigastric Artery Perforators—A Prospective Comparison Study. *J. Pers. Med.* **2021**, *11*, 1005. [CrossRef] [PubMed]
23. Prabha, S. Thermal Imaging Techniques for Breast Screening—A Survey. *Curr. Med. Imaging Rev.* **2020**, *16*, 855–862. [CrossRef]
24. Hakim, A.; Awale, R.N. Thermal Imaging—An Emerging Modality for Breast Cancer Detection: A Comprehensive Review. *J. Med. Syst.* **2020**, *44*, 136. [CrossRef] [PubMed]
25. Whatley, J.A.; Kay, S. Using thermal imaging to measure changes in breast cancer-related lymphoedema during reflexology. *Br. J. Community Nurs.* **2020**, *25* (Suppl. 10), S6–S11. [CrossRef]
26. Khavanin, N.; Qiu, C.; Darrach, H.; Kraenzlin, F.; Kokosis, G.; Han, T.; Sacks, J.M. Intraoperative Perfusion Assessment in Mastectomy Skin Flaps: How Close are We to Preventing Complications? *J. Reconstr. Microsurg.* **2019**, *35*, 471–478. [CrossRef]
27. Larson, D.L.; Basir, Z.; Bruce, T. Is Oncologic Safety Compatible with a Predictably Viable Mastectomy Skin Flap? *Plast. Reconstr. Surg.* **2011**, *127*, 27–33. [CrossRef] [PubMed]
28. Brigitte, W.F.Y.; Childs, C. A systematic review on the role of extremity skin temperature as a non-invasive marker for hypoperfusion in critically ill adults in the intensive care setting. *JBI Libr. Syst. Rev.* **2010**, *8* (Suppl. 34), 1–26. Available online: http://journals.lww.com/01583928-201008341-00007 (accessed on 2 February 2022).
29. Pereira, G.; Pereira, C. Skin edge debridement made easy. *Injury* **2003**, *34*, 954–956. [CrossRef]
30. Woerdeman, L.A.E.; Hage, J.J.; Hofland, M.M.I.; Rutgers, E.J.T. A Prospective Assessment of Surgical Risk Factors in 400 Cases of Skin-Sparing Mastectomy and Immediate Breast Reconstruction with Implants to Establish Selection Criteria. *Plast. Reconstr. Surg.* **2007**, *119*, 455–463. [CrossRef]
31. Davies, K.; Allan, L.; Roblin, P.; Ross, D.; Farhadi, J. Factors affecting post-operative complications following skin sparing mastectomy with immediate breast reconstruction. *Breast* **2011**, *20*, 21–25. [CrossRef]

# Article

# Improving the Safety of DIEP Flap Transplantation: Detailed Perforator Anatomy Study Using Preoperative CTA †

Katharina Frank [1], Armin Ströbel [2], Ingo Ludolph [1], Theresa Hauck [1], Matthias S. May [3], Justus P. Beier [1,4], Raymund E. Horch [1] and Andreas Arkudas [1,*]

1. Laboratory for Tissue Engineering and Regenerative Medicine, Department of Plastic and Hand Surgery, University Hospital Erlangen, Friedrich-Alexander University Erlangen-Nürnberg (FAU), 91054 Erlangen, Germany; frank_katharina@gmx.net (K.F.); ingo.ludolph@uk-erlangen.de (I.L.); theresa.hauck@uk-erlangen.de (T.H.); jbeier@ukaachen.de (J.P.B.); raymund.horch@uk-erlangen.de (R.E.H.)
2. Center for Clinical Studies, University Hospital Erlangen, Friedrich-Alexander University Erlangen-Nürnberg (FAU), 91054 Erlangen, Germany; armin.stroebel@uk-erlangen.de
3. Department of Radiology, University Hospital Erlangen, Friedrich-Alexander University Erlangen-Nürnberg (FAU), 91054 Erlangen, Germany; matthias.may@uk-erlangen.de
4. Department of Plastic Surgery, Hand Surgery–Burn Center, University Hospital RWTH Aachen, 52074 Aachen, Germany
* Correspondence: andreas.arkudas@uk-erlangen.de
† Parts of this work have been presented at the 50th annual meeting of the German society of plastic, reconstructive and aesthetic surgeons (DGPRÄC) and 24st annual meeting of the German Association of Aesthetic Plastic Surgeons (VDÄPC).

**Abstract:** Background: Deep inferior epigastric perforator and muscle sparing transverse rectus abdominis muscle flaps are commonly used flaps for autologous breast reconstruction. CT-angiography allows to analyse the perforator course preoperatively. Our aim was to compare the different aspects of perforator anatomy in the most detailed study. Methods: CT-angiographies of 300 female patients with autologous breast reconstruction of 10 years were analysed regarding the anatomy of the deep inferior epigastric artery and every perforator. Results: Overall, 2260 perforators were included. We identified correlations regarding the DIEA branching point and number of perforators and their intramuscular course. The largest perforator emerged more often from the medial branch of the DIEA than the smaller perforators (70% (416/595) vs. 54% (878/1634), $p < 0.001$) and more often had a direct connection to the SIEV (large 67% (401/595) vs. small 39% (634/1634), $p < 0.01$). Medial row perforators were larger than the laterals (lateral 1.44 mm ± 0.43 ($n = 941$) vs. medial 1.58 mm ± 0.52 ($n = 1304$) ($p < 0.001$)). The larger and more medial the perforator, the more likely it was connected to the SIEV: perforators with direct connection to the SIEV had a diameter of 1.65 mm ± 0.53 ($n = 1050$), perforators with indirect connection had a diameter of 1.43 mm ± 0.43 ($n = 1028$), perforators without connection had a diameter of 1.31 mm ± 0.37 ($n = 169$) ($p < 0.001$). Medial perforators were more often directly connected to the SIEV than lateral perforators (medial 56% (723/1302) vs. lateral 35% (327/941), $p < 0.001$). A lateral perforator more often had a short intramuscular course than medial perforators (69% (554/800) vs. 45% (474/1055), $p < 0.001$), which was also more often observed in the case of a small perforator and a caudal exit of the rectus sheath. Conclusion: The largest perforator emerges more often from the medial branch of the DIEA and frequently has a direct connection to the SIEV, making medial row perforators ideal for DIEP flap transplantation.

**Keywords:** CTA; autologous breast reconstruction; DIEP flap; MS-TRAM flap; perforator

## 1. Introduction

Breast cancer is the most common malignancy among women representing, depending on the literature, approximately 25% of all carcinomas and one of the leading causes of death [1–4]. If a mastectomy is necessary, breast reconstruction can be performed: implant-based or autologous reconstruction can be performed, the latter one in particular when radiotherapy is part of oncological treatment [5]. Autologous breast reconstruction can be performed using different pedicled or free flaps, which have been improved over the years even up to robot-assisted surgery [6–8]. Abdominal-based autologous breast reconstruction using the muscle-sparing transverse rectus abdominis myocutaneous (ms-TRAM), or the deep inferior epigastric perforator flap, is still the method of choice [9–15].

The perforator vessels are pivotal for a sufficient blood supply of the ms-TRAM/DIEP flap [16–18]. For raising such flaps, it is important to know the perforator's course through the rectus muscle, its characteristics, and any individual anatomy. The perforators originate with different patterns from the deep inferior epigastric artery (DIEA). For the DIEA itself several different branching patterns have also been described. Those aspects need to be collected by the surgeon before surgery so that a safe operation without an intraoperative time delay is possible [19].

Perforator mapping started in 1990 by using Doppler ultrasound [20] and later on by using MRI [21]. The CT angiography (CTA) has been introduced for evaluating these perforator and DIEA parameters prior to surgery in 2006 by Masia [22] and Alonso-Burgos [23] and was confirmed by others like Rozen in 2007 [24] and 2008 [19,25]. The CTA was shown to be superior regarding preoperative ms-TRAM/DIEP flap planning than Doppler ultrasound and MRI [16,19]. This led to better surviving rates of the flaps and a decreased operating time and therefore established CTA as the gold standard [22,23,25–29]. Therefore, preoperative decisions together with different kinds of intra- and postoperative monitoring are pivotal for optimizing postoperative outcome [30].

As an approach to gain a more detailed picture about the anatomic conditions, in this study, the data of 300 patients were collected and analysed especially regarding the number, calibre, course, and anastomosis to the superficial inferior epigastric vein (SIEV) of every single perforator and the branching pattern of the DIEAs. To the best of our knowledge, this is the largest and most detailed study including all perforators detected in the CTAs.

## 2. Materials and Methods

This is a retrospective study including all patients who underwent a single or bilateral autologous breast reconstruction using DIEP or ms-TRAM flaps between January 2010 and October 2019 at the Department of Plastic and Hand Surgery. CTA scans of the abdomen used for other flap planning were excluded. Since 2014, indocyanine green angiography was used for perfusion analysis of DIEP and ms-TRAM flaps. In total, 300 female patients (600 hemiabdominal walls) were evaluated. The patients' age ranged from 33 to 82 years (mean 63 ± 14 years). The mean body mass index (BMI) was 27.09 kg/m$^2$ (range 18.73–40.40 kg/m$^2$; SD 4.42). In 43 patients, a bilateral breast reconstruction was performed. Any incidentalomas were registered. All CTA scans were performed at the Radiology Department on a 128 slice multidetector CT (SOMATOM AS+, Siemens Healthcare GmbH, Forchheim, Germany) using a standardized protocol: collimation 64 × 2 × 0.6 mm by z-flying focal spot, rotation time 0.5 sec, spiral pitch factor 0.9, reference tube voltage 120 kV, reference tube current time product 200 mAs. A dose of 60 mL iodine-based contrast medium (Imeron 350, Bracco S.p.A., Milano, Italy) was injected in an antecubital vein in all patients with a flow rate of 5 mL/sec using a power injector (Accutron CT-D, Medtron AG, Saarbrücken, Germany). The CTA scans were reconstructed in thin slices (0.75 mm) with overlapping increments (0.5 mm) for 3D post processing purposes and in overlapping thick slice maximum intensity projections (10 mm/5 mm) in all three planes (transversal, sagittal, coronal) for clinical evaluation (Figure 1).

The relevant images were analysed from 4 cm above the umbilicus until the symphysis. The level of the umbilicus was always taken as a reference point to determine other parameters such as the perforator's exit out of the anterior rectus sheet as well as the branching of the DIEA. The localization of any branching or exit point was referred to the umbilicus as the y-axis and the midline for the x-axis. All assessed parameters regarding the DIEA branching, the perforator anatomy, and general parameters are summarized in Table 1.

Additionally, the connection to the SIEV was assessed for every perforator and classified as direct, indirect (drainage of superficial fat compartment), or no connection, respectively.

The mean operating time and any inflap anastomosis of the SIEV were noted. Furthermore, the number and DIEA row, i.e., medial vs. lateral row, of perforators included for flap transplantation were evaluated.

Statistical analysis:

The aims of the statistical analysis were: 1. a descriptive analysis of all collected variables and 2. to search for significant correlation between these variables.

The descriptive analysis used counts, percentages for categorical variables, and mean, median, and standard deviation for interval-scaled variables.

Correlation was evaluated by bivariate tests of all pairs of variables and subsequent post hoc tests with a correction for multiple testing. Software was GraphPad Prism 8 (GraphPad Software, San Diego, CA, USA) and R 3.6.1 (R Core Team (2019)).

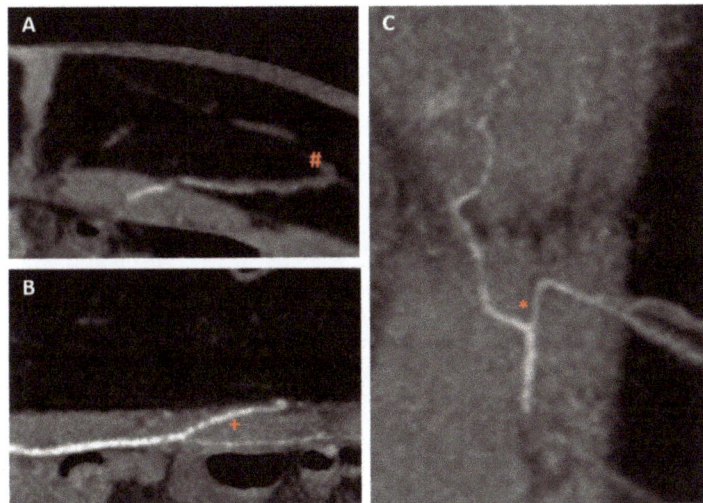

**Figure 1.** Perforator and DIEA mapping using computed tomographic angiography (CTA) in transversal (**A**), sagittal (**B**) and coronar (**C**) view (#: connection to SIEV, +: intramuscular course, *: branching of DIEA).

**Table 1.** Assessed parameters of CTAs.

| DIEA Branching | |
|---|---|
| Branching pattern | Type 0-IV according to Moon and Taylor classification (modified by Rozen et al.) |
| Branching pattern point | Localization on the x- and y-axis |
| **Perforator** | Sorted by diameter |
| Diameter | At the exit of the rectus sheath |
| Entrance of the perforator into the DIEA branch | Localization on the x- and y-axis |
| | Medial/lateral |
| Intramuscular course | Short (<1.5 cm), long (>1.5 cm), no intramuscular course (medially around the rectus muscle) |
| Exit of the rectus sheath | Localization on the x- and y-axis |
| SIEV | Direct connection, indirect connection, no connection to upper fat compartment |

Table 1. *Cont.*

| Subcutaneous fat | Thickness 3 cm to the right and left of the umbilicus |
|---|---|
| General information | - Operating time<br>- Incidentalomas<br>- Intraoperative SIEV anastomosis if necessary<br>- flap type<br>- Intraoperative used perforators<br>- BMI/height/weight |

## 3. Results

In total, 128 DIEP and 214 ms-TRAM flaps were performed, including 43 bilateral breast reconstructions. Out of those 214 ms-TRAM flaps, there were 2 ms0-, 164 ms1-, and 48 ms2-TRAM flaps. An amount of 600 hemiabdominal walls were analysed with 2260 perforators in total. The correlation of the thickness of the subcutaneous fat (mean 3.0 cm, SD 0.94 cm) and the flap choice indicated that ms-TRAM flaps were more often performed at higher BMIs.

In half of the cases (48.8%), there was a type II branching according to the Moon and Taylor Classification (modified by Rozen et al. [31]), followed by type I (37.8%), type III (12.7%), and IV (0.5%). Comparing the left to the right hemiabdomen there was a symmetry in most cases. Looking at the most common type II, the average branching point on the x-axis was 4.34 cm lateral and 5.73 cm on the y-axis caudal to the umbilicus. Only in ten cases was the branching cranial to the level of the umbilicus. Another significant observation was the correlation between branching type and the number of perforators: the higher the number of main DIEA branches, the more perforators were detected (correlation, $r = 0.2743; p < 0.0001$).

### 3.1. Diameter and Branching of Perforators

There were four perforators on each side of the abdomen on average (range 0–11; SD 2) with a diameter of 1.5 mm (SD 0.5 mm).

An amount of 58% of all perforators emerged off the medial branch of the DIEA and 42% were lateral branch perforators. The average entrance point of the rectus sheath was 3.5 cm lateral (SD 1.9 cm) and 0.94 cm caudal (SD 3.1 cm) of the umbilicus.

Statistical analysis showed that the diameter of medial row perforators (mean 1.58 mm; SD 0.52 mm) was significantly larger than the diameter of lateral row perforators (mean 1.44 mm; SD 0.43 mm) ($p < 0.001$) (Figure 2).

### 3.2. SIEV

There was a significant correlation between perforator diameter and SIEV connection. The larger the diameter of the perforator, the more likely a perforator had a connection to the SIEV or the superficial fat compartment (Figure 3).

Next to the diameter, the perforator exit of the rectus sheath on the x- and y-axis had a significant influence on SIEV connectivity ($p < 0.01$). A perforator with a close exit of the rectus sheath to the umbilicus on the x- and y-axis was more likely connected to the SIEV (Figure 4).

An amount of 46.9% of the perforators had a direct connection to the SIEV, 45.3% drained only the superficial fat compartment, whereas only 7.7% had no connection to the SIEV or superficial fat compartment at all. The medial row perforator more often showed a direct connection to the SIEV, whereas the lateral row perforator mainly drained the superficial compartment without direct connection to the SIEV ($p < 0.001$) (Figure 5).

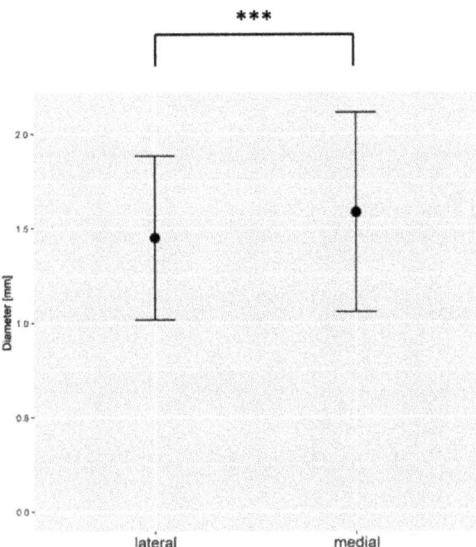

**Figure 2.** Medial row perforators have a statistically significantly larger diameter than lateral row perforators. *** = $p \leq 0.001$.

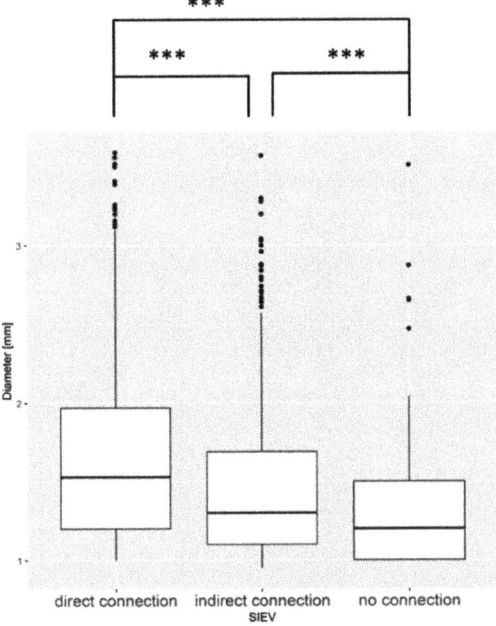

**Figure 3.** Boxplot of the diameter and different SIEV connections. SIEV = superficial inferior epigastric vein. The diameter of the perforator had a significant influence on the connection to the SIEV. The different connection types varied significantly among themselves. *** = $p \leq 0.001$.

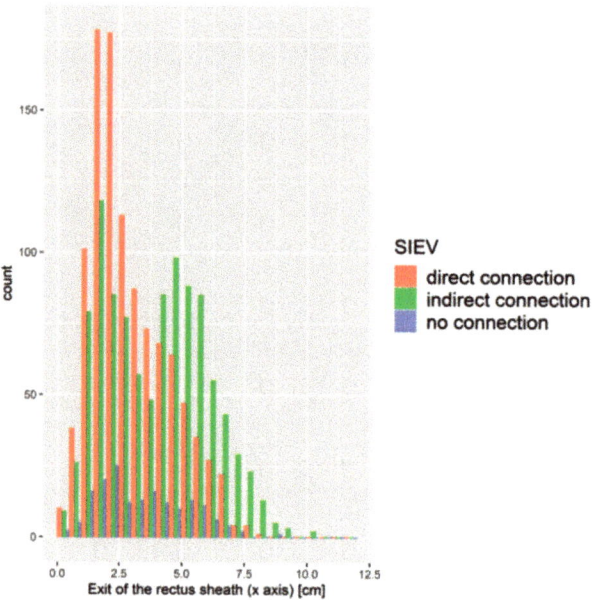

**Figure 4.** Absolute counts of different SIEV connection types regarding exit of the recuts sheath. Perforators close to the umbilicus were more likely connected to the SIEV.

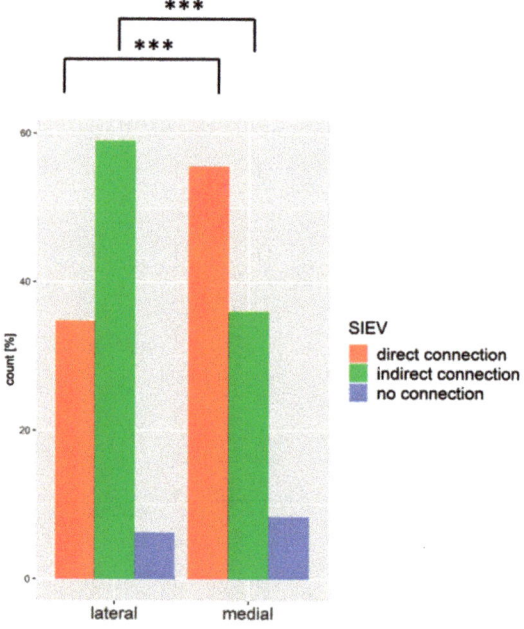

**Figure 5.** Medial row perforators were more often directly connected to the SIEV compared to lateral perforators. *** = $p \leq 0.001$.

## 3.3. Intramuscular Course

The intramuscular course of each perforator was categorized into "short" (<1.5 cm), "long" (>1.5 cm), and "no intramuscular course" (medially around the rectus muscle) regarding their cranial/caudal course through the rectus abdominis muscle. A total of 45.5% of all perforators showed a short course through the muscle, only 32.4% had a long course, and in only 100 perforators (4.5%) was a course medial around the muscle observed. In 17.7% of all perforators, there was no intramuscular course verifiable, thus making a classification not possible.

Comparing the medial and the lateral row perforators with regard to their intramuscular course, there was a significantly higher number of perforators with short course among the lateral row perforators as compared to medial row perforators (Figure 6).

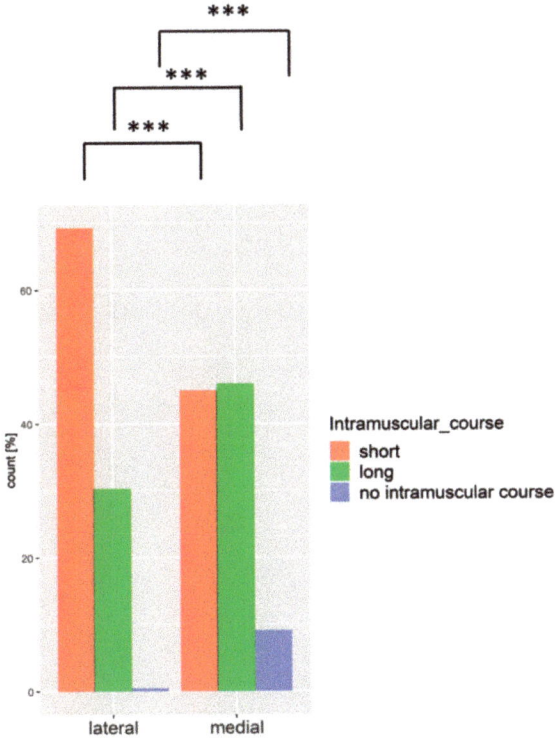

**Figure 6.** Medial row perforators had a more equally distributed intramuscular course, whereas lateral perforators more often had a short intramuscular course. *** = $p \leq 0.001$.

Also, the smaller the perforator in diameter, the less likely it had a long intramuscular course (one-way ANOVA, $p < 0.005$).

Furthermore, the course medially around the rectus muscle (also termed "septal", i.e., no intramuscular course at all) applied to 2/3 of the large perforators and to 1/3 of the small perforators.

## 3.4. Largest Perforator (No 1)

The largest perforator of every hemiabdomen was classified as the perforator no 1.

Comparing the perforator no 1 with a mean diameter of 2.0 mm (range 1–3.59 mm, SD 0.56 mm) with the remaining perforators (mean diameter of 1.4 mm, range 0.95–3.1 mm, SD 0.35 mm), it differed in all variables significantly. In 70%, the largest perforator originated from the medial branch of the DIEA, whereas the rest had a uniform distribution of the medial and lateral branch (Figure 7) and exited closer to the umbilicus. Furthermore, perforator no 1 was more often directly connected to the SIEV compared to the other perforators (Figure 8).

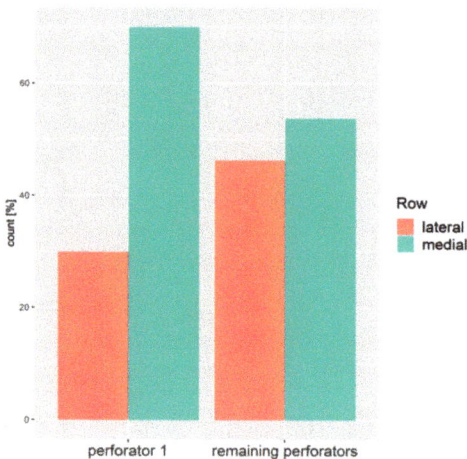

**Figure 7.** Distribution of the largest perforator versus the remaining perforators regarding the branch of the DIEA.

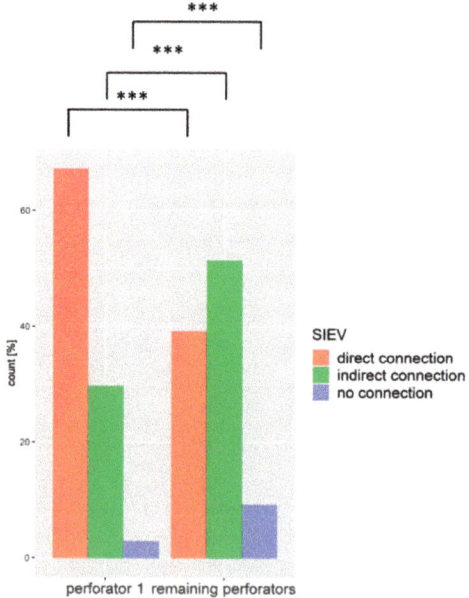

**Figure 8.** The largest perforator was significantly more often directly connected to the SIEV compared to the remaining perforators, whereas the remaining perforators were more often indirectly connected or without any connection. *** = $p \leq 0.001$.

## 4. Discussion

CTA has become the gold standard in preoperative diagnosis prior to autologous breast reconstruction using DIEP or ms-TRAM flaps [23] even though there is the disadvantage of radiation and higher costs compared to the Doppler ultrasound [32]. By knowing the course and characteristic of the perforators preoperatively, it allows the surgeon to reduce operating time and increase the safety of the operation. It also helps to decide whether a DIEP or ms-TRAM flap will be raised. In this retrospective study, we analysed every single perforator in 600 hemiabdominal walls to gain further insight into the perforators' characteristics and anatomy.

The main findings were that the largest perforator emerges in 2/3 of the medial row. Additionally, medial row perforators have a larger diameter than lateral row perforators. Furthermore, the closer the perforator leaves the rectus sheath to the umbilicus, the larger was the diameter. Additionally, medial row perforators are more likely connected to the SIEV than lateral row perforators. Regarding the perforator no 1, it differs significantly from the remaining perforators. The mean diameter of perforator no 1 was 2.0 mm compared to a diameter of 1.5 mm for perforator no 2, and 1.3 mm for perforator no 3. Schrögendorfer et al. noticed a mean diameter of 1.73 mm without splitting into different perforators [33]. In Masia et al., the dominant perforator's diameter ranged from 0.6 to 3.2 mm [34], which is similar to our range of 1–3.6 mm. Furthermore, perforator no 1 was almost twice as much as the remaining perforators connected to the SIEV, it was more equally distributed concerning short and long intramuscular course, it left the rectus sheath mainly medially, thus closer to the umbilicus on both axes. Therefore, we used a coordinate system that was already established in other studies [26,35,36]. Mohan et al. also detected that the larger dominant perforators arise mainly from the medial row around the umbilicus, calling it the "hot spot" [37]. Analysing the vascular territories using adult cadavers, Wong et al. even broke it down by comparing different flap types. The perfusion was found to be the largest in the full-width TRAM flap followed by the almost comparable medial row-perfused ms-TRAM and the medial row perforator DIEP flap [38].

Using the modified Moon and Taylor classification for grading the DIEA in a coronal view, we found a type II branching in 49%. The Moon and Taylor study showed 57% type II DIEAs, whereas Pellegrin only noticed a type II in 28% and mainly type I (65%) [39]. Masia et al. also included over 300 patients, but they analysed the perforators for only some patients in greater detail [34]. Regarding the branching pattern, they mainly detected a type II (right hemiabdomen: 58.8%, left hemiabdomen: 52.8%) and the rest showed a type I branching pattern. Rozen et al. showed a similar distribution to ours (I 29%, II 57%, III 14%). Masia's caudal point of the branching pattern was also closer to the umbilicus (5.05 cm) compared to our branching point, which was 5.73 cm caudal of the umbilicus. The Navarra conference led to the consensus that analysing the branching pattern in an anterior view is very helpful [32]. Almost every single branching point was caudal from the level of the umbilicus. We were able to show that the more branchings of the DIEA, the more perforators were detectable. Having four perforators on each side, the mean diameter for the largest perforator was 1.9 mm on the left and 2 mm on the right side [35]. Pellegrin et al. found fewer perforators [39] and differences between the left and the right side: three perforating branches on the right and two on the left side. This might be due to different inclusion criteria since in our study every single perforator that was found was analysed.

We also found that the closer the exit of the rectus sheath to the umbilicus on the x-axis, the larger the diameter of the largest perforator. Bailey et al. already confirmed this in a smaller study only analysing the largest perforator [26]. In several studies, it was also observed that those perforators that are located periumbilical show better perfusion of the elevated flaps [40,41]. While we decided to classify the cranial/caudal intramuscular course as "short" for distances under 1.5 cm, we found that mainly the lateral perforators more often had a short intramuscular course compared to a long intramuscular course. This was also detected by Rozen et al. in two studies but with fewer patients [25,29].

There is no standard yet for how to classify the intramuscular course and there are various options, whereas ours is only one of them. Navarra et al. analysed the intramuscular course in an axial MIP view [32]. This might lead to difficulties in comparing different studies. Comparing medial with lateral branch perforators, we found a distribution of 58% medial perforators versus 42% lateral perforators and significantly larger medial than lateral branch perforators. Similar results in Kukrek et al. confirm the occurrence of more medial perforators [42]. In their analysis, almost 50% of the perforators had a long intramuscular course, only 39% had a short intramuscular course, and 11% had a course medial around the rectus muscle, whereas in our study, the short course was predominate with 45%. This difference might depend on a different classification of the intramuscular course and fewer patients included in their study compared to ours.

The SIEV is an often undervalued topic in other studies, hence we analysed the connection of every perforator to the SIEV and found out that medial row perforators more often have a direct connection, whereas lateral row perforators often do not have a direct connection but drain the superficial fat compartment. Similarly, during the Navarra meeting, they found consensus that the venous system plays an immense role [32]. This was also mentioned by Zhang et al. without dealing in detail with the SIEV communicating with the perforators [43]. Between the right and left hemiabdomen, we did not find any statistically significant difference, thus it can be considered as symmetrically distributed. In this study, we have not evaluated the SIEA anatomy due to the focus on the DIEA anatomy and the arising perforators. We also did not correlate the CTA findings with intraoperative perforator choice and diameter and ICG flap viability due to the retrospective character of the study.

Bailey et al. compared the dominant medial row perforators on the right and left side and noticed symmetry as well [26]. Number and diameter were analysed in Rosson et al. and also identified as symmetric [28].

With a mean BMI of 27 kg/m$^2$, most of our patients were overweight. This matches the observations seen in other studies. Zang et al. had a smaller mean BMI of 23.6 kg/m$^2$ probably resulting from the fact that only Asian women were included [43]. Furthermore, the higher the BMI, the more likely a perforator emerges more lateral through the rectus sheath. A reason for this might also be a potential rectus diastase.

We acknowledge some limitations of our study. Due to the high number of perforators (>2000), pairwise statistical tests showed a significant result for almost everything irrespective of the strength of their connection. The enhanced artery and concomitant unenhanced veins run close together and are sometimes hard to distinguish making measurement of the perforator diameter difficult. Whereas this study dealt with the medical aspects concerning optimizing operative outcome, it is also important to consider the patient's perspective to gain the optimal result, for example, by using the BREAST-Q assessment [44–46]. Due to the retrospective character of the study, no correlation of the CTA findings with intraoperative findings was possible and therefore no outcome analysis like Breast-Q assessment was performed.

To the best of our knowledge, this is the largest anatomical study of CTAs prior autologous breast reconstruction.

## 5. Conclusions

The preoperative CTA provides multiple information regarding perforator anatomy, which were analysed in this study in great detail. We were able to show that the largest perforator emerges more often from the medial branch of the DIEA and more often has a direct connection to the SIEV. Large perforators were most likely found around the umbilicus and arising from the medial row. Additionally, medial row perforators showed more direct connections to the SIEV and larger diameters compared to lateral row perforators, making them ideal for DIEP flap transplantation.

**Author Contributions:** Conceptualization, A.A. and K.F.; methodology, A.A., M.S.M. and K.F.; statistical analysis, A.A., K.F. and A.S.; original draft preparation, K.F.; writing—review and editing, A.A., I.L., T.H., A.S., M.S.M., J.P.B., R.E.H. and K.F.; supervision, A.A. All authors have read and agreed to the published version of the manuscript.

**Funding:** We acknowledge financial support by Deutsche Forschungsgemeinschaft and Friedrich-Alexander-Universität Erlangen-Nürnberg within the funding programme "Open Access Publication Funding".

**Institutional Review Board Statement:** This study was approved by the ethical review committee of Friedrich-Alexander-Universität Erlangen-Nürnberg (registration number 29_20Bc).

**Informed Consent Statement:** Informed consent was obtained from all subjects involved in the study.

**Data Availability Statement:** Not applicable.

**Acknowledgments:** The present work was performed in (partial) fulfilment of the requirements for obtaining the degree of Katharina Frank.

**Conflicts of Interest:** The authors declare no conflict of interest.

## References

1. Bray, F.; Ferlay, J.; Soerjomataram, I.; Siegel, R.L.; Torre, L.A.; Jemal, A. Global cancer statistics 2018: GLOBOCAN estimates of incidence and mortality worldwide for 36 cancers in 185 countries. *CA Cancer J. Clin.* **2018**, *68*, 394–424. [CrossRef] [PubMed]
2. Robert Koch Institut. Krebs in Deutschland für 2015/2016. Available online: https://www.krebsdaten.de/Krebs/DE/Content/Publikationen/Krebs_in_Deutschland/kid_2019/krebs_in_deutschland_2019.pdf;jsessionid=ADE676158568FB2E31DD9F4EC7162474.2_cid372?__blob=publicationFile (accessed on 1 March 2020).
3. Francies, F.Z.; Hull, R.; Khanyile, R.; Dlamini, Z. Breast cancer in low-middle income countries: Abnormality in splicing and lack of targeted treatment options. *Am. J. Cancer Res.* **2020**, *10*, 1568–1591. [PubMed]
4. Chen, K.; Lu, P.; Beeraka, N.M.; Sukocheva, O.A.; Madhunapantula, S.V.; Liu, J.; Sinelnikov, M.Y.; Nikolenko, V.N.; Bulygin, K.V.; Mikhaleva, L.M.; et al. Mitochondrial mutations and mitoepigenetics: Focus on regulation of oxidative stress-induced responses in breast cancers. *Semin. Cancer Biol.* **2020**, in press. [CrossRef]
5. Alderman, A.K.; Wilkins, E.G.; Lowery, J.C.; Kim, M.; Davis, J.A. Determinants of patient satisfaction in postmastectomy breast reconstruction. *Plast. Reconstr. Surg.* **2000**, *106*, 769–776. [CrossRef]
6. Steiner, D.; Horch, R.E.; Ludolph, I.; Schmitz, M.; Beier, J.P.; Arkudas, A. Interdisciplinary Treatment of Breast Cancer After Mastectomy With Autologous Breast Reconstruction Using Abdominal Free Flaps in a University Teaching Hospital-A Standardized and Safe Procedure. *Front. Oncol.* **2020**, *10*, 177. [CrossRef]
7. Allen, R.J.; Treece, P. Deep inferior epigastric perforator flap for breast reconstruction. *Ann. Plast. Surg.* **1994**, *32*, 32–38. [CrossRef]
8. Chen, K.; Zhang, J.; Beeraka, N.M.; Sinelnikov, M.Y.; Zhang, X.; Cao, Y.; Lu, P. Robot-Assisted Minimally Invasive Breast Surgery: Recent Evidence with Comparative Clinical Outcomes. *J. Clin. Med.* **2022**, *11*, 1827. [CrossRef]
9. Ludolph, I.; Horch, R.E.; Harlander, M.; Arkudas, A.; Bach, A.D.; Kneser, U.; Schmitz, M.; Taeger, C.D.; Beier, J.P. Is there a Rationale for Autologous Breast Reconstruction in Older Patients? A Retrospective Single Center Analysis of Quality of life, Complications and Comorbidities after DIEP or ms-TRAM Flap Using the BREAST-Q. *Breast J.* **2015**, *21*, 588–595. [CrossRef]
10. Steiner, D.; Horch, R.E.; Ludolph, I.; Arkudas, A. Successful free flap salvage upon venous congestion in bilateral breast reconstruction using a venous cross-over bypass: A case report. *Microsurgery* **2020**, *40*, 74–78. [CrossRef]
11. Fritschen, U.V.; Grill, B.; Wagner, J.; Schuster, H.; Sukhova, I.; Giunta, R.E.; Heitmann, C.; Andree, C.; Horch, R.E.; Kneser, U.; et al. Quality assurance in breast reconstruction—Establishment of a prospective national online registry for microsurgical breast reconstructions. *Handchir. Mikrochir. Plast. Chir.* **2020**, *52*, 58–66. [CrossRef]
12. Cai, A.; Suckau, J.; Arkudas, A.; Beier, J.P.; Momeni, A.; Horch, R.E. Autologous Breast Reconstruction with Transverse Rectus Abdominis Musculocutaneous (TRAM) or Deep Inferior Epigastric Perforator (DIEP) Flaps: An Analysis of the 100 Most Cited Articles. *Med. Sci. Monit.* **2019**, *25*, 3520–3536. [CrossRef] [PubMed]
13. Hauck, T.; Horch, R.E.; Schmitz, M.; Arkudas, A. Secondary breast reconstruction after mastectomy using the DIEP flap. *Surg. Oncol.* **2018**, *27*, 513. [CrossRef] [PubMed]
14. Eisenhardt, S.U.; Momeni, A.; von Fritschen, U.; Horch, R.E.; Stark, G.B.; Bannasch, H.; Harder, Y.; Heitmann, C.; Kremer, T.; Rieger, U.M.; et al. Breast reconstruction with the free TRAM or DIEP flap—What is the current standard? Consensus Statement of the German Speaking Working Group for Microsurgery of the Peripheral Nerves and Vessels. *Handchir. Mikrochir. Plast. Chir.* **2018**, *50*, 248–255, Erratum in *Handchir. Mikrochir. Plast. Chir.* **2018**, *50*, E1. [CrossRef]
15. Blondeel, P.N. One hundred free DIEP flap breast reconstructions: A personal experience. *Br. J. Plast. Surg.* **1999**, *52*, 104–111. [CrossRef] [PubMed]
16. Casey, W.J., 3rd; Chew, R.T.; Rebecca, A.M.; Smith, A.A.; Collins, J.M.; Pockaj, B.A. Advantages of preoperative computed tomography in deep inferior epigastric artery perforator flap breast reconstruction. *Plast. Reconstr. Surg.* **2009**, *123*, 1148–1155. [CrossRef]

17. Salgarello, M.; Pagliara, D.; Rossi, M.; Visconti, G.; Barone-Adesi, L. Postoperative Monitoring of Free DIEP Flap in Breast Reconstruction with Near-Infrared Spectroscopy: Variables Affecting the Regional Oxygen Saturation. *J. Reconstr. Microsurg.* **2018**, *34*, 383–388. [CrossRef]
18. Chen, K.; Beeraka, N.M.; Sinelnikov, M.Y.; Zhang, J.; Song, D.; Gu, Y.; Li, J.; Reshetov, I.V.; Startseva, O.I.; Liu, J.; et al. Patient Management Strategies in Perioperative, Intraoperative, and Postoperative Period in Breast Reconstruction With DIEP-Flap: Clinical Recommendations. *Front. Surg.* **2022**, *9*, 729181. [CrossRef]
19. Rozen, W.M.; Ashton, M.W.; Stella, D.L.; Phillips, T.J.; Grinsell, D.; Taylor, G.I. The accuracy of computed tomographic angiography for mapping the perforators of the deep inferior epigastric artery: A blinded, prospective cohort study. *Plast. Reconstr. Surg.* **2008**, *122*, 1003–1009. [CrossRef]
20. Taylor, G.I.; Doyle, M.; McCarten, G. The Doppler probe for planning flaps: Anatomical study and clinical applications. *Br. J. Plast. Surg.* **1990**, *43*, 1–16. [CrossRef]
21. Ahn, C.Y.; Narayanan, K.; Shaw, W.W. In vivo anatomic study of cutaneous perforators in free flaps using magnetic resonance imaging. *J. Reconstr. Microsurg.* **1994**, *10*, 157–163. [CrossRef]
22. Masia, J.; Clavero, J.A.; Larranaga, J.R.; Alomar, X.; Pons, G.; Serret, P. Multidetector-row computed tomography in the planning of abdominal perforator flaps. *J. Plast. Reconstr. Aesthet. Surg.* **2006**, *59*, 594–599. [CrossRef] [PubMed]
23. Alonso-Burgos, A.; Garcia-Tutor, E.; Bastarrika, G.; Cano, D.; Martinez-Cuesta, A.; Pina, L.J. Preoperative planning of deep inferior epigastric artery perforator flap reconstruction with multislice-CT angiography: Imaging findings and initial experience. *J. Plast. Reconstr. Aesthet. Surg.* **2006**, *59*, 585–593. [CrossRef] [PubMed]
24. Rozen, W.M.; Stella, D.L.; Ashton, M.W.; Phillips, T.J.; Taylor, G.I. Three-dimensional CT angiography: A new technique for imaging microvascular anatomy. *Clin. Anat.* **2007**, *20*, 1001–1003. [CrossRef]
25. Rozen, W.M.; Phillips, T.J.; Ashton, M.W.; Stella, D.L.; Gibson, R.N.; Taylor, G.I. Preoperative imaging for DIEA perforator flaps: A comparative study of computed tomographic angiography and doppler ultrasound. *Plast. Reconstr. Surg.* **2008**, *121*, 1–8. [CrossRef] [PubMed]
26. Bailey, S.H.; Saint-Cyr, M.; Wong, C.; Mojallal, A.; Zhang, K.; Ouyang, D.; Arbique, G.; Trussler, A.; Rohrich, R.J. The single dominant medial row perforator DIEP flap in breast reconstruction: Three-dimensional perforasome and clinical results. *Plast. Reconstr. Surg.* **2010**, *126*, 739–751. [CrossRef] [PubMed]
27. Ghattaura, A.; Henton, J.; Jallali, N.; Rajapakse, Y.; Savidge, C.; Allen, S.; Searle, A.E.; Harris, P.A.; James, S.E. One hundred cases of abdominal-based free flaps in breast reconstruction. The impact of preoperative computed tomographic angiography. *J. Plast. Reconstr. Aesthet. Surg.* **2010**, *63*, 1597–1601. [CrossRef]
28. Rosson, G.D.; Williams, C.G.; Fishman, E.K.; Singh, N.K. 3D CT angiography of abdominal wall vascular perforators to plan DIEAP flaps. *Microsurgery* **2007**, *27*, 641–646. [CrossRef]
29. Rozen, W.M.; Ashton, M.W. Improving outcomes in autologous breast reconstruction. *Aesthetic Plast. Surg.* **2009**, *33*, 327–335. [CrossRef]
30. Salgarello, M.; Pagliara, D.; Visconti, G.; Barone-Adesi, L. Tissue Oximetry Monitoring for Free Deep Inferior Epigastric Perforator Flap Viability: Factors to be Considered toward Optimizing Postoperative Outcome. *J. Reconstr. Microsurg.* **2018**, *34*, e4. [CrossRef]
31. Rozen, W.M.; Ashton, M.W.; Grinsell, D. The branching pattern of the deep inferior epigastric artery revisited in-vivo: A new classification based on CT angiography. *Clin. Anat.* **2010**, *23*, 87–92. [CrossRef]
32. Rozen, W.M.; Garcia-Tutor, E.; Alonso-Burgos, A.; Acosta, R.; Stillaert, F.; Zubieta, J.L.; Hamdi, M.; Whitaker, I.S.; Ashton, M.W. Planning and optimising DIEP flaps with virtual surgery: The Navarra experience. *J. Plast. Reconstr. Aesthet. Surg.* **2010**, *63*, 289–297. [CrossRef] [PubMed]
33. Schrogendorfer, K.F.; Nickl, S.; Keck, M.; Lumenta, D.B.; Loewe, C.; Gschwandtner, M.; Haslik, W.; Nedomansky, J. Viability of five different pre- and intraoperative imaging methods for autologous breast reconstruction. *Eur. Surg.* **2016**, *48*, 326–333. [CrossRef] [PubMed]
34. Masia, J.; Kosutic, D.; Clavero, J.A.; Larranaga, J.; Vives, L.; Pons, G. Preoperative computed tomographic angiogram for deep inferior epigastric artery perforator flap breast reconstruction. *J. Reconstr. Microsurg.* **2010**, *26*, 21–28. [CrossRef]
35. Cina, A.; Barone-Adesi, L.; Rinaldi, P.; Cipriani, A.; Salgarello, M.; Masetti, R.; Bonomo, L. Planning deep inferior epigastric perforator flaps for breast reconstruction: A comparison between multidetector computed tomography and magnetic resonance angiography. *Eur. Radiol.* **2013**, *23*, 2333–2343. [CrossRef]
36. Karunanithy, N.; Rose, V.; Lim, A.K.; Mitchell, A. CT angiography of inferior epigastric and gluteal perforating arteries before free flap breast reconstruction. *Radiographics* **2011**, *31*, 1307–1319. [CrossRef] [PubMed]
37. Mohan, A.T.; Saint-Cyr, M. Anatomic and physiological fundamentals for autologous breast reconstruction. *Gland. Surg.* **2015**, *4*, 116–133. [CrossRef] [PubMed]
38. Wong, C.; Saint-Cyr, M.; Arbique, G.; Becker, S.; Brown, S.; Myers, S.; Rohrich, R.J. Three- and four-dimensional computed tomography angiographic studies of commonly used abdominal flaps in breast reconstruction. *Plast. Reconstr. Surg.* **2009**, *124*, 18–27. [CrossRef]
39. Pellegrin, A.; Stocca, T.; Belgrano, M.; Bertolotto, M.; Pozzi-Mucelli, F.; Marij Arnez, Z.; Cova, M.A. Preoperative vascular mapping with multislice CT of deep inferior epigastric artery perforators in planning breast reconstruction after mastectomy. *Radiol. Med.* **2013**, *118*, 732–743. [CrossRef]

40. Kelly, J.A.; Pacifico, M.D. Lateralising paraumbilical medial row perforators: Dangers and pitfalls in DIEP FLAP planning: A systematic review of 1116 DIEP flaps. *J. Plast. Reconstr. Aesthet. Surg.* **2014**, *67*, 383–388. [CrossRef]
41. Pennington, D.G.; Rome, P.; Kitchener, P. Predicting results of DIEP flap reconstruction: The flap viability index. *J. Plast. Reconstr. Aesthet. Surg.* **2012**, *65*, 1490–1495. [CrossRef]
42. Kuekrek, H.; Muller, D.; Paepke, S.; Dobritz, M.; Machens, H.G.; Giunta, R.E. [Preoperative CT angiography for planning free perforator flaps in breast reconstruction]. *Handchir. Mikrochir. Plast. Chir.* **2011**, *43*, 88–94. [CrossRef] [PubMed]
43. Zhang, X.; Mu, D.; Yang, Y.; Li, W.; Lin, Y.; Li, H.; Luan, J. Predicting the Feasibility of Utilizing SIEA Flap for Breast Reconstruction with Preoperative BMI and Computed Tomography Angiography (CTA) Data. *Aesthetic Plast. Surg.* **2020**, *45*, 100–107. [CrossRef] [PubMed]
44. Pusic, A.L.; Klassen, A.F.; Scott, A.M.; Klok, J.A.; Cordeiro, P.G.; Cano, S.J. Development of a new patient-reported outcome measure for breast surgery: The BREAST-Q. *Plast. Reconstr. Surg.* **2009**, *124*, 345–353. [CrossRef] [PubMed]
45. Cohen, W.A.; Mundy, L.R.; Ballard, T.N.; Klassen, A.; Cano, S.J.; Browne, J.; Pusic, A.L. The BREAST-Q in surgical research: A review of the literature 2009–2015. *J. Plast. Reconstr. Aesthet. Surg.* **2016**, *69*, 149–162. [CrossRef]
46. Pagliara, D.; Albanese, R.; Storti, G.; Barone-Adesi, L.; Salgarello, M. Patient-reported Outcomes in Immediate and Delayed Breast Reconstruction with Deep Inferior Epigastric Perforator Flap. *Plast. Reconstr. Surg. Glob. Open* **2018**, *6*, e1666. [CrossRef]

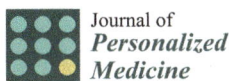

*Article*

# The Number of Surgical Interventions and Specialists Involved in the Management of Patients with Neurofibromatosis Type I: A 25-Year Analysis

Chih-Kai Hsu †, Rafael Denadai †, Chun-Shin Chang, Chuan-Fong Yao, Ying-An Chen, Pang-Yun Chou *, Lun-Jou Lo and Yu-Ray Chen

Department of Plastic and Reconstructive Surgery and Craniofacial Research Center, Chang Gung Memorial Hospital, Chang Gung University, Taoyuan 333, Taiwan; kkhsu0315@gmail.com (C.-K.H.); denadai.rafael@hotmail.com (R.D.); frankchang@cgmh.org.tw (C.-S.C.); chuanfongyao@gmail.com (C.-F.Y.); whysomimi@gmail.com (Y.-A.C.); lunjoulo@cgmh.org.tw (L.-J.L.); uraychen@cgmh.org.tw (Y.-R.C.)
* Correspondence: chou.asapulu@gmail.com
† These authors contributed equally in this study.

**Abstract:** *Objective:* In this study, we aim to present a single institution's 25-year experience of employing a comprehensive multidisciplinary team-based surgical approach for treating patients with NF-1. *Summary Background Data:* All patients ($n = 106$) with a confirmed diagnosis of NF-1 who were treated using a multidisciplinary surgical treatment algorithm at Chang Gung Memorial Hospital between 1994 and 2019 were retrospectively enrolled. Patients were categorized into groups according to the anatomy involved (craniofacial and noncraniofacial groups) and the type of clinical presentation (plexiform and cutaneous neurofibromas groups) for comparative analysis. *Methods:* The number of surgical interventions and number of specialists involved in surgical care were assessed. *Results:* Most of the patients exhibited craniofacial involvement (69.8%) and a plexiform type of NF-1 (58.5%), as confirmed through histology. A total of 332 surgical interventions ($3.1 \pm 3.1$ procedures per patient) were performed. The number of specialists involved in surgical care of the included patients was 11 ($1.6 \pm 0.8$ specialists per patient). Most of the patients (62.3%) underwent two or more surgical interventions, and 40.6% of the patients received treatment from two or more specialists. No significant differences were observed between the craniofacial and noncraniofacial groups in terms of the average number of surgical interventions ($3.3 \pm 3.2$ vs. $2.7 \pm 2.7$, respectively) and number of specialists involved ($1.7 \pm 0.9$ vs. $1.4 \pm 0.6$). Patients with plexiform craniofacial involvement underwent a significantly higher average number of surgical interventions ($4.3 \pm 3.6$ vs. $1.6 \pm 1.1$; $p < 0.001$) and received treatment by more specialists ($1.9 \pm 0.9$ vs. $1.2 \pm 0.5$; $p < 0.001$) compared with those having cutaneous craniofacial involvement. *Conclusions:* In light of the potential benefits of employing the multidisciplinary team-based surgical approach demonstrated in this study, such an approach should be adopted to provide comprehensive individualized care to patients with NF-1.

**Keywords:** neurofibromatosis; craniofacial; surgical treatment; multidisciplinary team; plexiform neurofibroma

**Citation:** Hsu, C.-K.; Denadai, R.; Chang, C.-S.; Yao, C.-F.; Chen, Y.-A.; Chou, P.-Y.; Lo, L.-J.; Chen, Y.-R. The Number of Surgical Interventions and Specialists Involved in the Management of Patients with Neurofibromatosis Type I: A 25-Year Analysis. *J. Pers. Med.* **2022**, *12*, 558. https://doi.org/10.3390/jpm12040558

**Academic Editors:** Andreas Arkudas and Raymund E. Horch

Received: 6 February 2022
Accepted: 24 March 2022
Published: 1 April 2022

**Publisher's Note:** MDPI stays neutral with regard to jurisdictional claims in published maps and institutional affiliations.

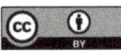

**Copyright:** © 2022 by the authors. Licensee MDPI, Basel, Switzerland. This article is an open access article distributed under the terms and conditions of the Creative Commons Attribution (CC BY) license (https:// creativecommons.org/licenses/by/ 4.0/).

## 1. Background

Neurofibromatosis type 1 (NF-1), also known as von Recklinghausen disease, is a hereditary condition with a worldwide incidence of 1 per 2500 to 3000 that predisposes an affected individual to tumor development and affects the central and peripheral nervous systems [1]. It is caused by pathogenic variants in the *NF1* gene and is characterized by *café au lait* macules, skin-fold freckling, Lisch nodules, optic glioma, and distinctive osseous lesions (such as sphenoid dysplasia or thinning of the long bone cortex) [1–6]. Patients with NF-1 are prone to numerous peripheral nerve sheath tumors [3–6]. Cutaneous and plexiform neurofibromas can grow to a large size, which considerably affects quality of life and has psychosocial implications because of itchiness, function impairment, physical disfigurement, and pain [7,8].

The wide range of clinical manifestations in neurofibromas, with varying anatomical location, number, size, progression, recurrence, local invasion, and compression of vital structures, necessitates multidisciplinary treatment and follow-up [8]. Although clinical trials have investigated the efficacy of various drugs (e.g., sirolimus, imatinib, tipifarnib, and pirfenidone) to treat particular features of NF1, surgical resection remains the standard procedure for the management of cutaneous and plexiform neurofibromas [9–12]. However, no single surgical algorithm is available to help clinicians in addressing the complexity and full spectrum of NF-1 abnormalities.

Because of the complexity due to the many regions and systems that may be affected, we applied an evolving multidisciplinary model of care that involves a range of health care professionals working in coordination at our center to provide comprehensive surgical treatment to complex and challenging conditions in patients presenting with NF-1. This long-term single-center study reports 25 years of evolving experience in implementing a multidisciplinary team-based surgical treatment approach for NF-1 management.

## 2. Methods

### 2.1. Patient Selection

This observational retrospective study included all patients with NF-1 who were surgically treated at a single institution (Linkou/Taoyuan Chang Gung Memorial Hospital) between 1994 and 2019. Patients with a confirmed diagnosis of NF-1, according to the cardinal criteria of consensus from the National Institutes of Health, who underwent surgical treatment performed by our multidisciplinary team were included. The exclusion criteria were patients with incomplete registration of treatment course, patients who received surgical treatment at another institution during the follow-up period, and replicated cases in the database. A total of 169 patients matches our inclusion criteria, and 53 patients were excluded. The remaining 106 cases, aged from 2 to 74, were enrolled for subsequent analysis.

### 2.2. Data Collection and Stratification

Demographic (age and sex), clinical (types of clinical presentation, disease involvement, and malignant transformation), and surgical (numbers and types of specialties and procedures) data were verified through review of electronic medical records and clinical photographs. On the basis of the type of clinical presentation, patients were categorized into either the plexiform neurofibroma or the cutaneous neurofibroma group. According to the anatomical region involved in the disease, patients were categorized into either the craniofacial (skull, face, orbit, brain, and cranial nerve) or the noncraniofacial (neck, chest wall, mediastinum, trunk, and extremities) group.

This study was approved by the Institutional Review Board of Chang Gung Medical Foundation (approval 202000258B0) and conducted in compliance with the 1975 Declaration of Helsinki, as amended in 1983. Singed consent forms for further academic use and publications were obtained from patients prior to every clinical photograph, including all of the cases presented in this article.

## 3. Statistical Analysis

Descriptive analysis was performed, and the data are presented as mean ± standard deviation for metric variables and percentages for categorical variables. Data distribution was verified using the Kolmogorov–Smirnov test. Independent $t$ tests were employed for comparative analysis (craniofacial versus noncraniofacial groups and plexiform versus cutaneous groups). Two-sided $p$ values of <0.05 were considered statistically significant. All analyses were performed using IBM SPSS software v22.0 (IBM Corp., Armonk, NY, USA).

## 4. Results

A total of 106 patients (57 men; mean age at initial evaluation of 24.44 ± 14.18 years; mean follow-up period of 9.71 ± 6.24 years) with NF-1 were enrolled in this study. Most of the patients had craniofacial involvement ($n$ = 74, 69.8%; Table 1) and histologically confirmed plexiform NF-1 ($n$ = 62, 58.5%). Most of the patients ($n$ = 47, 63.5%) with craniofacial involvement had a plexiform type of presentation.

Table 1. Distribution of patients ($n$ = 106) with neurofibromatosis type I according to anatomical region.

| Anatomical Region | Patients | Percentage |
|---|---|---|
| Skull | 18 | 17.0% |
| Face | 66 | 62.3% |
| Orbit | 28 | 26.4% |
| Brain | 11 | 10.4% |
| Cranial nerve | 1 | 0.9% |
| Neck | 25 | 23.6% |
| Trunk | 55 | 51.9% |
| Chest wall | 2 | 1.9% |
| Mediastinum | 4 | 3.8% |
| Lung | 2 | 1.9% |
| Extremities | 42 | 39.6% |
| Spine | 19 | 17.9% |
| Visceral | 1 | 0.9% |

A total of 332 surgical interventions (3.13 ± 3.05 (range, 1 to 19) procedures per patient) were performed. The number of specialties involved in surgical care of the included patients was 11 (1.57 ± 0.79 specialties (range, 1 to 4) per patient; Table 2). Most of the patients (62.3%) underwent two or more surgical interventions, and 40.6% of the patients received treatment by two or more specialists.

Table 2. Specialties involved in surgical care of patients ($n$ = 106) with neurofibromatosis type I.

| Specialty | Surgical Intervention (Number) | Patients (Number) | Patients (Percentage) |
|---|---|---|---|
| Plastic surgery | 160 | 60 | 56.6% |
| Ophthalmology | 48 | 25 | 23.6% |
| Neurosurgery | 31 | 22 | 20.8% |
| Orthopedics | 26 | 15 | 14.2% |
| Dermatology | 25 | 19 | 17.9% |
| Radiology | 22 | 13 | 12.3% |
| General surgery | 13 | 6 | 5.7% |
| Chest surgery | 2 | 2 | 1.9% |
| Otorhinolaryngology | 2 | 2 | 1.9% |
| Colorectal surgery | 1 | 1 | 0.9% |
| Pediatric surgery | 1 | 1 | 0.9% |

No significant differences were observed between the craniofacial and noncraniofacial groups in terms of the average number of surgical interventions (3.31 ± 3.21 vs. 2.72 ± 2.67, respectively; $p$ = 0.362) or the number of specialists involved in surgical care (1.65 ± 0.85 vs. 1.38 ± 0.61; $p$ = 0.065). Patients with plexiform craniofacial involvement had undergone a significantly higher average number of surgical interventions (4.28 ± 3.62 vs. 1.63 ± 1.08; $p$ < 0.001) and had been treated by more specialists (1.91 ± 0.91 vs. 1.19 ± 0.48; $p$ < 0.001) than those having cutaneous craniofacial involvement.

In our analysis, plastic surgeons and ophthalmologists were found to be the most common combination of specialists, being adopted to treat 10 patients. Other specialist teams comprised plastic surgeons, ophthalmologists, and neurosurgeons (employed to treat four patients); plastic surgeons and radiologists (employed to treat four patients);

plastic surgeons, ophthalmologists, neurosurgeons, and radiologists (employed to treat three patients); plastic surgeons and neurosurgeons (employed to treat three patients); and plastic surgeons, ophthalmologists, and radiologists (employed to treat three patients).

## 5. Multidisciplinary Approach

We have been using a comprehensive multidisciplinary team-based surgical approach in our center for managing patients with NF-1 for 25 years, with the approach evolving over time. Because of the progressive nature of NF-1 and the risk of it affecting multiple anatomical regions, the first professional who evaluates the patient has been responsible for general screening and referral to other specialists. Further referrals are made as needed according to further clinical findings made during the disease course. Additional professionals have been continually introduced when new clinical presentations are encountered by our team, and we have been updating the protocol on account of repeated observations of the same clinical presentation. At present, 11 specialties are engaged in providing a therapeutic algorithm at our center (Figure 1).

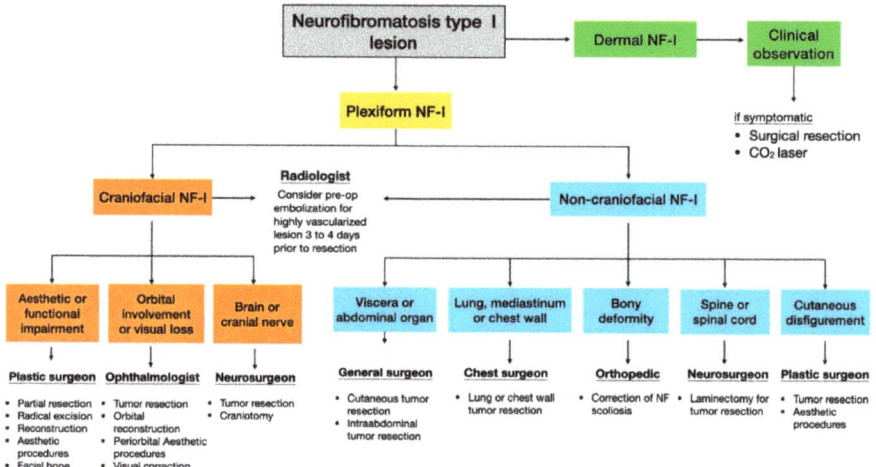

**Figure 1.** Multidisciplinary team-based treatment algorithm for neurofibromatosis type I (NF-1).

The psychological burden of a chronic and destructive disease associated with visible and stigmatizing skin lesions, which cause functional and aesthetic deficits in patients, is the main criteria for surgery. For cutaneous neurofibromas, which are characterized by superficial or dermal lesions, regular clinical follow-ups for the observation of each lesion is often sufficient [13]; surgical excision (scalpel- or laser-based removal) is indicated for symptomatic lesions (i.e., those exhibiting pain, bleeding, functional impairment, or disfigurement) or upon patient request [1,14,15]. For plexiform neurofibromas, which are characterized by deep lesions, the size, location, and symptomatic presentation serve as the influential factors to define the line of treatment. Targeted therapy can reduce tumor volume [16]; however, surgical excision remains the main therapeutic intervention for plexiform neurofibromas [8,15]. Imaging analysis (computed tomography, computed tomography angiography, and magnetic resonance imaging) can be used to help define the total size and depth of lesions as well as to reveal the involvement of adjacent structures; according to the imaging results, the appropriate specialist team can be assembled for surgical intervention [17].

## 6. Preoperative Embolization

Before surgical excision of plexiform neurofibromas, the necessity for preoperative embolization should be considered. A total of three patients with craniofacial NF-1 and histologically confirmed plexiform neurofibromas received preoperative embolization by a radiology team before radical resection of neurofibromas to prevent massive intraoperative blood loss. Most of the embolization procedures were performed 3 or 4 days prior to surgery. All of the embolized vessels were branches of the external and internal carotid arteries, which included the maxillary artery (100%), facial artery (75%), superficial temporal artery (37.5%), and superior thyroid artery (37.5%; Figure 2).

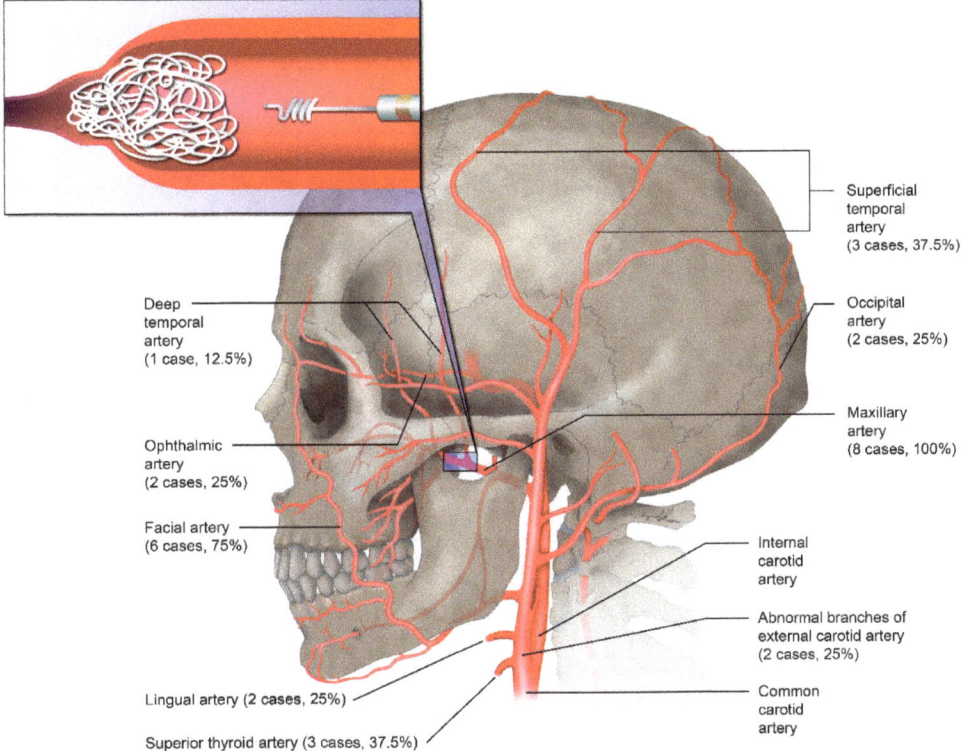

**Figure 2.** Target vessels of preoperative transarterial embolization ($n = 8$).

The possible role of embolization should be evaluated whenever radical excision with massive bleeding is anticipated and should be re-evaluated before secondary surgical interventions in each patient. Despite successful preoperative embolization, massive blood loss occurred during surgical intervention in our experience, which highlights the need for pre-emptive anesthesia (regional blocks plus hypotensive anesthesia) and proper surgical execution with careful soft tissue manipulation, systematic ligation of vessels, and blood transfusions as needed.

## 7. Malignant Transformation

In total, 19 (17.9%) patients were diagnosed as having neurofibromatosis-related malignancy, which included malignant peripheral nerve sheath tumors ($n = 17$), gastrointestinal stromal tumor (GIST; $n = 2$), and cerebellar astrocytoma ($n = 1$); one patient exhibited both malignant peripheral nerve sheath tumor and GIST. Malignant peripheral nerve sheath tumor was evident in various anatomical regions, namely the spine ($n = 6$), lung ($n = 4$), trunk (*n* = 4), liver (*n* = 2), peritoneum (*n* = 2), extremities (*n* = 2), scalp/face (*n* = 2), kidney (*n* = 1), brain (*n* = 1), and jejunum (*n* = 1). Despite the postoperative adjuvant radiotherapy performed on the patients to reduce the risk of local recurrence and as a salvage strategy after tumor resection, a high recurrence rate and disease progression were observed.

## 8. Complicated Cases

Seven patients with severe plexiform craniofacial neurofibroma-related functional and aesthetic impairment underwent surgical excisions that required microsurgical free flaps for reconstruction (Figures 3–5). Multi-stage and extensive revision procedures were necessarily required [18–21].

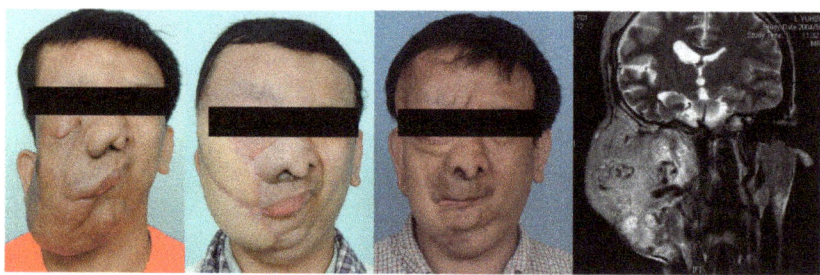

**Figure 3.** Clinical images of a 30-year-old man with hemifacial plexiform neurofibromatosis exhibiting no ipsilateral facial nerve function and vision. The patient was followed up by the multidisciplinary team for 12 years. Magnetic resonance imaging shows the extent of the plexiform tumor before surgical excision. Two sections of embolization of branches of the right external carotid artery, internal maxillary artery, and superficial temporal artery were completed before radical surgical excision. The distal right external carotid artery was ligated, and the tumor was extensively excised through scalp, preauricular, and submandibular incisions. Microsurgical free flaps (anterior lateral thigh flap and myocutaneous gracilis free flap) were transferred to reconstruct the facial defect. Additional procedures included orbitotomy, tumor resection (nasal and upper lip regions), labial suspension, canthopexies, eyelid reconstruction, and ocular prosthesis placement.

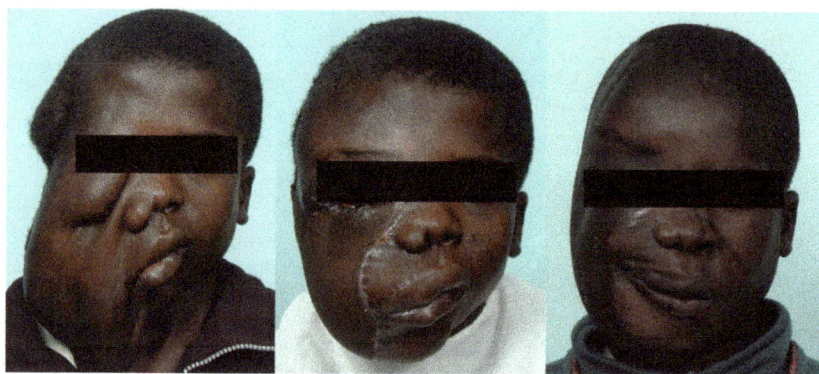

**Figure 4.** Clinical images of a 15-year-old adolescent boy from Africa who presented with diffuse plexiform craniofacial neurofibromatosis with no ipsilateral facial nerve function and no vision. After preoperative embolization (right superficial temporal, internal maxillary, and facial arteries) and intraoperative ligation of the right external carotid artery, a radical excision of the tumor with orbital repositioning was performed. Microsurgical free flaps (anterior lateral thigh flap and myocutaneous gracilis free flap) were transferred to reconstruct the facial defect. Additional procedures included orbitotomy, skull base tumor removal, and right fronto-orbital craniotomy, with orbital and craniofacial reconstruction and ocular prosthesis placement.

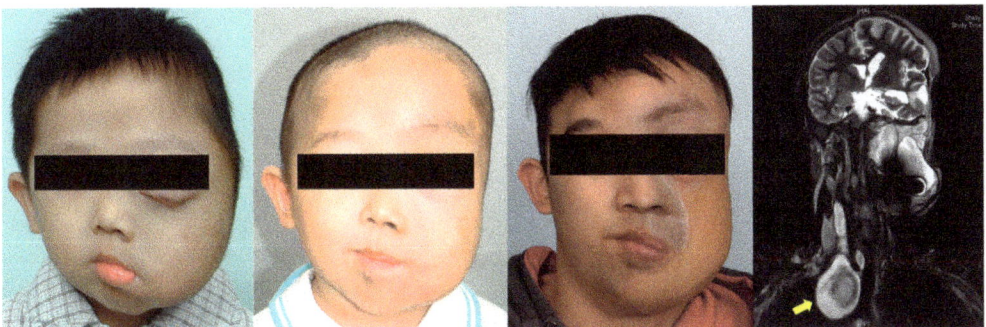

**Figure 5.** Clinical images of an 11-year-old boy with craniofacial plexiform neurofibromatosis who has been followed up with since the age of 2 and has been receiving orbital and zygomatic repositioning and reconstruction of the orbital roof and temporal bone. Owing to the disease progression, a radical excision was performed after preoperative embolization (branches of the left internal maxillary, lingual, and facial arteries) and total interruption of the left external carotid artery. The soft tissue defect was reconstructed with an anterior lateral thigh flap. Magnetic resonance imaging showed involvement of the left intraorbital, parasellar, parapharyngeal, and posterior pharyngeal regions and adjacent disorganized brain tissues and dural ectasia; craniotomy was performed for skull base and orbital tumor removal. Additional procedures included serial tumor excisions, lip repair, and canthoplasty. Magnetic resonance imaging indicated a mediastinal mass (yellow arrow) with neck swelling, and shortness of breath had developed in recent years. An additional neurofibroma compressing the cervical spine (C2 and C3 level) was also identified.

## 9. Discussion

The cohort in our study exemplified the wide spectrum of NF-1 presentation, with various anatomical sites affected by tumors, causing functional and aesthetic impairments in the patients [7,22]. Because NF-1 can be expressed clinically in various manners, differing even between members of the same family carrying the same NF1 mutation, treatment may range from clinical observation and isolated removal of cutaneous tumors to drug-centered therapy for neurological and endocrinological abnormalities and chemotherapy or targeted therapy for conditions such as optic gliomas, malignant peripheral nerve sheath tumors, and GIST [8,9,23–29]. This long-term study focused on the surgical treatment of patients with NF-1 by using a multidisciplinary team-based approach.

Overall, the number of affected anatomic regions and systems and the number of specialists involved in care were high in our study. We stratified the patients into craniofacial and noncraniofacial groups because it assisted us in surgical decision-making (Figure 1). Moreover, we tested the hypothesis that craniofacial involvement requires an intensive therapeutic approach to restore both functionality and aesthetics of craniofacial structures in the patients. Neurofibroma-related facial disfigurement strongly influences aesthetic appearance and interpersonal relationships, much more so than neurofibromas affecting the trunk or extremity regions [30–34]. Moreover, tumor lesions affecting the cranial nerves or orbital and brain regions can have a major effect on functional activities [5,23,24]. However, we observed no significant differences in the number of surgical interventions and specialists involved in care of patients with and without craniofacial involvement.

Patients with craniofacial plexiform neurofibromas underwent a higher number of surgical interventions and required more specialist treatment during the disease course than did those having craniofacial cutaneous neurofibromas. Plexiform neurofibromas occur less frequently than cutaneous neurofibromas, but plexiform lesions are considered the main source of morbidity in craniofacial NF-1 because these tumors can spread in size, eventually leading to soft tissue hypertrophy, and functional and aesthetic impairments. Therefore, patients with craniofacial plexiform neurofibromas require condition-specific planning for surgical treatment. This particular subset of patients with NF-1 experiences limited improvement after surgical excision of plexiform neurofibromas along with a high risk of perioperative complications and a high recurrence rate, which is frustrating for both the patients and clinicians [25,26].

The most common surgical approach for treating plexiform craniofacial neurofibroma that affects both patients functionality and aesthetics is en bloc translesional excision performed according to the facial aesthetic unit principle and without sacrificing the functional nerves [18]. In our analysis, plastic surgeons, ophthalmologists, neurosurgeons, and radiologists actively participated in the therapeutic management of these patients. Plastic surgeons were responsible for tumor resection and reconstruction. For patients with infiltrating tumors of the orbitotemporal region that cause ptosis, optic nerve compression, or blindness or even involve the brain or skull base, ophthalmologists and neurosurgeons provided the proper management [20,35–37]. Proper preoperative diagnosis and planning under the multidisciplinary team-based surgical approach permitted us to successfully maximize the risk-to-benefit ratio for treating these patients with plexiform craniofacial neurofibromatosis and to aim for maximal improvement in the functional and aesthetic outcomes with minimal complications and disruptions in the adjacent functional structures.

Microvascular free tissue transfer following radical resection of large neurofibromas was proven to be a safe and reliable method for the coverage of extensive soft tissue defects [38]. In our experience, despite the successful coverage of large, raw craniofacial wounds, functional reconstruction was not effective. Revision procedures were also required. Alternative forms of soft tissue coverage, including simple skin grafts, could also be considered [18]. In this setting, patients and parents should be advised of the limitations of surgical resection and reconstruction as well as the risk of relapse and malignant transformation [7,8,23]. Moreover, a shared decision-making process between patients, parents, and the members of the multidisciplinary team may assist in defining patients' expectations and in improving outcomes with treatment and follow-up.

According to a report, 8 to 12% of patients with NF-1 may develop malignant peripheral nerve sheath tumors during their lifetimes [3]. We documented a high incidence rate (16%) of malignant peripheral nerve sheath tumors in our study cohort and detected other malignancies (cerebellar astrocytoma and GIST) during the 25-year period. Because malignant peripheral nerve sheath tumors usually originate from a preexisting plexiform neurofibroma, patients with NF-1, particularly those with plexiform type, should receive regular follow-up to ensure early intervention if necessary.

The limitations of this study include an inherent bias associated with the retrospective design. We provided our current protocol that is the product of 25 years of development, but it should not be considered a unique or static protocol. Other centers engaged in the management of patients with NF-1 should publish their specific protocols and apply, refine, and adjust our protocol to their own environment of care. Future studies should assess further outcome metrics including patient-reported outcomes and total cost effectiveness of adopting a multidisciplinary team-based surgical approach in the management of patients with NF-1. The published protocols and results may provide a basis for enhancing the management of patients with NF-1.

## 10. Conclusions

In this long-term study, we assessed 25 years of surgical experience at a single institution in management of patients with NF-1. Our long-term experience suggests that the multidisciplinary team-based surgical approach should be adopted to provide comprehensive individualized care to patients with NF-1 and warrants its substantial role in treating the patients with complicated plexiform neurofibromas.

**Author Contributions:** C.-K.H. and R.D. were responsible for data collection, data interpretation, manuscript writing, and approval of final version. C.-S.C., C.-F.Y., Y.-A.C., P.-Y.C., L.-J.L. and Y.-R.C. were responsible for study conception and design, manuscript critical revisions, and approval of final version. All authors have read and agreed to the published version of the manuscript.

**Funding:** Part of this study was supported by grants from the Craniofacial Research Center, Taoyuan Chang Gung Memorial Hospital (CMRPG3L0361, CMRPG3J0823, CMRPG3K0391, and NRRPG3K0031).

**Institutional Review Board Statement:** The study (202000258B0) was approved by the Ethics Committee for Human Research, Taoyuan Chang Gung Memorial Hospital, Taiwan.

**Informed Consent Statement:** Informed consent was obtained from all subjects involved in the study.

**Acknowledgments:** This manuscript was edited by Wallace Academic Editing. The authors wish to thank Ingrid Kuo and the Center for Big Data Analytics and Statistics (Grant CLRPG3D0046) at Chang Gung Memorial Hospital for creating the illustrations used herein.

**Conflicts of Interest:** The authors declare that the article content was composed in the absence of any commercial or financial relationships.

## References

1. Williams, V.C.; Lucas, J.; Babcock, M.A.; Gutmann, D.H.; Korf, B.; Maria, B.L. Neurofibromatosis Type 1 Revisited. *Pediatrics* **2009**, *123*, 124–133. [CrossRef] [PubMed]
2. Awad, E.K.; Moore, M.; Liu, H.; Ciszewski, L.; Lambert, L.; Korf, B.R.; Popplewell, L.; Kesterson, R.A.; Wallis, D. Restoration of Normal NF1 Function with Antisense Morpholino Treatment of Recurrent Pathogenic Patient-Specific Variant c.1466A>G; p.Y489C. *J. Pers. Med.* **2021**, *11*, 1320. [CrossRef] [PubMed]
3. Boyd, K.P.; Korf, B.R.; Theos, A. Neurofibromatosis type 1. *J. Am. Acad. Dermatol.* **2009**, *61*, 1–14. [CrossRef] [PubMed]
4. Jensen, S.E.; Patel, Z.S.; Listernick, R.; Charrow, J.; Lai, J.-S. Lifespan Development: Symptoms Experienced by Individuals with Neurofibromatosis Type 1 Associated Plexiform Neurofibromas from Childhood into Adulthood. *J. Clin. Psychol. Med. Settings* **2018**, *26*, 259–270. [CrossRef] [PubMed]
5. Ortonne, N.; Wolkenstein, P.; Blakeley, J.O.; Korf, B.; Plotkin, S.R.; Riccardi, V.M.; Miller, D.C.; Huson, S.; Peltonen, J.; Rosenberg, A.; et al. Cutaneous neurofibromas: Current clinical and pathologic issues. *Neurology* **2018**, *91* (Suppl. S1), S5–S13. [CrossRef] [PubMed]
6. Stevenson, D.A.; Little, D.; Armstrong, L.; Crawford, A.H.; Eastwood, D.; Friedman, J.; Greggi, T.; Gutierrez, G.; Hunter-Schaedle, K.; Kendler, D.; et al. Approaches to treating NF1 tibial pseudarthrosis: Consensus from the Children's Tumor Foundation NF1 Bone Abnormalities Consortium. *J. Pediatr. Orthop.* **2013**, *33*, 269–275. [CrossRef] [PubMed]
7. Denadai, R.; Buzzo, C.L.; Takata, J.P.I.; Raposo-Amaral, C.A.; Raposo-Amaral, C.E. Comprehensive and Global Approach of Soft-Tissue Deformities in Craniofacial Neurofibromatosis Type 1. *Ann. Plast. Surg.* **2016**, *77*, 190–194. [CrossRef] [PubMed]
8. Hirbe, A.C.; Gutmann, D.H. Neurofibromatosis type 1: A multidisciplinary approach to care. *Lancet Neurol.* **2014**, *13*, 834–843. [CrossRef]
9. Falzon, K.; Drimtzias, E.; Picton, S.; Simmons, I. Visual outcomes after chemotherapy for optic pathway glioma in children with and without neurofibromatosis type 1: Results of the International Society of Paediatric Oncology (SIOP) Low-Grade Glioma 2004 trial UK cohort. *Br. J. Ophthalmol.* **2018**, *102*, 1367–1371. [CrossRef]
10. Gutmann, D.H.; Blakeley, J.O.; Korf, B.R.; Packer, R.J. Optimizing biologically targeted clinical trials for neurofibromatosis. *Expert Opin. Investig. Drugs* **2013**, *22*, 443–462. [CrossRef]
11. Kim, A.; Lu, Y.; Okuno, S.H.; Reinke, D.; Maertens, O.; Perentesis, J.; Basu, M.; Wolters, P.L.; De Raedt, T.; Chawla, S.; et al. Targeting Refractory Sarcomas and Malignant Peripheral Nerve Sheath Tumors in a Phase I/II Study of Sirolimus in Combination with Ganetespib (SARC023). *Sarcoma* **2020**, *2020*, 5784876. [CrossRef] [PubMed]
12. Stewart, D.R.; Korf, B.R.; Nathanson, K.L.; Stevenson, D.A.; Yohay, K. Care of adults with neurofibromatosis type 1: A clinical practice resource of the American College of Medical Genetics and Genomics (ACMG). *Genet. Med.* **2018**, *20*, 671–682. [CrossRef] [PubMed]
13. Méni, C.; Sbidian, E.; Moreno, J.C.; Lafaye, S.; Buffard, V.; Goldzal, S.; Wolkenstein, P.; Valeyrie-Allanore, L. Treatment of neurofibromas with a carbon dioxide laser: A retrospective cross-sectional study of 106 patients. *Dermatology* **2015**, *230*, 263–268. [CrossRef] [PubMed]
14. Verma, S.K.; Riccardi, V.M.; Plotkin, S.R.; Weinberg, H.; Anderson, R.R.; Blakeley, J.O.; Jarnagin, K.; Lee, J. Considerations for development of therapies for cutaneous neurofibroma. *Neurology* **2018**, *91* (Suppl. S1), S21–S30. [CrossRef]
15. Ly, K.I.; Blakeley, J.O. The Diagnosis and Management of Neurofibromatosis Type 1. *Med. Clin. N. Am.* **2019**, *103*, 1035–1054. [CrossRef]
16. Dombi, E.; Baldwin, A.; Marcus, L.J.; Fisher, M.J.; Weiss, B.; Kim, A.; Whitcomb, P.; Martin, S.; Aschbacher-Smith, L.E.; Rizvi, T.A.; et al. Activity of Selumetinib in Neurofibromatosis Type 1-Related Plexiform Neurofibromas. *N. Engl. J. Med.* **2016**, *375*, 2550–2560. [CrossRef]
17. Mautner, V.F.; Asuagbor, F.A.; Dombi, E.; Fünsterer, C.; Kluwe, L.; Wenzel, R.; Widemann, B.C.; Friedman, J. Assessment of benign tumor burden by whole-body MRI in patients with neurofibromatosis 1. *Neuro-oncology* **2008**, *10*, 593–598. [CrossRef]
18. Singhal, D.; Chen, Y.-C.; Fanzio, P.M.; Lin, C.H.; Chuang, D.C.-C.; Chen, Y.-R.; Chen, P.K.-T. Role of free flaps in the management of craniofacial neurofibromatosis: Soft tissue coverage and attempted facial reanimation. *J. Oral Maxillofac. Surg.* **2012**, *70*, 2916–2922. [CrossRef]

19. Singhal, D.; Chen, Y.-C.; Seselgyte, R.; Chen, P.K.-T.; Chen, Y.-R. Craniofacial neurofibromatosis and tissue expansion: Long-term results. *J. Plast. Reconstr. Aesthet. Surg.* **2012**, *65*, 956–959. [CrossRef]
20. Al-Otibi, M.; Rutka, J.T. Neurosurgical implications of neurofibromatosis Type I in children. *Neurosurg. Focus* **2006**, *20*, E2. [CrossRef]
21. Singhal, D.; Chen, Y.-C.; Tsai, Y.-J.; Yu, C.-C.; Chen, H.C.; Chen, Y.-R.; Chen, P.K.-T. Craniofacial neurofibromatosis: Treatment of the midface deformity. *J. Craniomaxillofac. Surg.* **2014**, *42*, 595–600. [CrossRef] [PubMed]
22. Farid, M.; Demicco, E.G.; Garcia, R.; Ahn, L.; Merola, P.R.; Cioffi, A.; Maki, R.G. Malignant peripheral nerve sheath tumors. *Oncologist* **2014**, *19*, 193–201. [CrossRef] [PubMed]
23. Chamseddin, B.H.; Hernandez, L.; Solorzano, D.; Vega, J.; Le, L.Q. Robust surgical approach for cutaneous neurofibroma in neurofibromatosis type 1. *JCI Insight* **2019**, *4*, e128881. [CrossRef] [PubMed]
24. Perrotta, R.; Tarico, M.S.; Virzì, D.; Manzo, G.; Currerí, S. Morpho-functional iterative surgery in a patient with von Recklinghausen disease. *G. Chir.* **2010**, *31*, 543–548. [PubMed]
25. Singhal, D.; Chen, Y.-C.; Chen, Y.-R.; Chen, P.K.-T.; Tsai, Y.-J. Soft tissue management of orbitotemporal neurofibromatosis. *J. Craniofac. Surg.* **2013**, *24*, 269–272. [CrossRef]
26. Thomson, S.A.; Fishbein, L.; Wallace, M.R. NF1 mutations and molecular testing. *J. Child Neurol.* **2002**, *17*, 555–561. [CrossRef]
27. Acosta, M.T.; Kardel, P.G.; Walsh, K.; Rosenbaum, K.N.; Gioia, G.A.; Packer, R.J. Lovastatin as treatment for neurocognitive deficits in neurofibromatosis type 1: Phase I study. *Pediatr. Neurol.* **2011**, *45*, 241–245. [CrossRef]
28. Fisher, M.J.; Loguidice, M.; Gutmann, D.; Listernick, R.; Ferner, R.; Ullrich, N.J.; Packer, R.J.; Tabori, U.; Hoffman, R.O.; Ardern-Holmes, S.L.; et al. Visual outcomes in children with neurofibromatosis type 1-associated optic pathway glioma following chemotherapy: A multicenter retrospective analysis. *Neuro-oncology* **2012**, *14*, 790–797. [CrossRef]
29. Fossali, E.; Signorini, E.; Intermite, R.C.; Casalini, E.; Lovaria, A.; Maninetti, M.M.; Rossi, L.N. Renovascular disease and hypertension in children with neurofibromatosis. *Pediatr. Nephrol.* **2000**, *14*, 806–810. [CrossRef]
30. Granstrom, S.; Langenbruch, A.; Augustin, M.; Mautner, V.-F. Psychological burden in adult neurofibromatosis type 1 patients: Impact of disease visibility on body image. *Dermatology* **2012**, *224*, 160–167. [CrossRef]
31. Wolkenstein, P.; Zeller, J.; Revuz, J.; Ecosse, E.; Leplège, A. Quality-of-Life Impairment in Neurofibromatosis Type 1: A Cross-sectional Study of 128 Cases. *Arch. Dermatol.* **2001**, *137*, 1421–1425. [CrossRef]
32. Page, P.Z.; Page, G.P.; Ecosse, E.; Korf, B.R.; Leplege, A.; Wolkenstein, P. Impact of neurofibromatosis 1 on Quality of Life: A cross-sectional study of 176 American cases. *Am. J. Med. Genet. A* **2006**, *140*, 1893–1898. [CrossRef]
33. Rumsey, N.; Harcourt, D. Body image and disfigurement: Issues and interventions. *Body Image* **2004**, *1*, 83–97. [CrossRef]
34. Latham, K.; Buchanan, E.P.; Suver, D.; Gruss, J.S. Neurofibromatosis of the head and neck: Classification and surgical management. *Plast. Reconstr. Surg.* **2015**, *135*, 845–855. [CrossRef]
35. Farmer, J.P.; Khan, S.; Khan, A.; Ortenberg, J.; Freeman, C.; O'Gorman, A.M.; Montes, J. Neurofibromatosis type 1 and the pediatric neurosurgeon: A 20-year institutional review. *Pediatr. Neurosurg.* **2002**, *37*, 122–136. [CrossRef]
36. Avery, R.A.; Katowitz, J.A.; Fisher, M.J.; Heidary, G.; Dombi, E.; Packer, R.J.; Widemann, B.C.; Hutcheson, K.A.; Madigan, W.P.; Listernick, R.; et al. Orbital/Periorbital Plexiform Neurofibromas in Children with Neurofibromatosis Type 1: Multidisciplinary Recommendations for Care. *Ophthalmology* **2017**, *124*, 123–132. [CrossRef]
37. Erb, M.H.; Uzcategui, N.; See, R.F.; Burnstine, M.A. Orbitotemporal neurofibromatosis: Classification and treatment. *Orbit* **2007**, *26*, 223–228. [CrossRef]
38. Uygur, F.; Chang, D.W.; Crosby, M.A.; Skoracki, R.J.; Robb, G.L. Free flap reconstruction of extensive defects following resection of large neurofibromatosis. *Ann. Plast. Surg.* **2011**, *67*, 376–381. [CrossRef]

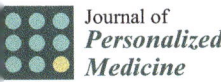

*Review*

# Defect Coverage after Forequarter Amputation—A Systematic Review Assessing Different Surgical Approaches

Denis Ehrl [1,†], Nikolaus Wachtel [1,*,†], David Braig [1], Constanze Kuhlmann [1], Hans Roland Dürr [2], Christian P. Schneider [3] and Riccardo E. Giunta [1]

1. Department of Hand, Plastic and Aesthetic Surgery, University Hospital, LMU Munich, Marchioninistraße 15, 81377 Munich, Germany; denis.ehrl@med.uni-muenchen.de (D.E.); david.braig@med.uni-muenchen.de (D.B.); constanze.kuhlmann@med.uni-muenchen.de (C.K.); riccardo.giunta@med.uni-muenchen.de (R.E.G.)
2. Orthopaedic Oncology, Department of Orthopaedics and Trauma Surgery, University Hospital, LMU Munich, Marchioninistraße 15, 81377 Munich, Germany; hans_roland.duerr@med.uni-muenchen.de
3. Department of Thoracic Surgery, University Hospital, LMU Munich, Marchioninistraße 15, 81377 Munich, Germany; christian.schneider@med.uni-muenchen.de
* Correspondence: nikolaus.wachtel@med.uni-muenchen.de
† These authors contributed equally to this work.

**Abstract:** Autologous fillet flaps are a common reconstructive option for large defects after forequarter amputation (FQA) due to advanced local malignancy or trauma. The inclusion of osseous structures into these has several advantages. This article therefore systematically reviews reconstructive options after FQA, using osteomusculocutaneous fillet flaps, with emphasis on personalized surgical technique and outcome. Additionally, we report on a case with an alternative surgical technique, which included targeted muscle reinnervation (TMR) of the flap. Our literature search was conducted in the PubMed and Cochrane databases. Studies that were identified were thoroughly scrutinized with regard to relevance, resulting in the inclusion of four studies (10 cases). FQA was predominantly a consequence of local malignancy. For vascular supply, the brachial artery was predominantly anastomosed to the subclavian artery and the brachial or cephalic vein to the subclavian or external jugular vein. Furthermore, we report on a case of a large osteosarcoma of the humerus. Extended FQA required the use of the forearm for defect coverage and shoulder contour reconstruction. Moreover, we performed TMR. Follow-up showed a satisfactory result and no phantom limb pain. In case of the need for free flap reconstruction after FQA, this review demonstrates the safety and advantage of osteomusculocutaneous fillet flaps. If the inclusion of the elbow joint into the flap is not possible, we recommend the use of the forearm, as described. Additionally, we advocate for the additional implementation of TMR, as it can be performed quickly and is likely to reduce phantom limb and neuroma pain.

**Keywords:** forequarter amputation; targeted muscle reinnervation; osteomusculocutaneous flap; fillet flap; epaulette flap; interscapulothoracic amputation; spare parts; microsurgery; reconstructive surgery

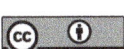

## 1. Introduction

The multimodal treatment of primary malignant bone or soft tissue tumors involves multiagent chemotherapy, radiotherapy, and wide surgical resection. Since the combination and enhancement of these regimes, long-term survival rates have improved significantly over the last decades and the operative treatment advanced from direct amputation to limb-sparing surgery [1]. However, for patients with locally advanced tumors of the limbs, amputation remains the only curative option.

With regard to the upper extremity, interscapulothoracic amputation (ISTA) or forequarter amputation (FQA) is the most radical ablative procedure [2]. It involves the amputation of the complete upper extremity, including the anatomic structures of the shoulder girdle, leading to the loss of the shoulder silhouette. Besides malignant bone tumors, post-radiation defects and traumatic scapulothoracic dissociation are the most common indications for this rare procedure [2–4]. Depending on the extent of FQA, direct wound closure is often not possible. A common reconstructive option for large defects after FQA are fillet flaps. These are harvested from the amputated limb and do not create any additional donor side morbidity. Depending on the surgical technique, different flap designs have been established for the upper extremity—the fasciocutaneous, the musculocutaneous, and the osteomusculocutaneous fillet flap [5–7]. While the first two techniques are viable options for the coverage of skin and soft-tissue defects, the inclusion of osseous structures can also stabilize the thoracic wall and reconstruct the shoulder contour. Hence, this flap is called the "epaulette" flap, similar to the ornamental shoulder piece of military uniforms [2]. Besides cosmetic advantages, the "epaulette" flap also creates a stable osseous and soft-tissue envelope that provides a socket for an upper-limb prosthesis [7,8].

Recent developments in prosthetic medicine have created devices that offer multi-functional joints with fine motor capabilities, as well as improved comfort and aesthetics [9]. With the aim to accelerate the cortical control of these advanced prosthetic systems, the concept of targeted muscle reinnervation (TMR) was presented in 2002. In TMR, transected peripheral nerves are transferred to recipient motor nerves of residual muscles in the amputated limb in order to avert muscle atrophy and reinitiate organized muscle innervation [10,11]. Prior studies revealed that TMR additionally significantly reduces the risk of developing neuromas and phantom limb pain [9,12,13]. These two characteristics make TMR a viable option for reconstructive procedures following curative or palliative FQA.

The aim of this article was to systematically review previous approaches for chest wall stabilization and shoulder contour reconstruction after FQA with osteomusculocutaneous free fillet flaps. Moreover, we report on a case with an alternative surgical technique that incorporates the forearm, wrist, and metacarpus of the amputated limb into the flap in combination with TMR. The simultaneous utilization of TMR provides the first results on feasibility and improved neuropathic pain management after FQA and osseous "spare-parts" reconstruction.

## 2. Methods

The identification of studies for this review was based on the Preferred Reporting Systems for Systematic Reviews and Meta-Analysis (PRISMA) statement [14]. The MeSH terms "fillet flap", "epaulette flap", "osteomusculocutaneous flap", "forequarter amputation", and "interscapulothoracic amputation" were used to search the PubMed and Cochrane databases for publications that focus on shoulder contour reconstruction and thoracic wall stabilization with osteomusculocutaneous free fillet flaps after FQA. The literature search was completed on 3 February 2022. In total, 387 articles were identified (Figure 1). All of the results were imported into the Covidence systematic review software (Veritas Health Innovation, Melbourne, Australia) for the removal of duplicates.

First, the titles and abstracts of the citations were individually scrutinized to determine which were relevant to the review. Subsequently, studies were excluded if they were not available in English or German, or if they described the usage of cutaneous and musculocutaneous (soft-tissue) fillet flaps or other reconstructive procedures (non-fillet flaps) after FQA. This resulted in the identification of six articles that describe the usage of osteomusculocutaneous fillet flaps for reconstruction following FQA. Two of these were excluded from the study as they did not provide enough details on the surgical technique used, as well as outcome measurements [7,15]. Four studies remained that met the inclusion criteria.

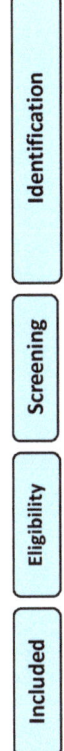
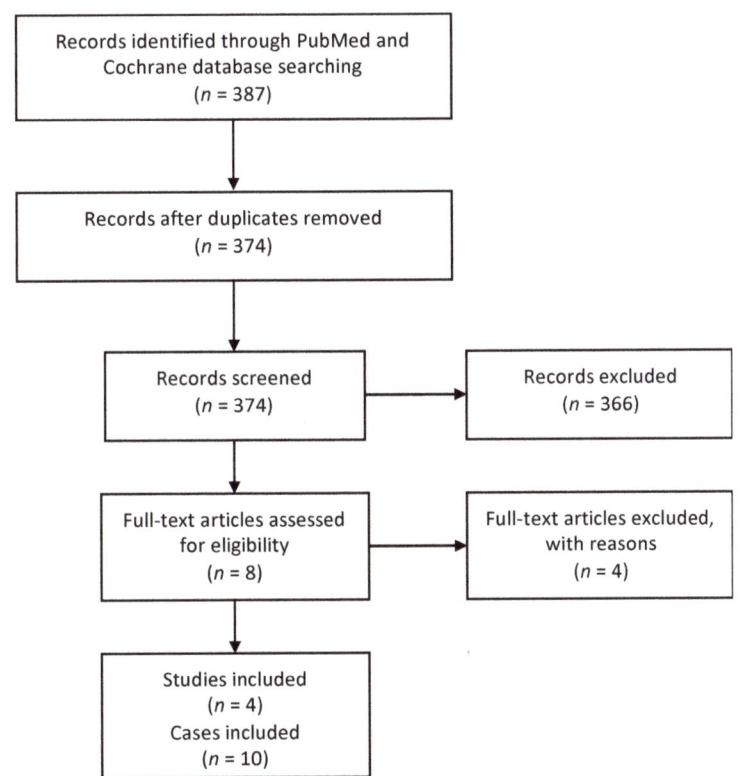

**Figure 1.** Study-selection algorithm based on the Preferred Reporting Systems for Systematic Reviews and Meta-Analysis (PRISMA) statement.

### 3. Results
*3.1. Literature Search*

Ten cases of shoulder contour reconstruction and thoracic wall stabilization with osteomusculocutaneous free fillet flaps after FQA were described in the four publications that were identified (Table 1). In 8 out of 10 cases, FQA was a consequence of a local malignancy, whereas two cases were due to prior trauma. Four patients required palliative FQA, the rest were treated in a curative intention ($n = 6$). All of the patients survived the initial surgery.

**Table 1.** Overview of all 10 cases that previously described free osteomusculocutaneous fillet flaps for thoracic wall stabilization and shoulder contour reconstruction after FQA.

| Ref. | Indication | Anastomosis | Reconstruction | Outcome |
|---|---|---|---|---|
| Steinau et al. (1992) [2] | 46 year old male with 8th local recurrence of a chondrosarcoma (T3 N0 M0 G2) with infiltration of the brachial plexus and the thoracic wall. Palliative FQA with resection of $\frac{3}{4}$ of ribs 1–5 and partial removal of the sternum | Brachial artery to subclavian artery; brachial and superficial vein to the bifurcation of the external jugular vein | Fixation of radius and ulna with interosseous wires to remaining parts of the sternum and the sixth rib for thoracic wall stabilization | Exitus letalis 13 months after surgery due to bilateral pulmonary metastases |

Table 1. Cont.

| Ref. | Indication | Anastomosis | Reconstruction | Outcome |
|---|---|---|---|---|
| Steinau et al. (1992) [2] | 22 year old male, recurrence of osteosarcoma (T3 N1 M0 G3), palliative FQA | Brachial artery to subclavian artery; brachial and superficial vein to the bifurcation of the external jugular vein | Radius and ulna were attached to the sternum and the thoracic wall with K-wires and strong circumferential wires | Revision due to an infected hematoma. Development of bilateral pulmonary metastases two months after surgery |
| | 30 year old male, traumatic interscapulothoracic avulsion accident | Brachial artery to subclavian artery; brachial vein to subclavian vein and a superficial vein to the external jugular vein | Fixation of the Olecranon to the stump of the clavicle and the radius and ulna to the thoracic wall. Both with K-wires | No complications; wears a passive prosthetic replacement |
| Kuhn et al. (1994) [16] | 21 year old male with an extensive recurrent desmoid tumor involving the chest wall from the clavicle to the 8th rib. Extensive FQA including ipsilateral hemithoracectomy and pneumectomy | Brachial artery to subclavian artery; cephalic vein to internal jugular vein and basilic vein to innominate vein | Free forearm fillet flap with attachment of the ulna to the 2nd and 9th rib with screws and miniplates. The radius was removed completely | No complications; returned to work three months after surgery |
| Osanai et al. (2005) [17] | 16 year old male with osteosarcoma, palliative FQA | Brachial artery to subclavian artery; brachial vein to subclavian vein | Plate osteosynthesis between the humerus and clavicle, 90° flexed elbow for shoulder contour reconstruction | Exitus letalis six months after surgery due to multiple pulmonary metastases |
| | 56 year old female, primary malignant cystosarcoma phyllodes of the breast with local progression, extensive FQA including chest wall and rib resection (ribs 2 to 4) | Brachial artery to suprascapular artery; brachial vein to suprascapular vein | Insertion of the end of the clavicle into the enlarged marrow cavity of the humerus and fixation with nonabsorbable sutures, 90° flexed elbow for shoulder contour reconstruction | No evidence of local recurrence 10 months after surgery |
| Koulaxouzidis et al. (2014) [18] | 46 year old male, traumatic FQA | Brachial artery to subclavian artery; Cubital vein to subclavian vein | Plate osteosynthesis between humerus and clavicle, 90° flexed elbow for shoulder contour reconstruction | Partial necrosis, three revision surgeries and split-thickness skin grafts |
| | 59 year old female, radiation induced soft tissue sarcoma (pT2a, N0, M0, G3) with infiltration of the brachial plexus and ulceration, extended FQA including the lateral third of the clavicle | Brachial artery to subclavian artery; cubital vein to subclavian vein | Cerclage wire osteosynthesis of the humerus to the middle third of the clavicle, 90° flexed elbow for shoulder contour reconstruction | Three revision surgeries due to arterial thrombosis, wound dehiscence, and partial necrosis of the flap. No local recurrence or metastasis in two-year follow up |

Table 1. Cont.

| Ref. | Indication | Anastomosis | Reconstruction | Outcome |
|---|---|---|---|---|
| Koulaxouzidis et al. (2014) [18] | 73 year old female, radiogenic sarcoma with invasion of the brachial and cervical plexus, the scapula, lateral clavicle, first three ribs and the apex of the lung, extended FQA including resection of the first three ribs and lung apex | Brachial artery to internal thoracic artery; brachial vein to internal thoracic vein | Cerclage wire osteosynthesis of the humerus to the middle third of the clavicle, 90° flexed elbow for shoulder contour reconstruction | No complications; the patient died 14 years after surgery from a sarcoma-unrelated causes |
| | 57 year old female, loco-regional persistence of an infiltrating lobular carcinoma of the breast 16 years after initial diagnosis and therapy. FQA was necessary due to infiltration of the brachial plexus and stenosis of the brachial vessels, infiltration of the biceps, triceps, and infraspinatus muscle as well as the scapula | Brachial artery to subclavian artery; cephalic vein to subclavian vein and brachial vein to external jugular vein | Plate osteosynthesis between humerus and clavicle, 90° flexed elbow for shoulder contour reconstruction | R1 resection, leading to re-excision with intraoperative radiation. Loco-regional recurrence after six years requiring another re-excision and adjuvant chemotherapy. Again, four years later the patient presented with cervical lymph node metastases leading to neck dissection. Subsequently, one year later, tumor recurrence at the thoracic wall |

Considering the vascular supply of the flap, the subclavian artery was predominantly anastomosed to the brachial artery ($n = 8$). Other options were the suprascapular artery ($n = 1$) and the internal thoracic artery ($n = 1$). In 5 out of 10 cases, two venous anastomoses were completed. In the majority of cases, the brachial or cephalic vein of the flap was connected to the subclavian or the external jugular vein ($n = 7$). Three cases required revision surgery due to an infected hematoma ($n = 1$), partial skin necrosis ($n = 2$), and/or arterial thrombosis ($n = 1$). Another case required tumor re-excision after the confirmation of a R1 tumor margin. Three out of a total of six sarcoma patients developed pulmonary metastases within the first 18 months after surgery, and two of these patients died within the observation period. Another patient died 13 years after the initial operation from a local recurrence of the sarcoma. Both patients with traumatic FQA survived the follow-up period.

*3.2. Case Report*

A 25-year-old male patient with a large chondroblastic osteosarcoma of the left upper humerus presented to our hospital and was treated by our multidisciplinary sarcoma team (Table 2). The patient was initially diagnosed eight months earlier but unfortunately decided to pursue an alternative treatment with a homeopathic practitioner for three months. When he returned to our hospital, the tumor had increased considerably in size and was staged as cT2 cN0, cM1, infiltrating the glenohumeral joint, the muscles of the upper arm and rotator cuff, as well as the latissimus dorsi and both pectoral muscles (Figure 2). Additionally, three suspect pulmonary lesions, thrombosis of the subclavian, axillar and brachial vein was observed on CT-Angio scans. Due to oligometastasis and the young age of the patient a curative treatment approach was initiated, including neoadjuvant chemotherapy followed by wide tumor resection. Oncological treatment following the protocol of the European and American Osteosarcoma Study Group (EURAMOS-1) was initiated [19,20].

After 6 weeks of chemotherapy, wide resection was conducted. The surgery was performed in an interdisciplinary collaboration of Tumor Orthopedics, Thoracic and Plastic Surgeons. Due to the extent of the sarcoma, an extended FQA, including an atypical lung segment resection and the resection of the first three ribs as well as the complete clavicle, was necessary to allow complete resection. Suspect pulmonary lesions were individually resected by atypical lung resections.

**Table 2.** Overview of the presented case using an osteomusculocutaneous fillet flap for defect coverage after FQA.

| Indication | Anastomosis | Reconstruction | TMR | Outcome |
| --- | --- | --- | --- | --- |
| 25 year old male with central chondroblastic osteosarcoma (cT2 cN0, cM1), extended FQA, including resection of the clavicle and the first three ribs | Brachial artery to thoracoacromial artery and cephalic vein to subclavian vein | Plate osteosynthesis between radius and sternum, 90° flexed wrist and fixation sutures between metacarpals and the lateral thoracic wall | Nerve coaptation between superior trunk and median nerve, middle trunk and radial nerve, and inferior trunk and ulnar nerve | Discharged after 11 days, stable osseous framework, Exitus letalis three months after surgery due to disseminated, primarily pulmonal, metastases |

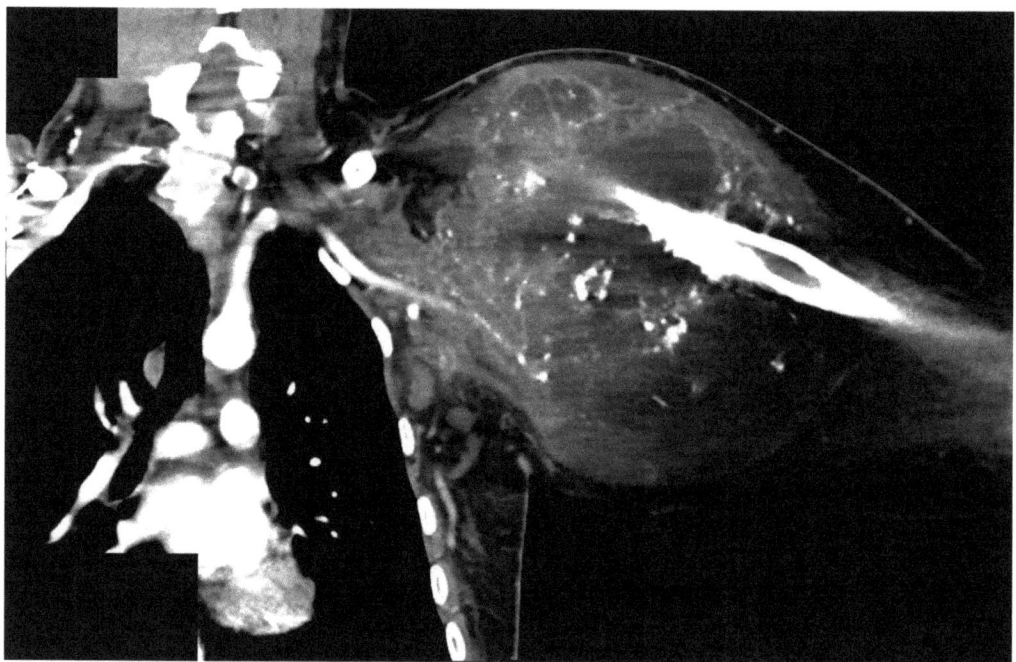

**Figure 2.** CT-Scan of a 25 year old male who presented with a chondroblastic osteosarcoma of the left proximal humerus, infiltrating the left glenohumeral joint and the muscles of the upper arm and rotator cuff, including latissimus dorsi and both pectoral muscles (staged at cT2 cN0, and cM1).

Tumor infiltration into the distal end of the humerus prohibited a reconstructive option that used the elbow joint [17,18]. We therefore decided to use an osteomusculocutaneous free fillet flap from the tumor-free forearm for defect coverage and shoulder contour reconstruction. The flexed wrist and metacarpal bones were incorporated into the flap to create a shoulder contour that would function as a prosthetic socket. The radius and ulna were shortened at the proximal end to a length of 14 cm and the skin and soft tissue were opened longitudinally on the ventral aspect of the forearm. The radius was then attached to the sternum with a plate. Subsequently, microsurgical anastomoses were performed between the brachial artery and thoracoacromial artery and between the cephalic vein and remaining stump of the subclavian vein in end-to-end technique with interrupted sutures (total time of ischemia: 165 min). The metacarpal bones were connected to the lateral thoracic wall using a non-resorbable suture to ensure lateral stability of the construct. TMR was performed by epineural coaptation of the three forearm motor-nerves (i.e., median, radial, and ulnar nerve) to the three trunks of the brachial plexus (Figure 3). The skin and soft tissue of the flap was fitted to the chest wall. The patient was transferred to the intensive-care unit after surgery and was extubated on the following day. Pathology confirmed R0-resection and complete wound healing occurred without infection or tissue loss. The patient was discharged 11 days after surgery.

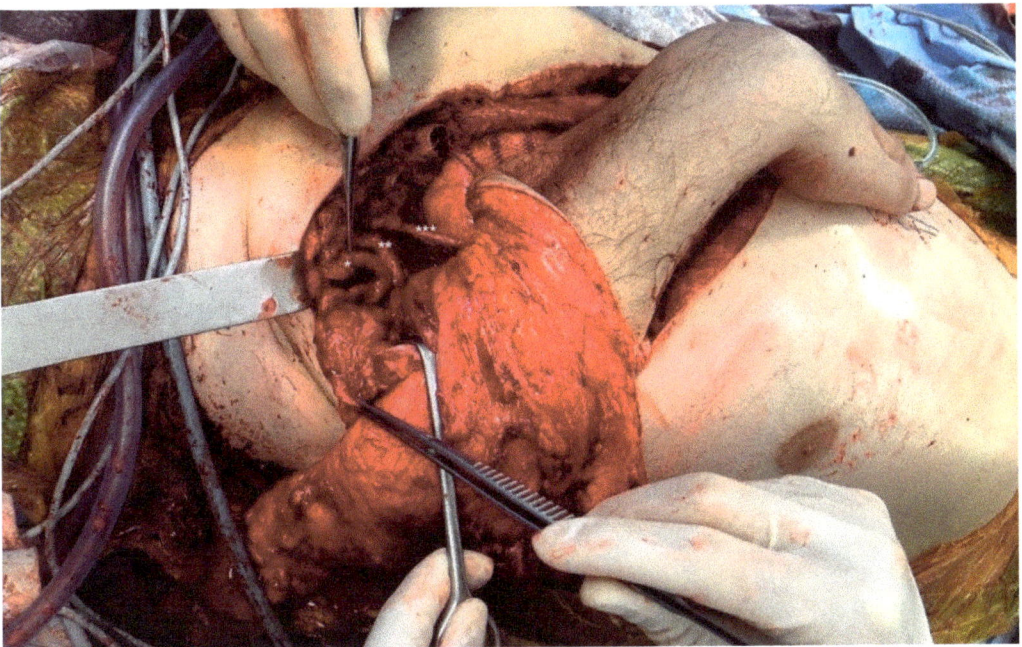

**Figure 3.** Intraoperative view of osteomusculocutaneous free fillet flap for defect coverage after forequarter amputation (FQA). The radius (and ulna) was shortened and attached to the sternum with a plate. Microsurgical anastomoses were performed between the brachial artery and thoracoacromial artery, and between the cephalic vein and the remaining stump of the subclavian vein. Subsequently, targeted muscle reinnervation (TMR) by epineural coaptation of the three forearm motor-nerves was performed: the superior trunk was connected to the median nerve (*), the middle trunk to the radial nerve (**), and the inferior trunk to the ulnar nerve (***).

Clinical follow-up showed a solid osseous framework with good protection of the thoracic organs (Figure 4) and an acceptable improvement of the shoulder contour (Figure 5). The patient did not suffer from phantom limb or neuroma pain. Moreover, neurological examination six weeks after surgery showed an increasing tactile sensation of the flap. However, pulmonary and lymph-node metastases occurred during follow-up, resulting in the continuous deterioration of the clinical condition. A palliative therapeutic concept commenced, and the patient died three months after tumor resection.

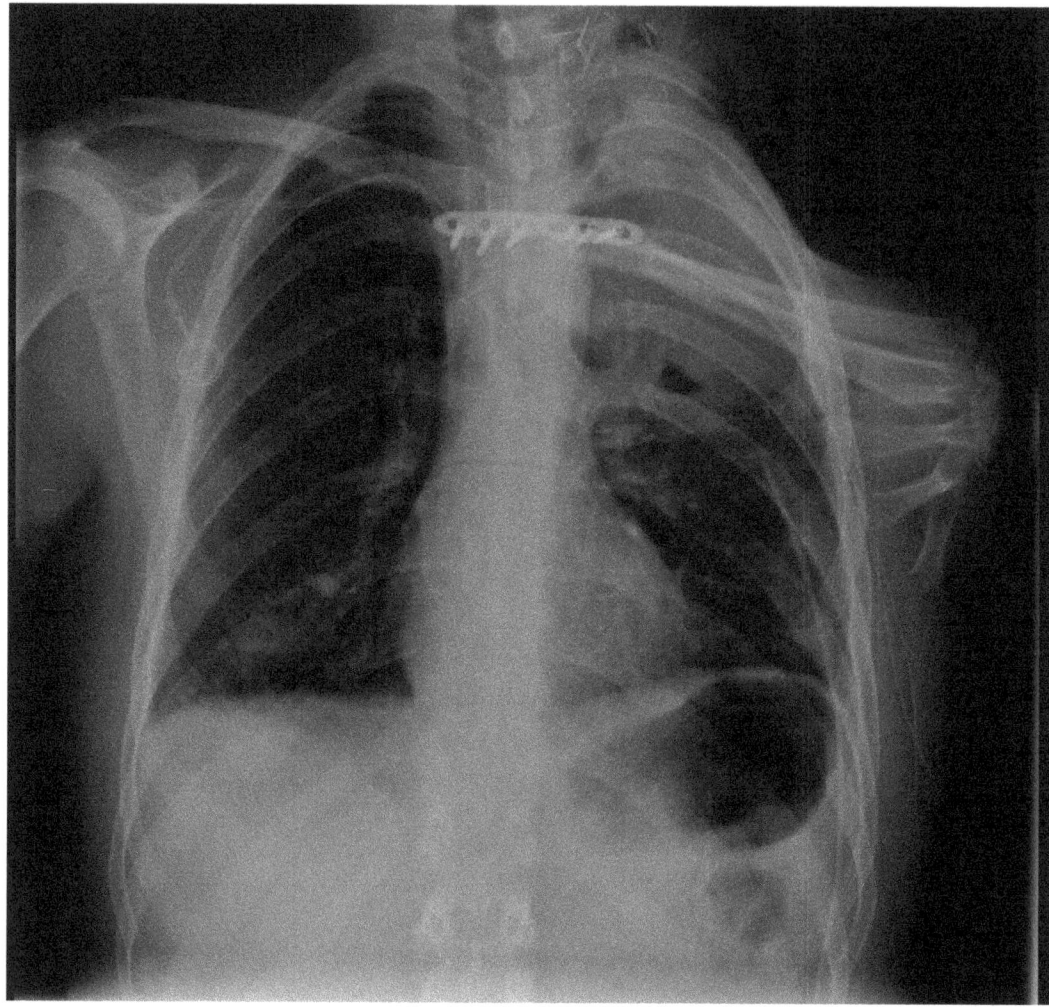

**Figure 4.** Osteomusculocutaneous free fillet flap including the tumor-free forearm for defect coverage and shoulder contour reconstruction (radiograph taken one week after surgery). The 90° flexed wrist, as well as the carpal and metacarpal bones, were incorporated into the flap to create a shoulder contour that would function as a prosthetic socket. Plate osteosynthesis was used to attach the sternum to the radius.

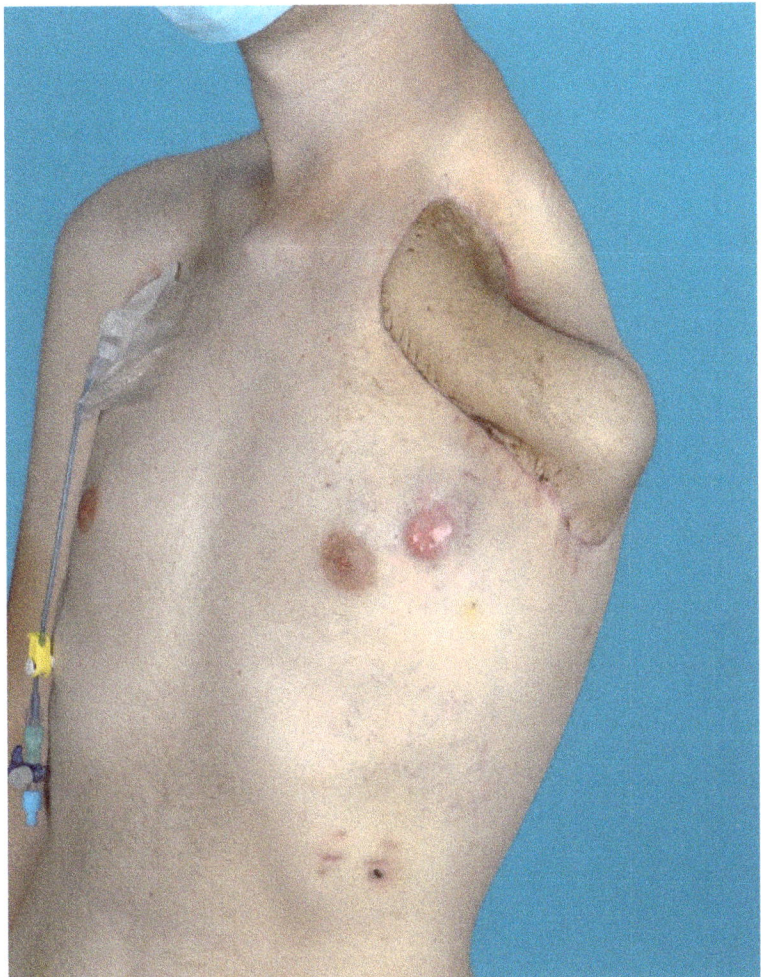

**Figure 5.** Clinical follow-up six weeks after osteomusculocutaneous free fillet flap defect coverage, including targeted muscle reinnervation (TMR). The results demonstrate an adequate reconstruction of the chest wall integrity, as a well as an improved appearance of the shoulder contour. The patient did not suffer from phantom limb or neuroma pain, and neurological examination showed an increasing tactile sensation of the flap. Due to disease progression in the course of treatment, cutaneous metastasis developed above the left breast.

## 4. Discussion

Improved reconstructive options and a multimodal treatment of mesenchymal tumors, such as osteosarcomas, enabled limb salvage in the majority of patients [21,22]. Nevertheless, radical tumor resection is usually necessary as inadequate surgical margins are significantly associated with higher local recurrence rates and decreased overall survival of patients [15,16,23]. With regard to locally progressed primary tumors of the proximal upper extremity, limb salvage is not always possible. In these cases, FQA allows for wide resection margins [24]. However, albeit technically feasible, the radical ablation of the arm and the anatomical structures of the shoulder girdle are associated with severe comorbidities, such as possible life-threatening intraoperative hemorrhage, as well as respiratory impairment or even failure [16,25], especially when including the resection of the chest wall and/or parts of the lung [16,26]. Nevertheless, while such a radical procedure has to be carefully assessed for its advisability for each individual patient, FQA allows for wide resection margins and, thus, a curative treatment concept [24,25].

A common consequence of the radical ablation of the arm and the anatomical structures of the shoulder girdle is the requirement of a subsequent microsurgical reconstruction in order to enable adequate defect coverage and wound closure. The "spare-parts concept", which utilizes tissue from the amputated limb to reconstruct a defect without creating additional donor side morbidity (i.e., fillet flap), is a recognized technique in reconstructive and traumatic surgery [7,15,27–29]. Küntscher and colleagues provided a thorough overview of this surgical technique in an extensive study on 104 fillet flaps. The authors classify fillet flaps into pedicled finger and toe, pedicled limb, and free filet flaps [15]. With regard to free fillet flaps used for reconstructive surgery after FQA, flaps have been predominantly described according to their tissue content (fasciocutaneous, musculocutaneous, and osteomusculocutaneous) [5,6]. In contrast to fasciocutaneous and musculocutaneous flaps, the inclusion of bones in the osteomusculocutaneous fillet flap enables restoration of the shoulder silhouette and provides additional stability, as well as protection of the thorax and its inner organs, when using this technique for reconstruction after FQA [5–7,30]. Indeed, the reconstruction of the chest wall integrity after extensive resection is of the highest priority as a reduced structural integrity of the chest is associated with paradox respiratory movement and therefore impaired ventilatory function [7,31]. Alternative methods that offer stability, such as the use of alloplastic materials (e.g., synthetic mesh), have been successfully described for the reconstruction of large chest wall defects [32,33]. These often require additional soft tissue coverage, commonly by extensive free flaps in the case of FQA. However, due to the risk of predominantly intraoperative bacterial contamination, these are associated with a higher rate of infection and impaired wound healing [34–38].

Instead of utilizing the amputated limb, local or free flap reconstructive options may be used for defect coverage after FQA. Indeed, several reports exist, which demonstrate the successful use of these techniques, such as the fasciocutaneous deltoid, the tensor fascia latae (TFL), or the TFL + rectus femoris flap [7,39,40]. Similarly, extensive studies have been published regarding the reconstruction of the chest wall using primarily local myocutaneous flaps [41–43]. However, in the case of FQA, where the subscapular system is often severed, pedicled flaps like latissimus dorsi, (para)scapular, and serratus flaps become unavailable local options. In addition, when compared to an osteomusculocutaneous fillet flap, these procedures involve additional donor site morbidity, as well as limited stability for the shoulder girdle.

Despite the potential physiological and psychological benefits for the patient, very few cases of osteomusculocutaneous free fillet flaps for chest wall and shoulder reconstruction have been described in previous publications. Our systematic literature search identified four articles that give detailed information on this technique in a total of ten cases (Table 1) [2,16–18]. Hitherto published surgical techniques on osteomusculocutaneous free fillet flaps after FQA can be separated into two main subgroups, depending on the choice of bones that were included into the flap—the approach by Steinau et al. as well as the one by Kuhn and colleagues, who described the utilization of the radius and/or ulna to stabilize the thoracic wall [2,16]. Thus, Steinau et al. reported on three cases in which the proximal forearm was fixated to the remaining parts of the clavicle or the sternum with the distal ends of the radius and ulna being attached to the thoracic wall [2]. Two years later, Kuhn et al. published a case report describing the use of the bones and soft-tissue of the forearm to reconstruct the thoracic wall and to allow for mediastinal protection after extended FQA, including complete anterior and posterior chest wall resection, as well as pneumectomy [16].

In contrast, in their subsequently published articles, Osanai and colleagues as well as Koulaxouzidis et al. described techniques that connect the distal humerus to the clavicle or the sternum (in cases where a complete resection of the clavicle was necessary) and created a lateral prominence that resembles the natural silhouette of the shoulder [17,18,37,44,45].

Thus, Osanai et al. included the flexed elbow joint into the flap to imitate the natural shoulder contour through the eminence of the olecranon [17]. Similarly, Koulaxouzidis et al. also used the elbow joint for shoulder contour reconstruction in a total of four patients [18]. Moreover, this technique also involved the reconstruction of the axillary fold in addition to the shoulder contour. The authors avoided large scale soft-tissue separation to preserve the outline of the elbow, and the cubital skin crease was thus used to recreate the axilla.

The results illustrate that the functional and cosmetic outcomes are highly dependent on the location and extent of the tumor or trauma. Local tumor progression of our patient required the resection of the complete clavicle, scapula, and the first three ribs. The upper arm had to be excluded from the flap to accomplish tumor free margins, permitting the previously published surgical approach that incorporates the elbow joint into the flap [17,18].

Thus, our surgical options were limited to the utilization of the forearm and the hand, as the osteomusculocutaneous free flap for the reconstruction of the thoracic wall and shoulder. Therefore, we decided to use a new surgical approach—by connecting the radius to the sternum, we were able to utilize the flexed wrist instead of the elbow joint to imitate the natural shoulder contour (Table 2). Short-term follow-up of the patient revealed limited appearance of the shoulder silhouette; however, sufficient protection of the thoracic organs through the osseous framework of the flap, and good anatomical conditions for attachment of a socket prosthesis. Consequently, we present a third subgroup of osteomusculocutaneous fillet flaps for reconstruction with "spare-parts" after FQA that incorporates the bones of the forearm, wrist, and metacarpus. Unfortunately, we cannot provide long-term results using this technique due to the rapid development of metastatic disease, resulting in the patient's death three months after surgery.

Common complications following extremity amputation are the occurrence of phantom limb pain and the development of neuromas [11]. The prevalence of phantom limb pain ranges between 45 and 85%, and typically displays two peaks in its incidence: one month and one year after amputation [46,47]. The concept of TMR was initially developed to enable advanced control of myoelectric prostheses, but has also shown to significantly reduce phantom pain and neuroma formation after limb amputation [13,47]. To exploit these features, we connected the trunks of the brachial plexus to the forearm nerves in the fillet flap. The epineural end-to-end coaptation required only a little extra time due to the large caliber of the peripheral nerves and was completed within 35 min. The patient did not develop any phantom limb or neuroma pain during the follow-up period. These findings provide new data on the feasibility and possible functional improvement of phantom pain management in patients who undergo fillet flap reconstruction after FQA. While the validity of our results is significantly limited due to the short observation period and single-case experience, previous studies have demonstrated the high effectiveness of TMR when performed as a preemptive measure, as well as when used as a treatment option for patients with postamputation pain [48–51]. Indeed, Mioton and colleagues demonstrated significant improvements of residual limb and phantom limb pain parameters in 33 patients with major limb amputations due to TMR one year after treatment [49]. Moreover, in a recent prospective randomized clinical trial, TMR was shown to reduce chronic pain in amputees when compared with the gold standard (excision and muscle burying) [48]. Similar results were shown by Valerio et al. when implementing TMR as a preemptive measure to reduce chronic postamputation pain [50]. In their multi-institutional cohort study, the authors demonstrated that patients who underwent TMR had less phantom and residual limb pain when compared with untreated amputee controls. This effect was shown across all subgroups. Considering these previous findings and also the outcome of our presented case, a high benefit to cost ratio of TMR along with fillet-flap reconstruction after FQA seems highly likely.

In the majority of reports, including our own case, tumor infiltration of the shoulder girdle or chest wall was the indication for FQA. Using the "spare-parts" of an extremity that was impaired by local cancerous progression asks the question of whether this procedure is a safe oncological approach. In this context, the fillet flap technique uses the identical principle of the resection–replantation technique reported by Windhager et al. [52]. The authors resected the tumor-bearing area of the upper extremity and replanted the distal part of the arm to the proximal stump. None of the 12 patients developed a local recurrence within the follow-up period. Furthermore, a different study by Ver Halen et al. described 27 soft tissue fillet flaps from the upper and lower extremity after soft tissue malignancies; none of the patients developed cancer recurrence within the flap itself, supporting the thesis that the fillet flap technique is oncologically safe [29].

However, in cases where FQA may be prevented or primary wound closure is possible, the overall prognosis of this special patient group must be taken into account, in particular when considering osteomusculocutaneous fillet flap reconstruction after FQA due to sarcoma. Even if primary tumor resection is successful, the disease-free five year survival of sarcoma patients requiring FQA is below 30% [53]. While Steinau et al. advocated that the use of osteomusculocutaneous fillet flaps even applies to a palliative reconstruction, the apparent limitations of ultra-radical interdisciplinary oncological surgery, albeit technically feasible, have to be critically reflected [2,25]. This holds true, in particular, when considering previously reported long-term impairment of respiratory function and of quality of life in patients with chest wall resection, as well as the significantly increased depressive symptoms of family members that often need to be consulted in the course of the intensive care treatment of critically ill patients [25,54,55].

Therefore, we advocate that the indication for FQA has to be individually considered and carefully evaluated with each patient after case discussion in a specialized interdisciplinary tumor board (if applicable, i.e., if FQA is considered to treat an underlying malignancy). However, if this process concludes that FQA is the best treatment option, radical tumor resections and subsequent osteomusculocutaneous fillet flap reconstruction, including TMR (when manageable in limited additional operating time), should be the first choice of surgical treatment.

## 5. Conclusions

In case of FQA and the need for free flap reconstruction, we consider the osteomusculocutaneous free fillet flap as the first choice. It enables the reconstruction of the chest wall integrity, provides support for a prosthesis socket, and improves the appearance of the shoulder contour. When using this technique, the remaining anatomical structures of the thorax, the vascular supply, and the distal resection margin of the amputated upper extremity are crucial components that have to be considered when the overall design of the flap is determined. If the inclusion of the elbow joint into the flap is not possible due to local tumor expansion or trauma, we recommend the use of the forearm and hand, as described. In general, we advocate for the additional implementation of TMR, as it can be performed quickly and is likely to reduce the occurrence of phantom limb and neuroma pain. However, the reviewed case series, as well as our own experience, emphasize that patients require careful evaluation of the benefit of FQA, as well as an individual solution for reconstructive surgery if the procedure is deemed to be the best possible option.

**Author Contributions:** Conceptualization, D.E., C.P.S., H.R.D., D.B. and R.E.G.; methodology, N.W. and C.K.; validation, D.E., D.B., C.K. and N.W.; investigation, N.W. and C.K.; resources, R.E.G., C.P.S. and H.R.D.; data curation, D.E., D.B., C.K. and N.W.; writing—original draft preparation, N.W., C.K. and D.B.; writing—review and editing, D.E. and R.E.G.; visualization, N.W.; supervision, R.E.G., C.P.S. and H.R.D. All authors have read and agreed to the published version of the manuscript.

**Funding:** This research received no external funding.

**Institutional Review Board Statement:** Ethical review and approval were waived for this study due to the anonymous case presentation in the article. A written consent was secured from the patient before publication.

**Informed Consent Statement:** Written informed consent has been obtained from the patient to publish this paper.

**Data Availability Statement:** Not applicable.

**Conflicts of Interest:** The authors declare no conflict of interest.

## References

1. Isakoff, M.S.; Bielack, S.S.; Meltzer, P.; Gorlick, R. Osteosarcoma: Current Treatment and a Collaborative Pathway to Success. *J. Clin. Oncol.* **2015**, *33*, 3029–3035. [CrossRef] [PubMed]
2. Steinau, H.U.; Germann, G.; Klein, W.; Roehrl, S.P.; Josten, C. The "Epaulette" Flap: Replantation of Osteomyocutaneous Forearm Segments in Interscapulothoracic Amputations. *Eur. J. Plast. Surg.* **1992**, *15*, 283–288. [CrossRef]
3. Anbarasan, A.; Mohamad, N.H.; Mariapan, S. Open Traumatic Scapulothoracic Dissociation: Case Report of a Rare Injury. *Trauma Case Rep.* **2018**, *18*, 42–45. [CrossRef] [PubMed]
4. Wittig, J.C.; Bickels, J.; Kollender, Y.; Kellar-Graney, K.L.; Meller, I.; Malawer, M.M. Palliative Forequarter Amputation for Metastatic Carcinoma to the Shoulder Girdle Region: Indications, Preoperative Evaluation, Surgical Technique, and Results. *J. Surg. Oncol.* **2001**, *77*, 105–113. [CrossRef]
5. Ayyala, H.S.; Mohamed, O.M.; Therattil, P.J.; Lee, E.S.; Keith, J.D. The Forearm Fillet Flap: 'Spare Parts' Reconstruction for Forequarter Amputations. *Case Rep. Plast. Surg. Hand Surg.* **2019**, *6*, 95–98. [CrossRef]
6. Cordeiro, P.G.; Cohen, S.; Burt, M.; Brennan, M.F. The Total Volar Forearm Musculocutaneous Free Flap for Reconstruction of Extended Forequarter Amputations. *Ann. Plast. Surg.* **1998**, *40*, 388–396. [CrossRef]
7. Tukiainen, E.; Barner-Rasmussen, I.; Popov, P.; Kaarela, O. Forequarter Amputation and Reconstructive Options. *Ann. Plast. Surg.* **2020**, *84*, 651–656. [CrossRef]
8. Pierrie, S.N.; Gaston, R.G.; Loeffler, B.J. Current Concepts in Upper-Extremity Amputation. *J. Hand Surg. Am.* **2018**, *43*, 657–667. [CrossRef]
9. Mioton, L.M.; Dumanian, G.A. Targeted Muscle Reinnervation and Prosthetic Rehabilitation after Limb Loss. *J. Surg. Oncol.* **2018**, *118*, 807–814. [CrossRef]
10. Bowen, J.B.; Ruter, D.; Wee, C.; West, J.; Valerio, I.L. Targeted Muscle Reinnervation Technique in Below-Knee Amputation. *Plast. Reconstr. Surg.* **2019**, *143*, 309–312. [CrossRef]
11. Bowen, J.B.; Wee, C.E.; Kalik, J.; Valerio, I.L. Targeted Muscle Reinnervation to Improve Pain, Prosthetic Tolerance, and Bioprosthetic Outcomes in the Amputee. *Adv. Wound Care* **2017**, *6*, 261–267. [CrossRef] [PubMed]
12. Cheesborough, J.E.; Smith, L.H.; Kuiken, T.A.; Dumanian, G.A. Targeted Muscle Reinnervation and Advanced Prosthetic Arms. *Semin. Plast. Surg.* **2015**, *29*, 62–72. [CrossRef] [PubMed]
13. Elmaraghi, S.; Albano, N.J.; Israel, J.S.; Michelotti, B.F. Targeted Muscle Reinnervation in the Hand: Treatment and Prevention of Pain After Ray Amputation. *J. Hand Surg. Am.* **2019**, *45*, 884.e1–884.e6. [CrossRef] [PubMed]
14. Moher, D.; Liberati, A.; Tetzlaff, J.; Altman, D.G.; Altman, D.; Antes, G.; Atkins, D.; Barbour, V.; Barrowman, N.; Berlin, J.A.; et al. Preferred Reporting Items for Systematic Reviews and Meta-Analyses: The PRISMA Statement. *Ann. Intern. Med.* **2009**, *151*, 264–269. [CrossRef]
15. Küntscher, M.V.; Erdmann, D.; Homann, H.H.; Steinau, H.U.; Levin, S.L.; Germann, G. The Concept of Fillet Flaps: Classification, Indications, and Analysis of Their Clinical Value. *Plast. Reconstr. Surg.* **2001**, *108*, 885–896. [CrossRef]
16. Kuhn, J.A.; Wagman, L.D.; Lorant, J.A.; Grannis, F.W.; Dunst, M.; Dougherty, W.R.; Jacobs, D.I. Radical Forequarter Amputation with Hemithoracectomy and Free Extended Forearm Flap: Technical and Physiologic Considerations. *Ann. Surg. Oncol.* **1994**, *1*, 353–359. [CrossRef]
17. Osanai, T.; Kashiwa, H.; Ishikawa, A.; Takahara, M.; Ogino, T. Improved Shoulder Contour Following Forequarter Amputation with an Osteomyocutaneous Free Flap from the Amputated Extremity: Two Cases. *Br. J. Plast. Surg.* **2005**, *58*, 165–169. [CrossRef]
18. Koulaxouzidis, G.; Simunovic, F.; Stark, G.B. Shoulder Silhouette and Axilla Reconstruction with Free Composite Elbow Tissue Transfer Following Interscapulothoracic Amputation. *J. Plast. Reconstr. Aesthet. Surg.* **2014**, *67*, 81–86. [CrossRef]
19. Bielack, S.S.; Werner, M.; Tunn, P.U.; Helmke, K.; Jürgens, H.; Calaminus, G.; Gerss, J.; Butterfass-Bahloul, T.; Reichardt, P.; Smeland, S.; et al. Methotrexate, Doxorubicin, and Cisplatin (MAP) plus Maintenance Pegylated Interferon Alfa-2b versus MAP Alone in Patients with Resectable High-Grade Osteosarcoma and Good Histologic Response to Preoperative MAP: First Results of the EURAMOS-1 Good Respons. *J. Clin. Oncol.* **2015**, *33*, 2279–2287. [CrossRef]
20. Marina, N.; Bielack, S.; Whelan, J.; Smeland, S.; Krailo, M.; Sydes, M.R.; Butterfass-Bahloul, T.; Calaminus, G.; Bernstein, M. International Collaboration Is Feasible in Trials for Rare Conditions: The EURAMOS Experience. *Cancer Treat. Res.* **2009**, *152*, 573–575. [CrossRef]
21. Lehnhardt, M.; Hirche, C.; Daigeler, A.; Goertz, O.; Ring, A.; Hirsch, T.; Drücke, D.; Hauser, J.; Steinau, H.U. Weichgewebssarkome Der Oberen Extremität: Analyse Prognoserelevanter Faktoren Bei 160 Patienten. *Chirurg* **2012**, *83*, 143–152. [CrossRef] [PubMed]
22. Zeller, J.; Kiefer, J.; Braig, D.; Winninger, O.; Dovi-Akue, D.; Herget, G.W.; Stark, G.B.; Eisenhardt, S.U. Efficacy and Safety of Microsurgery in Interdisciplinary Treatment of Sarcoma Affecting the Bone. *Front. Oncol.* **2019**, *9*, 1–9. [CrossRef] [PubMed]
23. Gomez-brouchet, A.; Mascard, E.; Siegfried, A.; De Pinieux, G.; Gaspar, N.; Bouvier, C.; Aubert, S.; Marec-bérard, P.; Piperno-neumann, S.; Marie, B.; et al. Assessment of Resection Margins in Bone Sarcoma Treated by Neoadjuvant Chemotherapy: Literature Review and Guidelines of the Bone Group ( GROUPOS ) of the French Sarcoma Group and Bone Tumor Study Group (GSF-GETO/RESOS). *Orthop. Traumatol. Surg. Res.* **2019**, *105*, 773–780. [CrossRef] [PubMed]

24. Elsner, U.; Henrichs, M.; Gosheger, G.; Dieckmann, R.; Nottrott, M.; Hardes, J.; Streitbürger, A. Forequarter Amputation: A Safe Rescue Procedure in a Curative and Palliative Setting in High-Grade Malignoma of the Shoulder Girdle. *World J. Surg. Oncol.* **2016**, *14*, 4–11. [CrossRef]
25. Dragu, A.; Hohenberger, W.; Lang, W.; Schmidt, J.; Horch, R.E. Forequarter amputation of the right upper chest: Limitations of ultra radical interdisciplinary oncological surgery. *Chirurg* **2011**, *82*, 834–838. [CrossRef]
26. O'Connor, B.; Collins, F.J. The Management of Chest Wall Resection in a Patient with Polyostotic Fibrous Dysplasia and Respiratory Failure. *J. Cardiothorac. Vasc. Anesth.* **2009**, *23*, 518–521. [CrossRef]
27. Jakubietz, R.G.; Jakubietz, M.G.; Kloss, D.F.; Gruenert, J.G. Combination of a Total Free Forearm Flap and a Sensate Local Flap for Preservation of the Shoulder Girdle in Massive, Nonreplantable Upper Extremity Injuries. *J. Trauma Acute Care Surg.* **2009**, *66*, 561–563. [CrossRef]
28. Scaglioni, M.F.; Lindenblatt, N.; Barth, A.A.; Fuchs, B.; Weder, W.; Giovanoli, P. Free Fillet Flap Application to Cover Forequarter or Traumatic Amputation of an Upper Extremity: A Case Report. *Microsurgery* **2016**, *36*, 700–704. [CrossRef]
29. Ver Halen, J.P.; Yu, P.; Skoracki, R.J.; Chang, D.W. Reconstruction of Massive Oncologic Defects Using Free Fillet Flaps. *Plast. Reconstr. Surg.* **2010**, *125*, 913–922. [CrossRef]
30. Steinau, H.U.; Germann, G.; Klein, W.; Josten, C. The Epaulette Flap: Replantation of Osteomyocutaneous Forearm Segments in Interscapulo-Thoracic Amputation. *Chirurg* **1992**, *63*, 368–372.
31. Netscher, D.T.; Baumholtz, M.A. Chest Reconstruction: I. Anterior and Anterolateral Chest Wall and Wounds Affecting Respiratory Function. *Plast. Reconstr. Surg.* **2009**, *124*, 240–252. [CrossRef] [PubMed]
32. Gonfiotti, A.; Santini, P.F.; Campanacci, D.; Innocenti, M.; Ferrarello, S.; Caldarella, A.; Janni, A. Malignant Primary Chest-Wall Tumours: Techniques of Reconstruction and Survival. *Eur. J. Cardio-Thorac. Surg.* **2010**, *38*, 39–45. [CrossRef] [PubMed]
33. Lardinois, D.; Müller, M.; Furrer, M.; Banic, A.; Gugger, M.; Krueger, T.; Ris, H.B. Functional Assessment of Chest Wall Integrity after Methylmethacrylate Reconstruction. *Ann. Thorac. Surg.* **2000**, *69*, 919–923. [CrossRef]
34. Arnold, P.G.; Pairolero, P.C. Chest-Wall Reconstruction: An Account of 500 Consecutive Patients. *Plast. Reconstr. Surg.* **1996**, *98*, 804–810. [CrossRef]
35. Hazel, K.; Weyant, M.J. Chest Wall Resection and Reconstruction: Management of Complications. *Thorac. Surg. Clin.* **2015**, *25*, 517–521. [CrossRef]
36. Huang, H.; Kitano, K.; Nagayama, K.; Nitadori, J.I.; Anraku, M.; Murakawa, T.; Nakajima, J. Results of Bony Chest Wall Reconstruction with Expanded Polytetrafluoroethylene Soft Tissue Patch. *Ann. Thorac. Cardiovasc. Surg.* **2015**, *21*, 119–124. [CrossRef]
37. Thomas, M.; Shen, K.R. Primary Tumors of the Osseous Chest Wall and Their Management. *Thorac. Surg. Clin.* **2017**, *27*, 181–193. [CrossRef]
38. Dietz, U.A.; Spor, L.; Germer, C.-T. Management of mesh-related infections. *Chirurg* **2011**, *82*, 208–217. [CrossRef]
39. Volpe, C.M.; Peterson, S.; Doerr, R.J.; Karakousis, C.P. Forequarter Amputation with Fasciocutaneous Deltoid Flap Reconstruction for Malignant Tumors of the Upper Extremity. *Ann. Surg. Oncol.* **1997**, *4*, 298–302. [CrossRef]
40. Ferrario, T.; Palmer, P.; Karakousis, C.P. Technique of Forequarter (Interscapulothoracic) Amputation. *Clin. Orthop. Relat. Res.* **2004**, *423*, 191–195. [CrossRef]
41. Skoracki, R.J.; Chang, D.W. Reconstruction of the Chestwall and Thorax. *J. Surg. Oncol.* **2006**, *94*, 455–465. [CrossRef] [PubMed]
42. Lasso, J.M.; Uceda, M.; Peñalver, R.; Moreno, N.; Casteleiro, R.; Cano, R.P. Large Posterior Chest Wall Defect Reconstructed with a De-Epithelised Trans-Thoracic TRAM Flap. *J. Plast. Reconstr. Aesthet. Surg.* **2010**, *63*, e458-62. [CrossRef] [PubMed]
43. Kishi, K.; Imanishi, N.; Ninomiya, R.; Okabe, K.; Ohara, H.; Hattori, N.; Nakajima, H.; Nakajima, T. A Novel Approach to Thoracic Wall Reconstruction Based on a Muscle Perforator. *J. Plast. Reconstr. Aesthet. Surg.* **2010**, *63*, 1289–1293. [CrossRef] [PubMed]
44. Hubmer, M.; Leithner, A.; Kamolz, L.P. Re: Shoulder Silhouette and Axilla Reconstruction with Free Composite Elbow Tissue Transfer Following Interscapulothoracic Amputation. *J. Plast. Reconstr. Aesthet. Surg.* **2014**, *67*, e232–e233. [CrossRef]
45. Wilks, D.J.; Hassan, Z.; Bhasker, D.; Kay, S.P.J. Re: Shoulder Silhouette and Axilla Reconstruction with Free Composite Elbow Tissue Transfer Following Interscapulothoracic Amputation. *J. Plast. Reconstr. Aesthet. Surg.* **2014**, *67*, 1162–1164. [CrossRef]
46. Kuffler, D.P. Coping with Phantom Limb Pain. *Mol. Neurobiol.* **2018**, *55*, 70–84. [CrossRef]
47. Luo, Y.; Anderson, T.A. Phantom Limb Pain A Review of the Literature. *Int. Anesthesiol. Clin.* **2016**, *54*, 121–139. [CrossRef]
48. Dumanian, G.A.; Potter, B.K.; Mioton, L.M.; Ko, J.H.; Cheesborough, J.E.; Souza, J.M.; Ertl, W.J.; Tintle, S.M.; Nanos, G.P.; Valerio, I.L.; et al. Targeted Muscle Reinnervation Treats Neuroma and Phantom Pain in Major Limb Amputees: A Randomized Clinical Trial. *Ann. Surg.* **2019**, *270*, 238–246. [CrossRef]
49. Mioton, L.M.; Dumanian, G.A.; Shah, N.; Qiu, C.S.; Ertl, W.J.; Potter, B.K.; Souza, J.M.; Valerio, I.L.; Ko, J.H.; Jordan, S.W. Targeted Muscle Reinnervation Improves Residual Limb Pain, Phantom Limb Pain, and Limb Function: A Prospective Study of 33 Major Limb Amputees. *Clin. Orthop. Relat. Res.* **2020**, *478*, 2161–2167. [CrossRef]
50. Valerio, I.L.; Dumanian, G.A.; Jordan, S.W.; Mioton, L.M.; Bowen, J.B.; West, J.M.; Porter, K.; Ko, J.H.; Souza, J.M.; Potter, B.K. Preemptive Treatment of Phantom and Residual Limb Pain with Targeted Muscle Reinnervation at the Time of Major Limb Amputation. *J. Am. Coll. Surg.* **2019**, *228*, 217–226. [CrossRef]
51. Souza, J.M.; Cheesborough, J.E.; Ko, J.H.; Cho, M.S.; Kuiken, T.A.; Dumanian, G.A. Targeted Muscle Reinnervation: A Novel Approach to Postamputation Neuroma Pain. *Clin. Orthop. Relat. Res.* **2014**, *472*, 2984–2990. [CrossRef] [PubMed]

52. Windhager, R.; Millesi, H.; Kotz, R. Resection-Replantation for Primary Malignant Tumours of the Arm. An Alternative to Fore-Quarter Amputation. *J. Bone Joint Surg. Br.* **1995**, *77*, 176–184. [CrossRef] [PubMed]
53. Rickelt, J.; Hoekstra, H.; Van Coevorden, F.; De Vreeze, R.; Verhoef, C.; Van Geel, A.N. Forequarter Amputation for Malignancy. *Br. J. Surg.* **2009**, *96*, 792–798. [CrossRef] [PubMed]
54. Heuker, D.; Lengele, B.; Delecluse, V.; Weynand, B.; Liistro, G.; Balduyck, B.; Noirhomme, P.; Poncelet, A.J. Subjective and Objective Assessment of Quality of Life after Chest Wall Resection. *Eur. J. Cardio-Thorac. Surg.* **2011**, *39*, 102–108. [CrossRef]
55. Hickman, R.L.J.; Daly, B.J.; Douglas, S.L.; Clochesy, J.M. Informational Coping Style and Depressive Symptoms in Family Decision Makers. *Am. J. Crit. Care* **2010**, *19*, 410–420. [CrossRef]

# Article

# Intraoperative Blood Flow Analysis of DIEP vs. ms-TRAM Flap Breast Reconstruction Combining Transit-Time Flowmetry and Microvascular Indocyanine Green Angiography

Alexander Geierlehner *, Raymund E. Horch, Ingo Ludolph and Andreas Arkudas

Department of Plastic and Hand Surgery and Laboratory for Tissue Engineering and Regenerative Medicine, University Hospital Erlangen, Friedrich Alexander University Erlangen-Nürnberg (FAU), 91054 Erlangen, Germany; raymund.horch@uk-erlangen.de (R.E.H.); ingo.ludolph@uk-erlangen.de (I.L.); andreas.arkudas@uk-erlangen.de (A.A.)
* Correspondence: alexander.geierlehner@uk-erlangen.de; Tel.: +49-9131-85-33277

**Abstract:** Background: Vascular patency is the key element for high flap survival rates. The purpose of this study was to assess and compare the blood flow characteristics of deep inferior epigastric perforator (DIEP) and muscle-sparing transverse rectus abdominis musculocutaneous (ms-TRAM) flaps for autologous breast reconstruction. Methods: This prospective clinical study combined Transit-Time Flowmetry and microvascular Indocyanine Green Angiography for the measurement of blood flow volume, vascular resistance, and intrinsic transit time. Results: Twenty female patients (mean age, 52 years) received 24 free flaps (14 DIEP and 10 ms-TRAM flaps). The mean arterial blood flow of the flap in situ was $7.2 \pm 1.9$ mL/min in DIEP flaps and $11.5 \pm 4.8$ mL/min in ms-TRAM flaps ($p < 0.05$). After anastomosis, the mean arterial blood flow was $9.7 \pm 5.6$ mL/min in DIEP flaps and $13.5 \pm 4.2$ mL/min in ms-TRAM flaps ($p = 0.07$). The arterial vascular resistance of DIEP flaps was significantly higher than that of ms-TRAM flaps. The intrinsic transit time of DIEP flaps was $52 \pm 18$ s, and that of ms-TRAM flaps was $33 \pm 11$ s ($p < 0.05$). The flap survival rate was 100%. One DIEP flap with the highest intrinsic transit time (77 s) required surgical revision due to arterial thrombosis. Conclusion: In this study, we established the blood flow characteristics of free DIEP and ms-TRAM flaps showing different blood flow rates, vascular resistances, and intrinsic transit times. These standard values will help to determine the predictive values for vascular compromise, hence improving the safety of autologous breast reconstruction procedures.

**Keywords:** microsurgery; flap imaging; perforator flaps; autologous breast reconstruction; free tissue transfer; indocyanine green angiography; transit-time flowmetry

## 1. Introduction

Nowadays, abdominal tissue as the main source for breast reconstruction is preferably harvested either as a complete muscle-preserving deep inferior epigastric perforator (DIEP) flap or as a muscle-sparing transverse rectus abdominis musculocutaneous (ms-TRAM) flap [1,2]. The ability to reconstruct the female breast in a like-with-like fashion with low donor site morbidity has led to its widespread use [3]. Some of the latest tissue engineering and regenerative medicine methods aiming to overcome donor site sequelae are promising but not yet clinically feasible [4,5]. Although both DIEP and ms-TRAM flaps have overall low complication rates, partial flap necrosis and total flap loss due to vascular compromise remain imminent postoperative risks [6]. Sufficient vascular perfusion remains a key aspect for the overall outcome and flap survival. In the last few years, numerous clinical studies assessed the intra- and postoperative perfusion of free flaps using different technologies [7–14]. However, several studies aiming to understand the hemodynamics of free flaps showed methodological flaws such as a heterogeneous study population, small sample sizes of the included flap types in terms of tissue composition, the sole assessment of arterial flow characteristics, or the use of nowadays outdated technologies [15–19]. This study measures and compares intraoperative arterial and venous blood flow and perfusion characteristics of DIEP and ms-TRAM flaps for breast reconstruction combining Transit-Time Flowmetry (TTFM) and Indocyanine Green Angiography at a microscopic level (mICG-A). TTFM, an ultrasound-based technology for the assessment of vascular blood flow, was originally introduced into clinical practice for cardiac surgery [20,21]. Validation studies showed highly accurate and reproducible measurements which enabled its extension towards other surgical specialties such as vascular surgery and microsurgery [22–24]. The intravenous application of Indocyanine Green in combination with microscope-integrated fluorescence-based video angiography (IR800) and the analysis tool FLOW800 (Carl Zeiss, Oberkochen, Germany) enables the recording, measurement, and assessment of the microvascular patency and blood flow characteristics of vessels just a few millimeters in diameter [25,26]. The assembly of these two state-of-the art technologies is considered a novel approach. We believe that an advanced understanding of their hemodynamic properties will improve the safety of the two most commonly used free flaps for autologous breast reconstruction. This study further aimed to establish normative blood flow and perfusion values as groundwork for the determination of predictive values for postoperative thrombotic events.

## 2. Materials and Methods

Patients receiving DIEP or ms-TRAM flaps for breast reconstruction were enrolled in this prospective mono-centered clinical study. The study was approved by the Ethical Committee in accordance with the Declaration of Helsinki. Prior to study inclusion, written consent was given by each patient.

*2.1. Surgical Technique*

Autologous breast reconstructions were performed by three experienced surgeons. All patients received a standardized computed tomography angiography (CTA) of the abdomen for perforator mapping prior to surgery. Depending on the anatomy of the selected perforators (size, course, and number), the patients included in this study received DIEP or ms-TRAM free flaps for autologous breast reconstruction. Our postoperative anticoagulation regimen usually consists of low-molecular-weight heparin application subcutaneously until full mobilization is achieved. If contraindications for low-molecular-weight heparin exist, patients usually receive weight-adjusted unfractionated heparin. Patients suffering from hyperthyroidism, thyroid adenoma or autonomy, and known allergies/hypersensitivity to Indocyanine green or sodium iodide were excluded. The patient body temperature was kept stable by using a warming mattress (37 °C) and maintaining the ambient temperature between 20 °C and 22 °C. All patients received a balanced intraoperative crystalloid volume substitution of, on average, 53 mL/kg (mean: 3780 ± 1710 mL) in order to maintain stable hemodynamic conditions. The average intraoperative blood loss was 140 ± 100 mL. The internal mammary artery (IMA) and vein (IMV) were used as recipient vessels in all cases. Each flap was harvested in a standardized fashion with the inferior epigastric artery and the inferior epigastric vein as vascular pedicle dissected towards their origin at the external iliac artery and vein. Each vascular pedicle consisted of one artery and one vein. DIEP and ms-TRAM flaps with more than one venous anastomosis were excluded from this study. All arterial and venous anastomoses were performed end to end. Arterial anastomoses were hand-sewn with interrupted nylon sutures, whereas all venous anastomoses were performed using a venous coupler device (Synovis Micro Companies Alliance, Inc., Birmingham, AL, USA).

*2.2. Transit-Time Flow Measurement (TTFM)*

MiraQ™ Vascular (Medistim ASA, Oslo, Norway) was used for intraoperative blood flow measurements. The probe diameter ranged from 1.5 to 4 mm depending on the vessel size. Blood flow values were recorded for several minutes until a steady curve of blood flow occurred (Figure 1). Arterial and venous blood flow volume measurements were performed at three predefined time points during surgery:

- Measurement F was taken after flap elevation and isolation on its vascular pedicle prior to free flap transfer
- Measurement R was performed at the recipient vessel prior to anastomosis.
- Measurement AA was taken at the vascular pedicle after anastomosis and flap reperfusion.

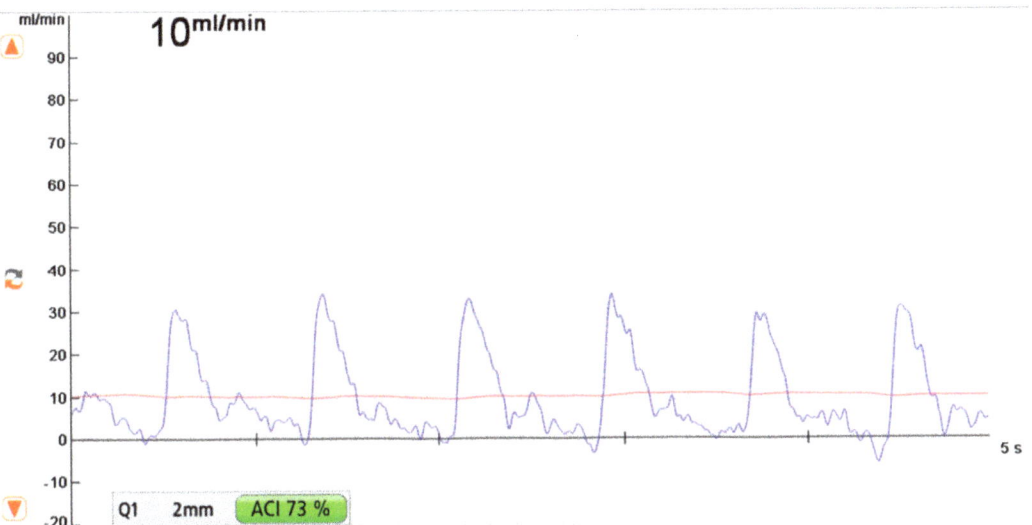

**Figure 1.** Transit-Time Flow Volume Measurement (TTFM) showing a flow volume of 10 mL/min with an Acoustic Coupling Index (ACI) of 73% using a 2 mm probe.

The mean arterial pressure was measured and documented at each measurement time point.

*2.3. Microvascular Indocyanine Green Angiography (mICG-A)*

In this clinical study, Indocyanine Green (ICG) was administered as an intravenous bolus (3 mL VERDYE 5 mg/mL) after arterial and venous anastomosis and flap reperfusion. The anastomosed flap pedicle was placed below the microscope (KINEVO 900, Carl Zeiss, Oberkochen, Germany). Recordings of the supplying artery and draining vein started immediately after intravenous ICG application and were continued until the intensity of the ICG markedly decreased in the artery and vein. Intraoperative fluorescence analysis requires the selection of certain regions of interest (ROI). Two ROIs were placed at the flap pedicle, one at the supplying artery, and the other at the draining vein close to the anastomosis, uncovered from any surrounding tissue (Figure 2). FLOW800 measures the intensity of ICG in the regions of interest for a time period and enables the instant visualization of blood flow variations within small vessels. The time between the maximum ICG intensity of arterial inflow and venous outflow is defined as Intrinsic Transit Time (ITT), which is considered as a parameter of blood flow velocity within the flap (Figure 2) [27].

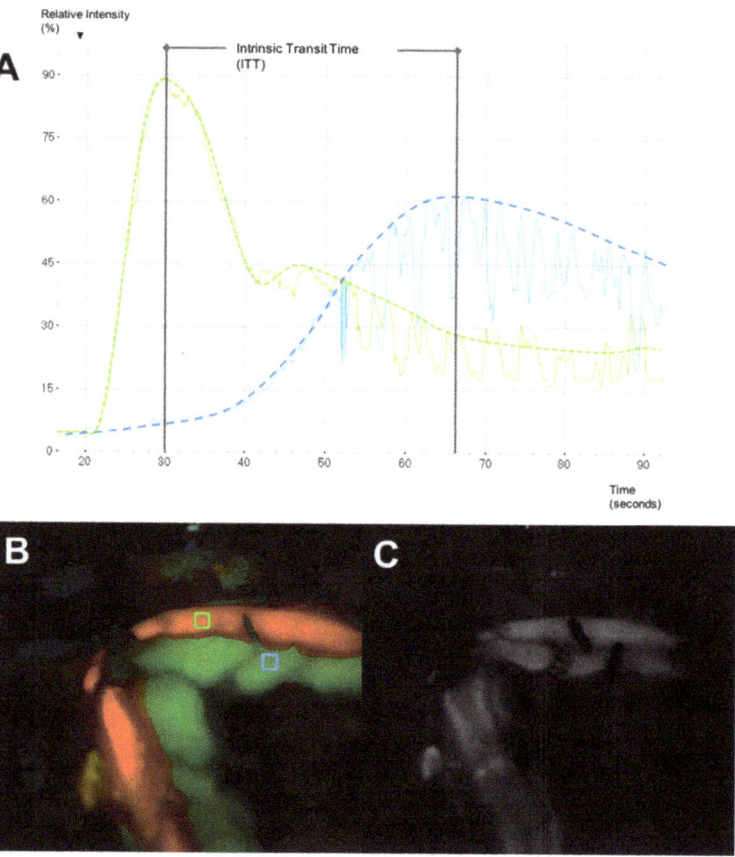

**Figure 2.** (**A**) Microvascular Indocyanine Green Angiography (mICG-A) flow curves in two selected regions of interest (ROI) (green curve: arterial flow, blue curve: venous flow). The spikes are artefacts caused by respiratory movements. (**B**) Delay Map obtained with FLOW800 illustrating both ROIs (green ROI placed at the artery, blue ROI placed at the vein) and picturing the two flow curves. (**C**) Gray-scale map of fluorescence intensity (Intensity Map) illustrating both artery and vein after anastomosis.

*2.4. Vascular Resistance*

Arterial vascular Resistance ($aVR$) was calculated as millimeters of mercury per milliliter per minute (mmHg/mL/min) based on a previously reported method in adherence to the Poiseuille's Law, using the following formula: [28,29]

$$R = \Delta P / Q$$

$R = aVR$ = arterial vascular resistance, $\Delta P$ = blood pressure gradient = mean arterial blood pressure ($MAP$)–mean venous blood pressure ($MVP$). The mean venous blood pressure ($MVP$) is estimated to be close to 0 and, as a result, disregarded in the calculation of vascular resistances. This results in the following formula: [28–31]

$$aVR = MAP / aBF$$

*2.5. Data Analysis and Synthesis*

Descriptive analysis was performed for patient demographics. Data are shown as mean ± standard deviation. Changes in blood flow and vascular resistance between the different time points within one group were calculated using the paired Student's $t$-test. Blood flow and vascular resistance between DIEP and ms-TRAM flaps at different time points was analyzed using an unpaired Student's $t$-test. Nonparametric data were analyzed with the Wilcoxon matched-pairs rank test within one group, whereas the Mann–Whitney U test was used for analyses of nonparametric data between DIEP and ms-TRAM flaps. The correlation of data assuming Gaussian distribution was calculated using the Pearson correlation coefficient. The Spearman's rank correlation coefficient was used for data not passing a test for normality. The significance level was set at $p < 0.05$. Three outliers (one arterial and two venous blood flow values at the recipient site (Measurement R) before anastomosis) were identified using the ROUT method ($Q = 1\%$) and appropriately excluded from statistical analysis. Statistical analyses and graphic illustrations were performed using GraphPad Prism (GraphPad Software, Inc., San Diego, CA, USA).

## 3. Results

A total of 20 female patients receiving 24 DIEP or ms-TRAM flaps for breast reconstruction were included in this prospective study. Patients' average age was 52 years, ranging from 39 to 68 years. Fourteen flaps were harvested as DIEP (57%), and 10 as ms-TRAM (43%). Seven ms-TRAM flaps were classified as ms1-TRAM flap, and three as ms2-TRAM flap, according to the classification by Nahabedian et al. (Table 1) [32]. The median flap weight was 435 g, ranging from 299 to 1169 g. The median weight of DIEP flaps (390 g) was not significantly different from that of ms-TRAM flaps (491 g). The average flap ischemia time was 46 min. The venous coupler size ranged from 2.5 to 3.5 mm.

*3.1. Blood Flow Volume (mL/min)*

The average blood flow of the flap artery isolated as pedicle prior to free tissue transfer (F) was $9 \pm 4$ mL/min (mean ± SD). Its venous outflow was lower ($7.5 \pm 3.5$ mL/min), resulting in an artery-to-vein (A/V) flow ratio of $1.4 \pm 0.7$. The mean blood flow of the recipient internal mammary artery and vein prior to flap anastomosis (R) was $16.9 \pm 6.3$ and $9.4 \pm 8$ mL/min, respectively. After anastomosis (AA), the arterial and venous blood flow volume was $11.3 \pm 5.3$ and $7.4 \pm 4.1$ mL/min, respectively, with an A/V flow ratio of $1.8 \pm 1.3$. The arterial blood flow of the intact recipient artery (R) significantly decreased after anastomosis with the flap artery (AA) ($p = 0.002$). However, the arterial and venous blood flow of the included flaps did not significantly change after flap transfer. (Figure 3) The blood flow of the intact recipient artery (R) did not alter the blood flow of the flaps after anastomosis. There was a significant positive correlation between the arterial inflow and the venous outflow both before (F) and after anastomosis (AA) ($p < 0.05$). The arterial and venous blood flow rates before and after anastomosis in DIEP flaps were lower than in ms-TRAM flaps (Table 2). There was no correlation between the arterial blood flow volume and the flap weight. The flap ischemia time did not change the blood flow rates of the examined flaps.

*3.2. Vascular Resistance (mmHg/mL/min)*

The mean arterial vascular resistance (aVR) of the included flaps prior to tissue transfer ($10 \pm 4.2$ mmHg/mL/min) did not significantly change after anastomosis ($9.2 \pm 5.2$ mmHg/mL/min). The vascular resistance of the recipient artery, however, significantly increased from $5.4 \pm 2.6$ to $9.2 \pm 5.2$ mmHg/mL/min after anastomosis to the flap ($p < 0.001$). The average arterial vascular resistance (aVR) of DIEP flaps prior to (F) and after flap transfer (AA) was $12 \pm 3.8$ and $11.2 \pm 5.8$ mmHg/mL/min, respectively. By contrast, ms-TRAM flaps had significantly lower arterial vascular resistance values prior to ($7.2 \pm 3$ mmHg/mL/min; $p = 0.004$) and after flap reperfusion ($6.5 \pm 2.3$ mmHg/mL/min;

$p$ = 0.02) (Figure 4 and Table 3). There was no correlation between the arterial vascular resistance and the weight of the included flaps before or after flap transfer.

**Table 1.** Characteristics of the included patients. Abbreviations: DIEP: deep inferior epigastric perforator; ms-TRAM: muscle-sparing transverse rectus abdominis musculocutaneous.

| Patient Number | Age (Years) | Type of Flap | Flap Weight (g) | Ischemia Time (min) | Intrinsic Transit Time (s) | Hemodynamic Postoperative Complications |
|---|---|---|---|---|---|---|
| 1 | 46 | DIEP | 459 | 70 | 37 | - |
| 2 | 55 | ms-TRAM | 340 | 49 | 46 | - |
|   |    | DIEP | 314 | 53 | 36 | - |
| 3 | 57 | DIEP | 1036 | 45 | 27 | - |
| 4 | 46 | ms-TRAM | 344 | 46 | 50 | - |
| 5 | 39 | ms-TRAM | 1169 | 35 | 22 | - |
| 6 | 62 | DIEP | 309 | 37 | 60 | - |
| 7 | 49 | DIEP | 370 | 56 | 14 | - |
|   |    | ms-TRAM | 310 | 64 | 25 | - |
| 8 | 47 | DIEP | 514 | 42 | 76 | - |
| 9 | 57 | ms-TRAM | 328 | 56 | 30 | - |
| 10 | 55 | DIEP | 591 | 54 | 59 | - |
| 11 | 51 | DIEP | 352 | 50 | 77 | Arterial Thrombosis |
| 12 | 55 | ms-TRAM | 464 | 42 | 28 | - |
|    |    | ms-TRAM | 517 | 32 | 27 | - |
| 13 | 44 | DIEP | 365 | 44 | 72 | - |
| 14 | 56 | DIEP | 310 | 48 | 48 | - |
| 15 | 49 | DIEP | 688 | 44 | 63 | - |
| 16 | 43 | DIEP | 299 | 41 | 51 | - |
| 17 | 64 | ms-TRAM | 691 | 41 | 20 | - |
|    |    | ms-TRAM | 810 | 40 | 44 | - |
| 18 | 68 | DIEP | 713 | 43 | 57 | - |
| 19 | 42 | ms-TRAM | 631 | 38 | 39 | - |
| 20 | 51 | DIEP | 410 | 42 | 52 | - |

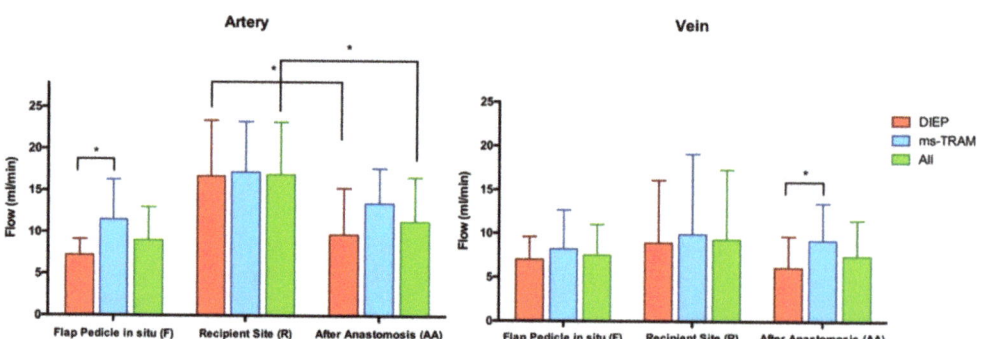

**Figure 3.** Arterial and venous blood flows (mL/min) at three predefined time points (F, R, AA). The bars represent means ± standard error (* indicates significant differences).

**Table 2.** Comparison of the Blood flow (mL/min) of the Flap Pedicle in situ (F), of the Recipient Artery (R), and After Anastomosis (AA).

| Type of Flap | No. of Flaps | Flow in mL/in (Mean ± SD) | | | | | | | | p-Value | | |
|---|---|---|---|---|---|---|---|---|---|---|---|---|
| | | Flap Pedicle In Situ (F) | | | Recipient Vessel (R) | | After Anastomosis (AA) | | | | | |
| | | Artery | Vein | Ratio A/V | Artery | Vein | Artery | Vein | Ratio A/V | Artery vs. Vein | F vs. AA | R vs. AA |
| All | 24 | 9 ± 4 | 7.5 ± 3.5 | 1.4 ± 0.7 | 16.9 ± 6.3 | 9.4 ± 8 | 11.3 ± 5.3 | 7.4 ± 4.1 | 1.8 ± 1.3 | 0.07 (F); **0.0001** (AA) | 0.1 (A); 0.9 (V) | **0.002** (A); 0.4 (V) |
| DIEP | 14 | 7.2 ± 1.9 | 7 ± 2.6 | 1.1 ± 0.3 | 16.7 ± 6.7 | 8.9 ± 7.2 | 9.7 ± 5.6 | 6.1 ± 3.6 | 1.9 ± 1.6 | 0.5 (F); **0.002** (AA) | 0.2 (A); 0.5 (V) | **0.01** (A); 0.2 (V) |
| ms-TRAM | 10 | 11.5 ± 4.8 | 8.2 ± 4.5 | 1.8 ± 1 | 17.2 ± 6.1 | 9.9 ± 9.2 | 13.5 ± 4.2 | 9.2 ± 4.3 | 1.7 ± 0.8 | **0.04** (F); **0.02** (AA) | 0.1 (A); 0.5 (V) | 0.1 (A); 0.9 (V) |
| p-value (DIEP vs. ms-TRAM) | | **0.02** | 0.5 | 0.06 | 0.85 | 0.96 | 0.07 | **0.04** | 0.8 | | | |

Bold numbers indicate significant differences.

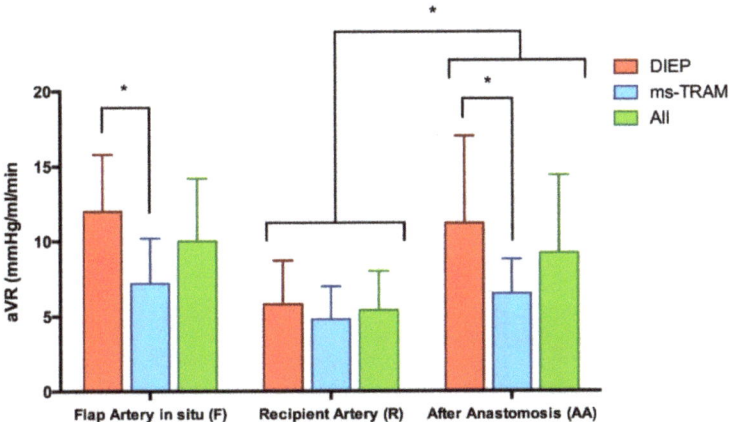

**Figure 4.** Arterial Vascular Resistance (aVR) at three predefined time points (F, R, AA). The bars represent means ± standard error (* indicates significant differences).

**Table 3.** Comparison of Arterial Vascular Resistances (mmHg/mL/min) of the flap pedicle in situ (F), of the Recipient Artery (R) and After Anastomosis (AA).

| Type of Flap | Arterial Vascular Resistance (aVR) in mmHg/mL/min (Mean ± SD) | | | p-Value | |
|---|---|---|---|---|---|
| | Flap Artery (FA) | Recipient Artery (RA) | After Anastomosis (AA) | FA vs. AA | RA vs. AA |
| All | 10 ± 4.2 | 5.4 ± 2.6 | 9.2 ± 5.2 | 0.5 | **0.0002** |
| DIEP | 12 ± 3.8 | 5.8 ± 2.9 | 11.2 ± 5.8 | 0.7 | **0.005** |
| ms-TRAM | 7.2 ± 3 | 4.8 ± 2.2 | 6.5 ± 2.3 | 0.5 | **0.02** |
| p-value (DIEP vs. ms-TRAM) | **0.004** | 0.4 | **0.02** | | |

The bold numbers indicate significant differences.

### 3.3. Intrinsic Transit Time

The mean Intrinsic Transit Time (ITT) after flap reperfusion was 44 ± 18 s (s), ranging from 14 to 77 s. The average ITT of DIEP flaps (52 ± 18 s) was significantly higher than the average ITT of ms-TRAM flaps (33 ± 11 s) ($p = 0.005$). The average vascular resistance at the time of ITT measurements was 9 ± 4.7 mmHg/mL/min. There was a significant negative correlation between the arterial blood flow and the ITT after anastomosis ($p = 0.001$)

(Figure 5). By contrast, a significant positive correlation was seen between the arterial vascular resistance (aVR) and the ITT after anastomosis ($p = 0.0006$) (Figure 6). There was no correlation between the ITT and flap ischemia time, flap weight, or mean arterial pressure (MAP).

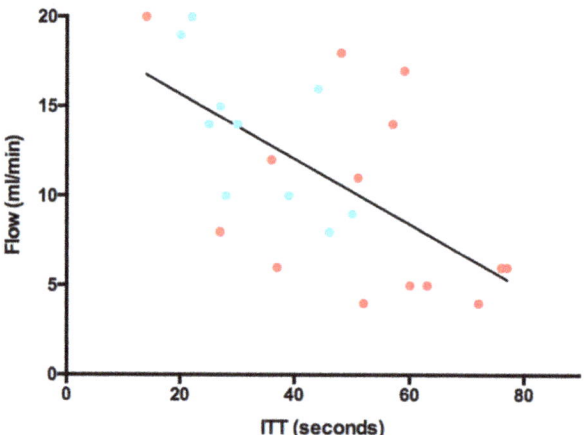

**Figure 5.** Arterial blood flow (mL/min) versus Intrinsic Transit Time (ITT, seconds); $y = -0.182x + 19.33$; $p = 0.001$; $r2 = 0.3875$; red dots = DIEP flaps; blue dots = ms-TRAM flaps.

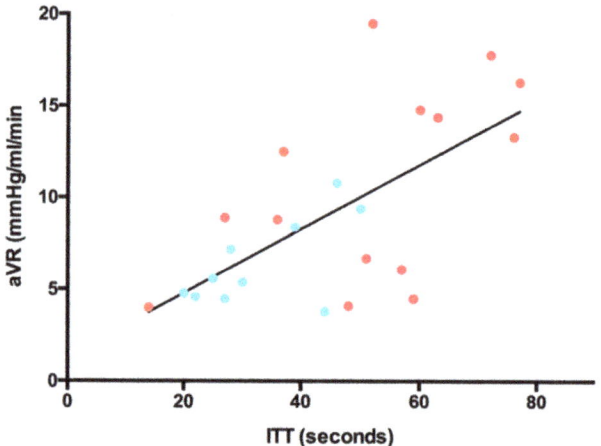

**Figure 6.** Arterial Vascular Resistance (aVR, mmHg/mL/min) versus Intrinsic Transit Time (ITT, seconds); $y = 0.1744x + 1.308$; $p = 0.0006$; $r2 = 0.4196$; red dots = DIEP flaps; blue dots = ms-TRAM flaps.

Of all included free flaps, one DIEP flap required surgical revision due to a thrombotic event occurring on the fourth day after autologous breast reconstruction. The ITT of this flap was 77 s. After emergency thrombectomy, no further complication occurred. The overall flap survival rate was 100%.

## 4. Discussion

Numerous recently developed technologies enable the illustration and measurement of vascularity and perfusion in free flaps at a pre-, intra, or postoperative stage, with the ultimate goal to increase their safety and efficacy [7,11,12,18,33–36]. The combination of Transit-Time Flowmetry (TTFM) and microvascular Indocyanine Green Angiography (mICG-A) is considered a unique approach aiming to meticulously evaluate and compare the intraoperative blood flow characteristics of DIEP and ms-TRAM flaps. A recent study successfully established this combination for the detection of early venous congestion in an animal flap model [37]. However, no study so far assessed the combined potential of these techniques in a clinical setting for autologous breast reconstructions. Our results show that the overall arterial blood flow of both DIEP and ms-TRAM flaps did not significantly increase after anastomosis with the recipient internal mammary vessel. The blood flow of the intact recipient artery did not influence the arterial blood flow of the included flaps. In fact, it seemed to be the opposite. In this study, both DIEP and ms-TRAM flaps downregulated the recipient artery flow towards blood flow values of the in situ flap prior to tissue transfer. These observations are supported by other studies showing that the flow of the recipient artery can either be down- or upregulated after flap anastomosis, approximating blood flow values of the flap isolated on its pedicle before tissue transfer [19,38–40]. Lorenzetti et al. measured the blood flow of the thoracodorsal artery before and after anastomosis with ms-TRAM flaps and reported an upregulation of the recipient artery. Before anastomosis, the thoracodorsal artery had relatively low blood flow values (4.9 ± 3 mL/min) in situ. However, after anastomosis with the ms-TRAM flap, the blood flow increased (13.7 ± 5 mL/min) towards the original blood flow rate of the isolated flap pedicle in situ before tissue transfer [38]. This phenomenon was observed not only in fasciocutaneous but also in musculocutaneous and muscle free flaps and therefore seems to be irrespective of the tissue composition [40]. Previous studies reported generally different blood flow rates and vascular resistances in fasciocutaneous, musculocutaneous, muscle, and intraperitoneal flaps [31,38]. These findings support the notion that both blood flow and vascular resistance depend on the type of tissue and its relative proportion. The tissue composition determines the vascularity of each flap, which at the same time, reflects the vascular resistance. Free flaps mainly composed of muscle tissue contain a rich vascular network connected by resistance vessels, resulting in a lower vascular resistance than fasciocutaneous flaps with a rather sparse network of much smaller vessels [30,31]. In our study, ms-TRAM flaps had an average arterial blood flow of 13.5 mL/min and a vascular resistance of 6.4 mmHg/mL/min after anastomosis. By contrast, DIEP flaps showed significantly lower blood flow values and consequently a higher vascular resistance. Although both flaps were, apart from a small segment of the rectus abdominis muscle in ms-TRAM flaps, grossly composed of the same tissue, the difference in vascular resistance seemed to be a matter of vascularity. We theorize that a larger number of perforators in ms-TRAM flaps was the main reason for a lower vascular resistance, hence providing a higher overall and weight-adjusted arterial blood flow in comparison to DIEP flaps. The overall arterial inflow of the included flaps was about 1.4 to 1.8 times greater than the venous outflow. Selber et al. reported similar results in ms-TRAM and other fasciocutaneous flaps [41]. We theorize that the peripheral leakage of small blood vessels at the flap edges caused the disparity between arterial inflow and venous outflow. An A/V ratio of more than 1 seems to a certain level inevitable and needs to be considered by surgeons during free flap flow measurements.

Microvascular Indocyanine Green Angiography (mICG-A) combined with the microscope-integrated software FLOW800 provides valuable information on vascular patency and enables the real-time visualization of arterial in- and venous outflow in free flaps [42–44]. It is a matter of common pathophysiological knowledge that the alteration in blood flow, as part of the Virchow's triad, is a main contributor to thrombus formation in blood vessels [45,46]. Previous studies have already theorized that a prolonged ITT might be an indicator of low blood flow velocities, hence accounting for increased vascular resistances [27]. The combination of TTFM with mICG-A enabled to measure and detect a positive correlation of ITT with vascular resistance in free flaps. ITT, similar to blood flow, seems to depend on the flap tissue composition. In our study, the DIEP flap, which was composed of fasciocutaneous tissue, had a significantly higher average ITT (52 s) than the ms-TRAM flap (33 s), classified as musculocutaneous flap. These observations are supported by a previous study measuring a shorter ITT in muscle flaps (27.7 s) than in fasciocutaneous flaps (47.5 s) [26]. Holm et al. reported that an ITT of more than 50 s was associated with an increased risk for vascular compromise and surgical revision in free tissue transfer procedures [27]. The study, however, showed essential methodological flaws such as a heterogenous study population with varying free flap entities. In our study, eight flaps surpassed the threshold of 50 s without any hemodynamic postoperative complication. Only one DIEP flap with an ITT of 77 s required surgical revision due to a thrombotic event several days after flap transplantation. Although this was the highest ITT of all included flaps, the scarce occurrence of just a single hemodynamic complication several days after autologous breast reconstruction did not allow drawing any correlation between a prolonged ITT and the increased risk of postoperative hemodynamic complications. To the best of our knowledge, this is the first study that measures, compares, and detects hemodynamic differences between DIEP and ms-TRAM flaps. The clinical relevance of this study is the establishment of standard values of intraoperative hemodynamic and perfusion properties of DIEP and ms-TRAM flaps. We could detect significant differences in hemodynamics properties between DIEP and ms-TRAM flaps. Flaps with abnormally high or low blood flow values, according to our newly established standard hemodynamic characteristics, made a closer intraoperative assessment of anastomotic patency necessary. We are aware that these techniques do not replace a clinical examination but rather help to improve our intraoperative decision-making process. The results of this study, however, do not provide any recommendation in terms of favoring one or the other free flap type for autologous breast reconstruction. Historically, the choice between DIEP and ms-TRAM flap has been a far more extensive topic that needs to take numerous other variables into account. Our meticulous assessment of arterial and venous blood flow, arterial vascular resistance, and ITT at crucial intraoperative time points enables the establishment of normative values. This should help to assess vascular patency especially in cases where the surgeon or devices such as a regular hand-held Doppler fail to detect a more subtle vascular compromise.

## 5. Conclusions

In this study, we evaluated the hemodynamic characteristics of free DIEP and ms-TRAM flaps. The combination of Transit-Time Flowmetry and microvascular Indocyanine Green Angiography enabled the qualitative and quantitative intraoperative assessment of anastomotic patency. Our study serves as fundamental work for the determination of predictive values for postoperative thrombotic events and of cut-off values that will ease intraoperative decision making in the future.

**Author Contributions:** Conceptualization: A.G., R.E.H. and A.A.; Investigation: A.G., R.E.H., I.L. and A.A.; Methodology: A.G., I.L. and A.A.; Project administration: A.G., R.E.H. and A.A.; Resources: R.E.H.; Supervision: R.E.H. and A.A.; Validation: A.G. and A.A.; Visualization: A.G.; Writing—original draft: A.G.; Writing—review & editing: A.G., R.E.H., I.L. and A.A. All authors have read and agreed to the published version of the manuscript.

**Funding:** We acknowledge financial support by Deutsche Forschungsgemeinschaft and Friedrich-Alexander-Universität Erlangen-Nürnberg within the funding programme "Open Access Publication Funding".

**Institutional Review Board Statement:** The study was conducted according to the guidelines of the Declaration of Helsinki and approved by the Ethics Committee of Friedrich-Alexander-University of Erlangen-Nuremberg, Germany (registration number: 447_19B).

**Informed Consent Statement:** Informed consent was obtained from all subjects involved in the study.

**Data Availability Statement:** The datasets generated during the current study are available from the corresponding author on reasonable request.

**Acknowledgments:** The present work was performed in fulfillment of the requirements for obtaining the degree "Dr. med." for the author A.G.

**Conflicts of Interest:** The authors declare no conflict of interest.

## References

1. Eisenhardt, S.U.; Momeni, A.; von Fritschen, U.; Horch, R.E.; Stark, G.B.; Bannasch, H.; Harder, Y.; Heitmann, C.; Kremer, T.; Rieger, U.M.; et al. Breast reconstruction with the free TRAM or DIEP flap—What is the current standard? Consensus Statement of the German Speaking Working Group for Microsurgery of the Peripheral Nerves and Vessels. *Handchirurgie Mikrochirurgie Plastische Chirurgie* **2018**, *50*, 248–255. [CrossRef]
2. Cai, A.; Suckau, J.; Arkudas, A.; Beier, J.P.; Momeni, A.; Horch, R.E. Autologous Breast Reconstruction with Transverse Rectus Abdominis Musculocutaneous (TRAM) or Deep Inferior Epigastric Perforator (DIEP) Flaps: An Analysis of the 100 Most Cited Articles. *Med. Sci. Monit.* **2019**, *25*, 3520–3536. [CrossRef] [PubMed]
3. Fritschen, U.V.; Grill, B.; Wagner, J.; Schuster, H.; Sukhova, I.; Giunta, R.E.; Heitmann, C.; Andree, C.; Horch, R.E.; Kneser, U.; et al. Quality assurance in breast reconstruction—Establishment of a prospective national online registry for microsurgical breast reconstructions. *Handchirurgie Mikrochirurgie Plastische Chirurgie* **2020**, *52*, 58–66. [CrossRef]
4. Kengelbach-Weigand, A.; Tasbihi, K.; Strissel, P.L.; Schmid, R.; Marques, J.M.; Beier, J.P.; Beckmann, M.W.; Strick, R.; Horch, R.E.; Boos, A.M. Plasticity of patient-matched normal mammary epithelial cells is dependent on autologous adipose-derived stem cells. *Sci. Rep.* **2019**, *9*, 10722. [CrossRef]
5. Tong, J.; Mou, S.; Xiong, L.; Wang, Z.; Wang, R.; Weigand, A.; Yuan, Q.; Horch, R.E.; Sun, J.; Yang, J. Adipose-derived mesenchymal stem cells formed acinar-like structure when stimulated with breast epithelial cells in three-dimensional culture. *PLoS ONE* **2018**, *13*, e0204077. [CrossRef] [PubMed]
6. Jeong, W.; Lee, S.; Kim, J. Meta-analysis of flap perfusion and donor site complications for breast reconstruction using pedicled versus free TRAM and DIEP flaps. *Breast* **2018**, *38*, 45–51. [CrossRef]
7. Beier, J.P.; Horch, R.E.; Arkudas, A.; Dragu, A.; Schmitz, M.; Kneser, U. Decision-making in DIEP and ms-TRAM flaps: The potential role for a combined laser Doppler spectrophotometry system. *J. Plast. Reconstr. Aesthetic Surg. JPRAS* **2013**, *66*, 73–79. [CrossRef]
8. Wechselberger, G.; Rumer, A.; Schoeller, T.; Schwabegger, A.; Ninkovic, M.; Anderl, H. Free-flap monitoring with tissue-oxygen measurement. *J. Reconstr. Microsurg.* **1997**, *13*, 125–130. [CrossRef]
9. Machens, H.G.; Mailänder, P.; Pasel, J.; Lutz, B.S.; Funke, M.; Siemers, F.; Berger, A.C. Flap perfusion after free musculocutaneous tissue transfer: The impact of postoperative complications. *Plast. Reconstr. Surg.* **2000**, *105*, 2395–2399. [CrossRef]
10. Udesen, A.; Løntoft, E.; Kristensen, S.R. Monitoring of free TRAM flaps with microdialysis. *J. Reconstr. Microsurg.* **2000**, *16*, 101–106. [CrossRef]
11. Ludolph, I.; Arkudas, A.; Schmitz, M.; Boos, A.M.; Taeger, C.D.; Rother, U.; Horch, R.E.; Beier, J.P. Cracking the perfusion code?: Laser-assisted Indocyanine Green angiography and combined laser Doppler spectrophotometry for intraoperative evaluation of tissue perfusion in autologous breast reconstruction with DIEP or ms-TRAM flaps. *J. Plast. Reconstr. Aesthetic Surg. JPRAS* **2016**, *69*, 1382–1388. [CrossRef]
12. Ludolph, I.; Horch, R.E.; Arkudas, A.; Schmitz, M. Enhancing Safety in Reconstructive Microsurgery Using Intraoperative Indocyanine Green Angiography. *Front. Surg.* **2019**, *6*, 39. [CrossRef]
13. Yuen, J.C.; Feng, Z. Monitoring free flaps using the laser Doppler flowmeter: Five-year experience. *Plast. Reconstr. Surg.* **2000**, *105*, 55–61. [CrossRef]
14. Salmi, A.M.; Tierala, E.K.; Tukiainen, E.J.; Asko-Seljavaara, S.L. Blood flow in free muscle flaps measured by color Doppler ultrasonography. *Microsurgery* **1995**, *16*, 666–672. [CrossRef]
15. Figus, A.; Mosahebi, A.; Ramakrishnan, V. Microcirculation in DIEP flaps: A study of the haemodynamics using laser Doppler flowmetry and lightguide reflectance spectrophotometry. *J. Plast. Reconstr. Aesthetic Surg. JPRAS* **2006**, *59*, 604–612, discussion 613. [CrossRef]
16. Heitland, A.S.; Markowicz, M.; Koellensperger, E.; Schoth, F.; Feller, A.M.; Pallua, N. Duplex ultrasound imaging in free transverse rectus abdominis muscle, deep inferior epigastric artery perforator, and superior gluteal artery perforator flaps: Early and long-term comparison of perfusion changes in free flaps following breast reconstruction. *Ann. Plast. Surg.* **2005**, *55*, 117–121. [CrossRef]
17. Sekido, M.; Yamamoto, Y.; Sugihara, T. Arterial blood flow changes after free tissue transfer in head and neck reconstruction. *Plast. Reconstr. Surg.* **2005**, *115*, 1547–1552. [CrossRef]
18. Nasir, S.; Baykal, B.; Altuntas, S.; Aydin, M.A. Hemodynamic differences in blood flow between free skin and muscles flaps: Prospective study. *J. Reconstr. Microsurg.* **2009**, *25*, 355–360. [CrossRef]
19. Malagon, P.; Carrasco, C.; Vila, J.; Priego, D.; Higueras, C. Intraoperative hemodynamic changes in the arterial blood flow measured by transit time flowmetry (TTFM) during breast reconstruction with free diep flap. *J. Plast. Reconstr. Aesthetic Surg. JPRAS* **2020**, *73*, 1775–1784. [CrossRef]
20. Groom, R.; Tryzelaar, J.; Forest, R.; Niimi, K.; Cecere, G.; Donegan, D.; Katz, S.; Weldner, P.; Quinn, R.; Braxton, J.; et al. Intra-operative quality assessment of coronary artery bypass grafts. *Perfusion* **2001**, *16*, 511–518. [CrossRef]
21. D'Ancona, G.; Karamanoukian, H.L.; Ricci, M.; Schmid, S.; Bergsland, J.; Salerno, T.A. Graft revision after transit time flow measurement in off-pump coronary artery bypass grafting. *Eur. J. Cardio-Thorac. Surg. Off. J. Eur. Assoc. Cardio-Thorac. Surg.* **2000**, *17*, 287–293. [CrossRef]
22. Albäck, A.; Mäkisalo, H.; Nordin, A.; Lepäntalo, M. Validity and reproducibility of transit time flowmetry. *Ann. Chir. Gynaecol.* **1996**, *85*, 325–331.

23. Laustsen, J.; Pedersen, E.M.; Terp, K.; Steinbrüchel, D.; Kure, H.H.; Paulsen, P.K.; Jørgensen, H.; Paaske, W.P. Validation of a new transit time ultrasound flowmeter in man. *Eur. J. Vasc. Endovasc. Surg. Off. J. Eur. Soc. Vasc. Surg.* **1996**, *12*, 91–96. [CrossRef]
24. Beldi, G.; Bosshard, A.; Hess, O.M.; Althaus, U.; Walpoth, B.H. Transit time flow measurement: Experimental validation and comparison of three different systems. *Ann. Thorac. Surg.* **2000**, *70*, 212–217. [CrossRef]
25. Holm, C.; Mayr, M.; Höfter, E.; Dornseifer, U.; Ninkovic, M. Assessment of the patency of microvascular anastomoses using microscope-integrated near-infrared angiography: A preliminary study. *Microsurgery* **2009**, *29*, 509–514. [CrossRef]
26. Holzbach, T.; Artunian, N.; Spanholtz, T.A.; Volkmer, E.; Engelhardt, T.O.; Giunta, R.E. Microscope-integrated intraoperative indocyanine green angiography in plastic surgery. *Handchirurgie Mikrochirurgie Plastische Chirurgie* **2012**, *44*, 84–88. [CrossRef]
27. Holm, C.; Dornseifer, U.; Sturtz, G.; Basso, G.; Schuster, T.; Ninkovic, M. The intrinsic transit time of free microvascular flaps: Clinical and prognostic implications. *Microsurgery* **2010**, *30*, 91–96. [CrossRef]
28. Mahabir, R.C.; Williamson, J.S.; Carr, N.J.; Courtemanche, D.J. Vascular resistance in human muscle flaps. *Ann. Plast. Surg.* **2001**, *47*, 148–152. [CrossRef]
29. Warren, J.V.; Gorlin, R. Calculation of vascular resistance. *Methods Med. Res.* **1958**, *7*, 98–99. [PubMed]
30. Sasmor, M.T.; Reus, W.F.; Straker, D.J.; Colen, L.B. Vascular resistance considerations in free-tissue transfer. *J. Reconstr. Microsurg.* **1992**, *8*, 195–200. [CrossRef] [PubMed]
31. Takanari, K.; Kamei, Y.; Toriyama, K.; Yagi, S.; Torii, S. Differences in blood flow volume and vascular resistance between free flaps: Assessment in 58 cases. *J. Reconstr. Microsurg.* **2009**, *25*, 39–45. [CrossRef] [PubMed]
32. Nahabedian, M.Y.; Momen, B.; Galdino, G.; Manson, P.N. Breast Reconstruction with the free TRAM or DIEP flap: Patient selection, choice of flap, and outcome. *Plast. Reconstr. Surg.* **2002**, *110*, 466–475, discussion 467–476. [CrossRef] [PubMed]
33. Steiner, D.; Horch, R.E.; Ludolph, I.; Schmitz, M.; Beier, J.P.; Arkudas, A. Interdisciplinary Treatment of Breast Cancer After Mastectomy with Autologous Breast Reconstruction Using Abdominal Free Flaps in a University Teaching Hospital—A Standardized and Safe Procedure. *Front. Oncol.* **2020**, *10*, 177. [CrossRef]
34. Hembd, A.S.; Yan, J.; Zhu, H.; Haddock, N.T.; Teotia, S.S. Intraoperative Assessment of DIEP Flap Breast Reconstruction Using Indocyanine Green Angiography: Reduction of Fat Necrosis, Resection Volumes, and Postoperative Surveillance. *Plast. Reconstr. Surg.* **2020**, *146*, 1e–10e. [CrossRef]
35. Akita, S.; Mitsukawa, N.; Tokumoto, H.; Kubota, Y.; Kuriyama, M.; Sasahara, Y.; Yamaji, Y.; Satoh, K. Regional Oxygen Saturation Index: A Novel Criterion for Free Flap Assessment Using Tissue Oximetry. *Plast. Reconstr. Surg.* **2016**, *138*, 510e–518e. [CrossRef]
36. Rother, U.; Muller-Mohnssen, H.; Lang, W.; Ludolph, I.; Arkudas, A.; Horch, R.E.; Regus, S.; Meyer, A. Wound closure by means of free flap and arteriovenous loop: Development of flap autonomy in the long-term follow-up. *Int. Wound J.* **2020**, *17*, 107–116. [CrossRef]
37. Ritschl, L.M.; Schmidt, L.H.; Fichter, A.M.; Hapfelmeier, A.; Wolff, K.D.; Mucke, T. Multimodal analysis using flowmeter analysis, laser-Doppler spectrophotometry, and indocyanine green videoangiography for the detection of venous compromise in flaps in rats. *J. Cranio-Maxillo-Fac. Surg. Off. Publ. Eur. Assoc. Cranio-Maxillo-Fac. Surg.* **2018**, *46*, 905–915. [CrossRef]
38. Lorenzetti, F.; Suominen, S.; Tukiainen, E.; Kuokkanen, H.; Suominen, E.; Vuola, J.; Asko-Seljavaara, S. Evaluation of blood flow in free microvascular flaps. *J. Reconstr. Microsurg.* **2001**, *17*, 163–167. [CrossRef]
39. Lorenzetti, F.; Kuokkanen, H.; von Smitten, K.; Asko-Seljavaara, S. Intraoperative evaluation of blood flow in the internal mammary or thoracodorsal artery as a recipient vessel for a free TRAM flap. *Ann. Plast. Surg.* **2001**, *46*, 590–593. [CrossRef]
40. Lorenzetti, F.; Giordano, S.; Tukiainen, E. Intraoperative hemodynamic evaluation of the latissimus dorsi muscle flap: A prospective study. *J. Reconstr. Microsurg.* **2012**, *28*, 273–278. [CrossRef]
41. Selber, J.C.; Garvey, P.B.; Clemens, M.W.; Chang, E.I.; Zhang, H.; Hanasono, M.M. A prospective study of transit-time flow volume measurement for intraoperative evaluation and optimization of free flaps. *Plast. Reconstr. Surg.* **2013**, *131*, 270–281. [CrossRef]
42. Preidl, R.H.; Schlittenbauer, T.; Weber, M.; Neukam, F.W.; Wehrhan, F. Assessment of free microvascular flap perfusion by intraoperative fluorescence angiography in craniomaxillofacial surgery. *J. Cranio-Maxillo-Fac. Surg. Off. Publ. Eur. Assoc. Cranio-Maxillo-Fac. Surg.* **2015**, *43*, 643–648. [CrossRef]
43. Eguchi, T.; Kawaguchi, K.; Basugi, A.; Kanai, I.; Hamada, Y. Intraoperative real-time assessment of blood flow using indocyanine green angiography after anastomoses in free-flap reconstructions. *Br. J. Oral Maxillofac. Surg.* **2017**, *55*, 628–630. [CrossRef]
44. Hitier, M.; Cracowski, J.L.; Hamou, C.; Righini, C.; Bettega, G. Indocyanine green fluorescence angiography for free flap monitoring: A pilot study. *J. Cranio-Maxillo-Fac. Surg. Off. Publ. Eur. Assoc. Cranio-Maxillo-Fac. Surg.* **2016**, *44*, 1833–1841. [CrossRef]
45. Aschoff, L. *Thrombosis. Lectures on Pathology*; Paul, B., Ed.; Hoeber, Inc.: New York, NY, USA, 1924; pp. 253–278.
46. Bagot, C.N.; Arya, R. Virchow and his triad: A question of attribution. *Br. J. Haematol.* **2008**, *143*, 180–190. [CrossRef]

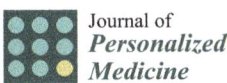

Article

# Microsurgical Transplantation of Pedicled Muscles in an Isolation Chamber—A Novel Approach to Engineering Muscle Constructs via Perfusion-Decellularization

Aijia Cai [1,*], Zengming Zheng [1], Wibke Müller-Seubert [1], Jonas Biggemann [2], Tobias Fey [2,3], Justus P. Beier [4], Raymund E. Horch [1], Benjamin Frieß [1,†] and Andreas Arkudas [1,†]

1 Department of Plastic and Hand Surgery and Laboratory for Tissue Engineering and Regenerative Medicine, University Hospital of Erlangen, Friedrich-Alexander University of Erlangen-Nürnberg (FAU), Krankenhausstraße 12, 91054 Erlangen, Germany; zhengzengming@163.com (Z.Z.); wibke.mueller-seubert@uk-erlangen.de (W.M.-S.); raymund.horch@uk-erlangen.de (R.E.H.); bennifriess@gmx.de (B.F.); andreas.arkudas@uk-erlangen.de (A.A.)
2 Department of Materials Science and Engineering, Institute of Glass and Ceramics, Friedrich-Alexander-University Erlangen-Nürnberg (FAU), Martensstr. 5, 91058 Erlangen, Germany; jonas.biggemann@fau.de (J.B.); tobias.fey@fau.de (T.F.)
3 Frontier Research Institute for Materials Science, Nagoya Institute of Technology, Gokiso-cho, Showa-ku, Nagoya 466-8555, Japan
4 Department of Plastic Surgery, Hand Surgery, Burn Center, University Hospital RWTH Aachen, Pauwelsstr. 30, 52074 Aachen, Germany; jbeier@ukaachen.de
\* Correspondence: aijia.cai@uk-erlangen.de; Tel.: +49-9131-85-33296; Fax: +49-9131-85-39327
† These authors contributed equally to this work.

**Abstract:** Decellularized whole muscle constructs represent an ideal scaffold for muscle tissue engineering means as they retain the network and proteins of the extracellular matrix of skeletal muscle tissue. The presence of a vascular pedicle enables a more efficient perfusion-based decellularization protocol and allows for subsequent recellularization and transplantation of the muscle construct in vivo. The goal of this study was to create a baseline for transplantation of decellularized whole muscle constructs by establishing an animal model for investigating a complete native muscle isolated on its pedicle in terms of vascularization and functionality. The left medial gastrocnemius muscles of 5 male Lewis rats were prepared and raised from their beds for in situ muscle stimulation. The stimulation protocol included twitches, tetanic stimulation, fatigue testing, and stretching of the muscles. Peak force, maximum rate of contraction and relaxation, time to maximum contraction and relaxation, and maximum contraction and relaxation rate were determined. Afterwards, muscles were explanted and transplanted heterotopically in syngeneic rats in an isolation chamber by microvascular anastomosis. After 2 weeks, transplanted gastrocnemius muscles were exposed and stimulated again followed by intravascular perfusion with a contrast agent for μCT analysis. Muscle constructs were then paraffin embedded for immunohistological staining. Peak twitch and tetanic force values all decreased significantly after muscle transplantation while fatigue index and passive stretch properties did not differ between the two groups. Vascular analysis revealed retained perfused vessels most of which were in a smaller radius range of up to 20 μm and 45 μm. In this study, a novel rat model of heterotopic microvascular muscle transplantation in an isolation chamber was established. With the assessment of in situ muscle contraction properties as well as vessel distribution after 2 weeks of transplantation, this model serves as a base for future studies including the transplantation of perfusion-decellularized muscle constructs.

**Keywords:** muscle transplantation; rat gastrocnemius; in situ stimulation; muscle contraction; perfusion-decellularization

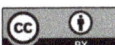

## 1. Introduction

Tissue engineering of skeletal muscle holds great promise for the treatment of volumetric muscle loss. It can help to circumvent substantial donor site morbidity, resulting from donor tissue transfer, including free autologous muscle flaps [1–3]. Common tissue engineering approaches have attempted to create three-dimensional (3D) constructs by combining scaffolds with stem cells and growth factors [3,4]. However, the production of biocompatible and stable scaffolds can be time consuming and expensive and cell adherence, invasion, and differentiation can be demanding in this synthetic 3D environment [5,6].

Decellularized extracellular matrix scaffolds have been a popular platform for regenerating skeletal muscle, as they contain structural proteins and molecules of skeletal muscle tissue, which is difficult to mimic by artificial means [6,7]. Established protocols have mostly applied diffusion techniques on skeletal muscle so far, although perfusion-decellularization through a vascular pedicle seems more beneficial by retaining the complex 3D architecture of the native tissue while effectively removing all cells [8]. The presence of a vascular pedicle enables subsequent transplantation of the decellularized and possibly recellularized construct in vivo.

Critical size defects necessitate volumetric tissue constructs for reconstruction, which on the other hand depend on adequate blood supply for survival [9]. Thus, a functional blood vessel network is a prerequisite for the growth of tissues and organs in vivo. The arteriovenous (AV) loop model contains a vein graft anastomosed to an artery and a vein, creating a loop that is transferred to an enclosed implantation chamber [10]. This creates an isolated microenvironment, which is connected to the living organism only by means of the vascular axis. Any disturbing influences from the surroundings are shielded off and the tissue with its vascularization can be analyzed in the controlled environment.

Perfusion-decellularization of a whole muscle via its main vascular pedicle, subsequent recellularization of the skeletal muscle matrix, and transplantation of the whole construct in vivo have the potential to generate new functional muscle tissue. An isolation chamber allows for analysis of the newly generated and vascularized tissue independent of external factors similar to the AV-loop model. Prior to establishing such a model, baseline values concerning vascularization and functionality of such transplanted muscle constructs are needed.

The principal contribution of this work is a novel in vivo animal model for investigating a transplanted complete native muscle isolated on its pedicle in terms of vascularization and functionality.

## 2. Methods

### 2.1. Experimental Animals

Animal experiments were carried out following the German regulations for the care of laboratory animals at all times. Experiments were approved by the local Animal Care Committee (approval number RUF 55.2.2-2532.2-658-48).

Gastrocnemius muscles were taken from the left hindlimb of 5 male Lewis donor rats (Charles River Laboratories, Sulzfeld, Germany) and transplanted into the left hindlimb of 5 syngenic recipient rats.

All animals were anesthetized during the surgical procedures through the administration of gaseous isoflurane (op-pharma, Burgdorf, Germany) at concentrations between 1.5–5% under spontaneous breathing. For analgesia, animals received intravenous meloxicam (2 mg/kg) and butorphanol (1.5 mg/kg), whereas butorphanol was substituted every 2 h.

### 2.2. Muscle Preparation

Donor animals were placed in the supine position on a heating plate. Dissection through the adductor muscles of the left hind limb was carried out under aseptic conditions until the medial gastrocnemius muscle was reached and freed from all muscular and tendon attachments. All vessels branching off the muscle except for the popliteal artery and vein, representing the main pedicle, were ligated. Popliteal vessels were tracked proximally up to their origin from the femoral vessels until the gastrocnemius muscle was solely attached in situ via its vascular pedicle and the tibial nerve (Figure 1). The distal tendon was then tied with a 4-0 Vicryl suture (Ethicon, Somerville, NJ, USA) and connected to a servomotor lever arm (model 305C Dual-Mode Lever Arm System; Aurora Scientific Inc, Aurora, Ontario, Canada), while the proximal tendon was fixed in a clamp on a self-constructed metal frame, placed under the heating plate (Figure 2). After stimulation of the gastrocnemius, the rat receiving the gastrocnemius muscle as a transplant was surgically prepared (see Section 2.4 for details).

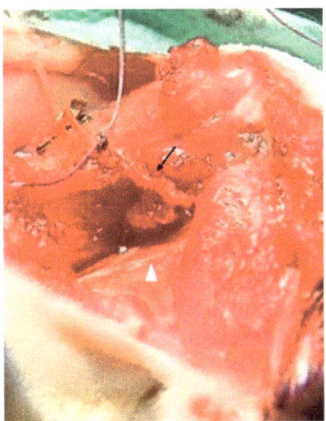

**Figure 1.** After surgical preparation, the gastrocnemius muscle was attached in situ via its vascular pedicle (arrow) and the tibial nerve (white arrowhead).

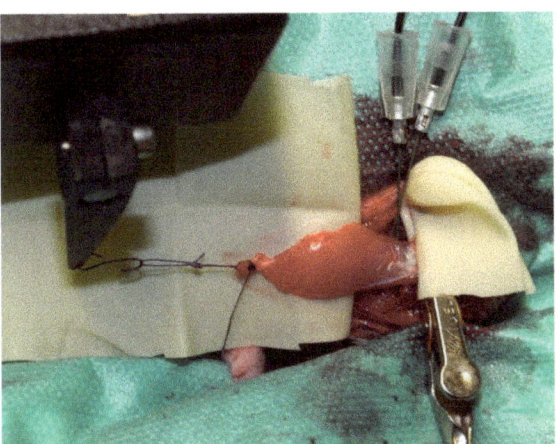

**Figure 2.** For electrical stimulation, the muscle was connected to a servomotor lever arm distally and fixed with a clamp proximally. Electrodes ware placed near the entry of the tibial nerve.

### 2.3. Muscle Stimulation

Prior to transplantation and perfusion, the gastrocnemius muscle was stimulated via electrodes placed into the muscle close to where the tibial nerve enters the muscle. A stimulation and recording system (150 A and 615A Dynamic Muscle Control and High-Throughput Analysis software suite; Aurora Scientific Inc., Aurora, ON, Canada), was used to stimulate the muscle after optimal length was determined as described by Tamayo et al. [11]. For twitches, the muscle was stimulated every 3 s with 1 ms pulses for 10 repetitions. The maximum force (i.e., peak force), maximum rate of contraction and relaxation, time to maximum contraction and relaxation, and maximum contraction and relaxation rate were measured. This was followed by 80 Hz, 100 Hz, and 120 Hz tetanic stimulation. Peak force, maximum contraction rate, and time to maximum contraction were assessed. For fatigue testing, a 150 Hz burst of stimulation was applied to the muscle every 3 s for 7.5 min. The fatigue index was determined as the ratio between the maximum and minimum force difference and the maximum force. A break of at least 1 min was taken between each measurement. For passive tension properties, the muscle was stretched to 110% of its original length in 1% steps. During each stretch, contractile forces to gain the length of the muscle were measured.

### 2.4. Muscle Transplantation

After stimulation of the donor rat muscle, a second rat was prepared for surgery in the supine position. The left hind limb was incised and the saphenous artery and superficial inferior epigastric vein were dissected and prepared for vascular anastomosis.

The dissected gastrocnemius muscle was harvested from the donor animal by cutting the femoral vessels. The muscle was flushed with heparine (50 I.U.) via the femoral artery until a clear heparine solution came out of the femoral vein. The wet weight of the muscle was determined. The donor rat was sacrificed and the gastrocnemius muscle was transplanted into the recipient rat by anastomosing the femoral artery to the saphenous artery and femoral vein to the superficial inferior epigastric vein (SIEV) with 11-0 interrupted sutures (Figure 3). The patency of anastomoses was confirmed via the milking patency test [12]. The revascularized muscle was placed into an isolation chamber made out of polylactide via 3D printing by fused deposition modeling (FDM) using an Ultimater 2+ (Ultimaker B.V., Utrecht, The Netherlands). The isolation chamber consisted of two parts: one bottom part, which was sutured to the anterior muscle of the hind leg (Figure 4A,C), and a lid that enclosed the transplanted muscle while avoiding squeezing of the muscle (Figure 4B,D). Anastomoses were fixed with fibrin glue to avoid kinking of the vessels. The skin was closed in 2 layers. Antibiotics (7.5 mg/kg enrofloxacin) were administered perioperatively intravenously and continued subcutaneously for 5 days. Animals received 10 mg/kg low molecular weight heparin and meloxicam (2 mg/kg) subcutaneously for 5 days.

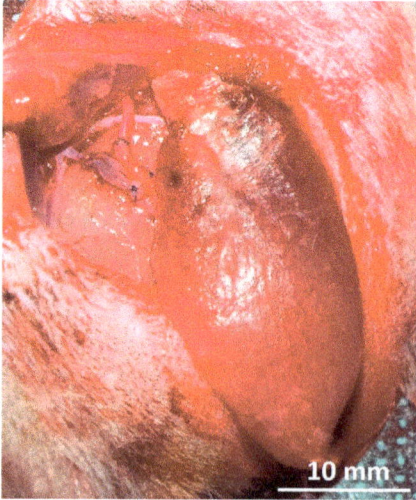

**Figure 3.** Gastrocnemius muscle was transplanted via anastomosis of the femoral artery to the saphenous artery and femoral vein to the superficial inferior epigastric vein.

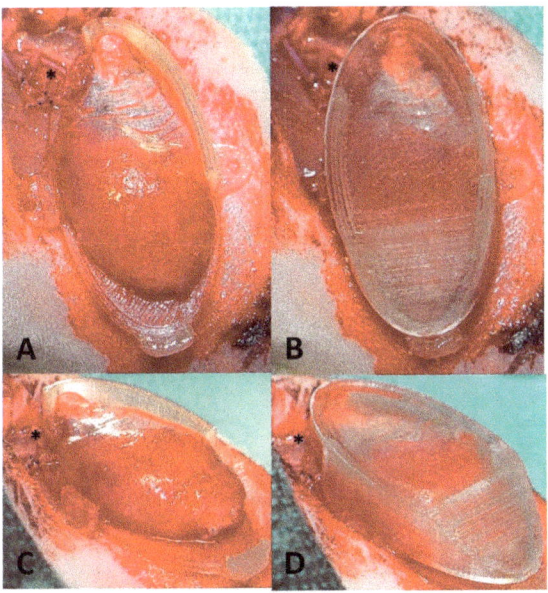

**Figure 4.** Different perspectives showing transplanted gastrocnemius muscle placed onto bottom part of isolation chamber (**A,C**) and into isolation chamber with lid on top (**B,D**). Note the opening of the chamber for the vascular pedicle (asterisk).

*2.5. Perfusion and Explantation of Constructs*

After two weeks of implantation, rats were again anesthetized as described above and placed in the supine position. The left hind limb was dissected and the isolation chamber was opened to expose the transplanted gastrocnemius muscle (Figure 5A). The muscles were taken out of the chamber and stimulation was carried out as described above. After that, muscles were perfused with the contrast agent Microfil® as described previously [13]. Briefly, laparotomy incision was performed and animals were perfused by flushing the aorta with 150 mL of heparine solution and afterward with 20 mL yellow Microfil® (MV-122) containing 2.5% of MV Curing Agent (both Flowtech, Carver, MA, USA) (Figure 5B). Finally, the aorta and inferior vena cava were ligated, and the rats were placed at 7 °C for 24 h. Constructs were explanted in toto and fixed in 3.5% formalin solution overnight and placed in PBS solution for microtomography (µCT) analysis.

*2.6. Micro-Computed Tomography*

High-resolution µCT scans were performed using Skyscan 1172 with an 11-MP detector and a tungsten tube at a voltage of 80 kV and a current of 100 mA (Skyscan B.V., Leuven, Belgium) as described previously [14]. Briefly, after scanning at 180° with a rotation step of 0.25° and a resolution of 4.47 µm/voxel, the data were reconstructed with Radeon back Transformation using the tomographic reconstruction software (NRecon Client and Server 1.7.42 with GPU support; Skyscan Leuven, Belgium) while adjusting the X/Y shift and alignment during measurement. The visualization and vessel radius evaluation was carried out by imaging software (Amira 2021.1; Thermo Fisher Scientific, Berlin, Germany).

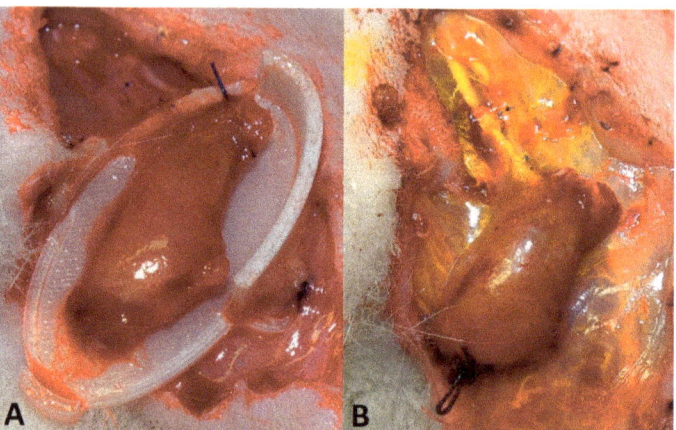

**Figure 5.** After 2 weeks of implantation, the gastrocnemius muscle has shrunken to approximately half its original size (**A**). After electrical stimulation, the muscle was perfused with a contrast agent (Microfil® = yellow) (**B**).

*2.7. Immunohistochemical Analysis*

After µCT analysis, constructs were processed for paraffin embedding. The feasibility of histologic analysis after Microfil® perfusion has been demonstrated before [14–16]. Three-micrometer cross-sections were obtained from the middle of the gastrocnemius muscles perpendicular to the main vascular axis with a microtome (Leica Microsystems, Wetzlar, Germany). Hematoxylin and eosin (HE) were performed according to standard protocols. For myosin heavy chain (MHC) staining, sections were blocked with 10% goat serum (Vector Laboratories, Burlingame, CA, USA) and incubated with anti-fast myosin skeletal heavy chain (MHC) antibody (ab91506, Abcam, Cambridge, UK) at a concentration of 5 µg/mL overnight at 4 °C. After washing with TBS-T (1 mL Tween20 per 1 L of 100 mM Tris and NaCl in $H_2O$, pH 7.4), Alexa Fluor 647 goat anti-rabbit IgG (H + L) cross-adsorbed secondary antibody (A-21244) was used at a concentration of 4 µg/mL for 30 min at room temperature. Probes were counterstained with DAPI 1 µg/mL (diamidine-phenylindole-dihydrochloride, Thermo Fisher Scientific Inc.) for 5 min. For visualizing neuromuscular junctions, deparaffinized sections were stained with recombinant anti-Synaptophysin antibody [YE269] (ab32127, Abcam) at a concentration of 0.5 µg/mL and incubated overnight. Afterwards, sections were incubated with Alexa Fluor 488 anti-rabbit (A11008, Thermofisher Scientific Inc.) at a concentration of 4 µg/mL for 30 min followed by α-Bungarotoxin, Alexa Fluor 647 conjugated (B35450, Thermo Fisher Scientific Inc., Waltham, MA, USA) for 1 h and counterstaining with DAPI as described above. For macrophage detection, CD68 staining was performed with anti-CD68 antibody (BIO-RAD, Hercules, CA, USA) in a dilution of 1:300 overnight on deparaffinized and blocked sections. For enzymatic detection, an alkaline phosphate-labeled anti-mouse-antibody and Fast Red TR/Naphthol AS (Sigma-Aldrich, Missouri, USA) were applied. Haemalaun was used for counterstaining.

*2.8. Vessel Quantification*

Reconstructed two-dimensional cross-sections from µCT scans were exported as 256 grey value level images and used for segmentation of the vessels, as previously described [14]. Additional shrink and grow image calculation operations were carried out to ensure filled blood vessels for analysis to prevent misleading results from e.g., bubbles in the Microfil®. Accumulated vessel lengths were calculated for each vessel radius starting from 5 µm at histogram class widths of 10 µm. To exclude material that did not belong to the muscle, the cut-off was set at 335 µm. This agrees with the maximum diameter of

500–600 µm of the vascular pedicle of the gastrocnemius muscle. Values are summarized for every radius range of 40 µm, e.g., 5–45 µm.

HE stained sections were used for vessel counting in ImageJ 1.53e (National Institutes of Health, Bethesda, MD, USA). After setting a scale, the lumen of all vessels with a clearly visible lumen or lumen filled with Microfil® was outlined using the freehand tool in the ROI manager. The radius was calculated using the resulting area of the vessel lumen, and the number of radius ranges of 20 µm, e.g., 0.1–20 µm, 20.1–40 µm was depicted.

*2.9. Statistical Analysis*

Data are expressed as the mean ± standard deviation (SD). Data normality of force values was verified by the Shapiro–Wilk test. Pairwise comparisons between muscles before and after transplantation were carried out using paired $t$-test or Mann–Whitney test, as appropriate. Statistical analysis was performed using GraphPad Prism version 8.3, La Jolla, CA, USA. A $p$-value $\leq 0.05$ was considered statistically significant.

## 3. Results

*3.1. Surgery and Animals*

All animals tolerated surgeries well. Weight properties of the involved rats and muscles with the corresponding ischemia time are listed in Table 1.

**Table 1.** Animal data.

| Rat | Donor Rat Weight (g) | Gastrocnemius Muscle Weight (g) | Recipient Rat Weight (g) | Ischemia Time (min) |
| --- | --- | --- | --- | --- |
| 1 | 285 | 1 | 410 | 120 |
| 2 | 240 | 0.87 | 440 | 100 |
| 3 | 260 | 0.94 | 400 | 85 |
| 4 | 290 | 1 | 370 | 90 |
| 5 | 320 | 1.03 | 410 | 90 |

Four out of 5 animals developed postoperative seroma, that were punctured once (2 animals) or twice (2 animals) under sterile conditions. At the time of explantation after 2 weeks, all muscles were vital but had shrunken to approximately half their original size (Figure 5A).

*3.2. Muscle Function*

Peak force after twitch decreased significantly by 95.5% 2 weeks after the gastrocnemius muscle was transplanted within the isolation chamber ($p = 0.0041$) (Figure 6). Time to peak force, maximum contraction, and relaxation rate all decreased after transplantation ($p = 0.011$, $p = 0.0018$, and $p = 0.0042$, respectively). Time to 50% and 100% relaxation did not differ between the two groups ($p = 0.0735$ and $p = 0.7621$, respectively) (Figure 7). Peak force and contraction rate after tetanic stimulation decreased after transplantation for all frequencies ($p = 0.0014$ and $p = 0.001$, respectively, for 80 Hz, $p = 0.0028$ and $p = 0.0003$, respectively, for 100 Hz, $p = 0.0058$ and $p = 0.0035$, respectively, for 120 Hz). Time to peak force decreased at 80 Hz ($p = 0.0115$), 100 Hz ($p = 0.0035$), and 120 Hz ($p < 0.0001$). Detailed values for twitch and tetanus are listed in Table 2.

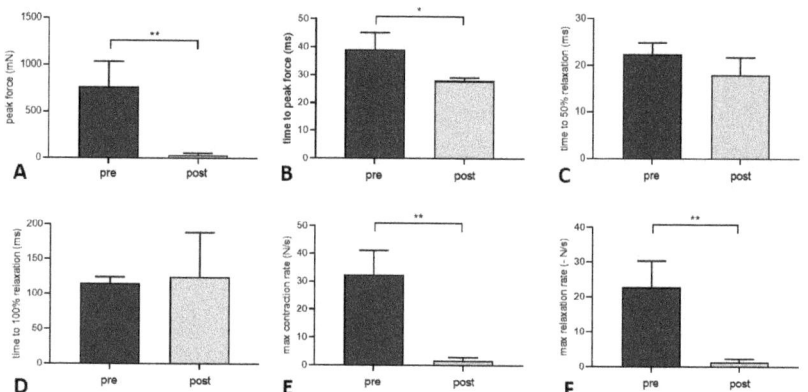

**Figure 6.** Force values before and 2 weeks after transplantation of the gastrocnemius muscle. Peak force (**A**), time to peak force (**B**), and maximum contraction and relaxation rate (**E,F**) decreased after transplantation while time to 50% and 100% relaxation (**C,D**) did not change (paired *t*-test). Level of significance was * $p < 0.05$, ** $p < 0.01$.

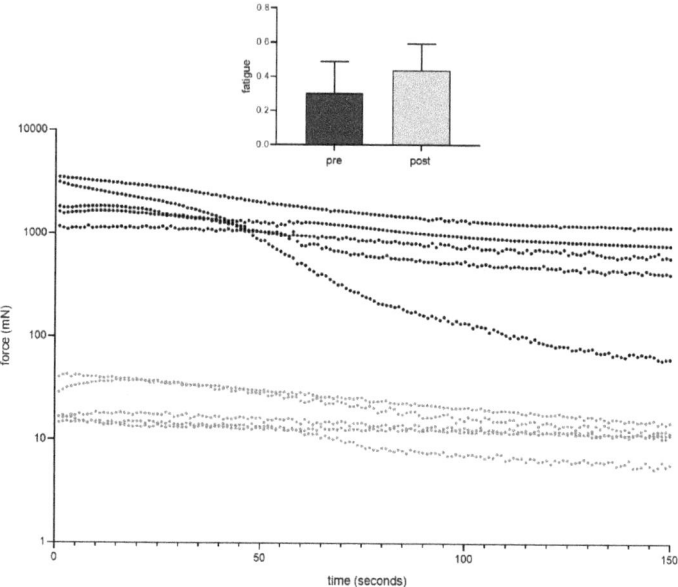

**Figure 7.** Fatigue index was similar before (dark grey) and 2 weeks after muscle transplantation (light grey) (paired *t*-test).

During fatigue testing, there was an obvious difference between pre and post transplantation groups (Figure 7). Nevertheless, fatigue index was similar between the two groups ($p = 0.287$). Passive stretch properties did not change after transplantation (Figure 8). For each % increase in length from 100–110%, contractile forces needed to maintain the respective length of the muscle did not differ between the two groups: 1% ($p = 0.641$), 2% ($p = 0.707$), 3% ($p = 0.878$), 4% ($p = 0.832$), 5% ($p = 0.708$), 6% ($p = 0.631$), 7% ($p = 0.550$), 8% ($p = 0.437$), 9% ($p = 0.395$), 10% ($p = 0.323$).

**Table 2.** Force values before and after transplantation.

|  | Pre Transplantation | Post Transplantation |
|---|---|---|
| Peak twitch force (mN) | 768.5 ± 266.6 | 34.7 ± 19.7 (**) |
| Time to peak twitch force (ms) | 39.2 ± 6.0 | 28.1 ± 1.0 (*) |
| Time to 50% relaxation (twitch force) (ms) | 22.5 ± 2.4 | 18.0 ± 3.7 |
| Time to 100% relaxation (twitch force) (ms) | 115.6 ± 8.3 | 124.5 ± 63.9 |
| Maximum contraction rate (twitch) (N/s) | 32.5 ± 8.6 | 1.9 ± 1.1 (**) |
| Maximum relaxation rate (twitch) (-N/s) | 22.8 ± 7.5 | 1.4 ± 0.9 (**) |
| Maximum tetanic force (at 80 Hz) (mN) | 2771 ± 772.7 | 28.6 ± 14.7 (**) |
| Maximum contraction rate (tetanus at 80 Hz) (N/s) | 57.8 ± 14.7 | 1.0 ± 0.5 (**) |
| Time to peak force (tetanus at 80 Hz) (ms) | 33.7 ± 7.1 | 19.6 ± 2.2 (*) |
| Maximum tetanic force (at 100 Hz) (mN) | 2920 ± 981.9 | 32.1 ± 14.2 (**) |
| Maximum contraction rate (tetanus at 100 Hz) (N/s) | 59.1 ± 10.5 | 1.1 ± 0.5 (***) |
| Time to peak force (tetanus at 100 Hz) (ms) | 32.2 ± 4.6 | 19.7 ± 2.2 (**) |
| Maximum tetanic force (at 120 Hz) (mN) | 2970 ± 1172 | 34.5 ± 13.4 (**) |
| Maximum contraction rate (tetanus at 120 Hz) | 56.3 ± 19.7 | 1.2 ± 0.5 (**) |
| Time to peak force (tetanus at 120 Hz) (ms) | 32.5 ± 2.8 | 19.6 ± 1.9 (***) |

All values are mean ± SD; */**/*** indicate differences between muscles forces of gastrocnemius muscles pre and post transplantation (paired *t*-test); * $p < 0.05$; ** $p < 0.01$; *** $p < 0.001$.

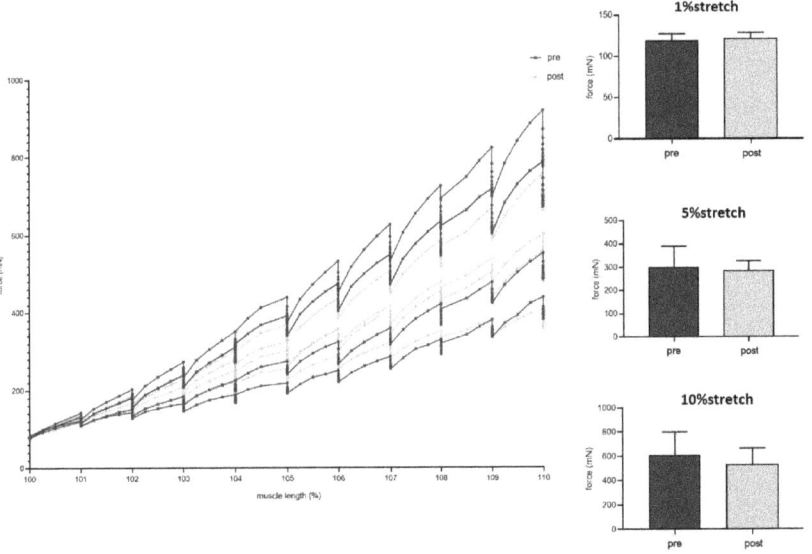

**Figure 8.** Passive stretch properties were similar before (dark grey) and 2 weeks after muscle transplantation (light grey). Exemplary data are shown for forces needed for 1%, 5%, and 10% length gain (paired *t*-test).

*3.3. Vessel Quantification*

Three-dimensional (3D) μCT scans showed the cumulative lengths for different vessel radius ranges (Table 3 and Figure 9). Vessels with smaller radii (measuring 5–45 μm and 55–95 μm) were the highest in number and cumulative length. The larger the radius of the vessels the lower was the cumulative length.

Table 3. Vessel distribution depicted from µCT analysis.

| Vessel Radius (µm) | Number of Vessels | Cumulative Length (mm) |
|---|---|---|
| 5–45 | 4168 ± 1110 | 595.4 ± 112.1 |
| 55–95 | 3007 ± 1858 | 266.2 ± 122.9 |
| 105–145 | 1017 ± 794.1 | 155.7 ± 111.2 |
| 155–195 | 444.2 ± 372.2 | 96.3 ± 88.1 |
| 205–245 | 243.2 ± 188.4 | 61.5 ± 51.5 |
| 255–295 | 157 ± 90.7 | 45.6 ± 33.5 |
| 305–335 | 68.8 ± 42.9 | 24.9 ± 16.8 |

All values are the mean ± SD.

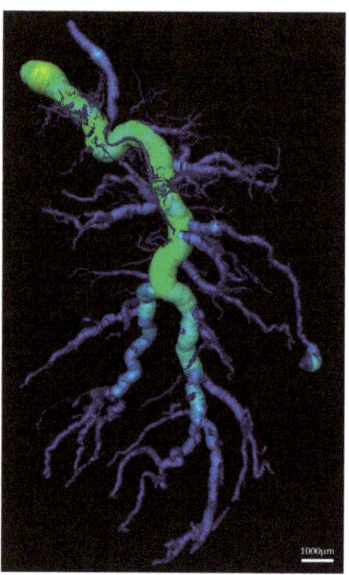

**Figure 9.** Exemplary 3D µCT scan of a gastrocnemius muscle perfused with contrast agent after 2 weeks of transplantation.

Vessel analysis of immunohistochemical sections revealed a similar trend (Table 4): the smallest vessels, ranging from 0.1–20 µm, were the most prevalent while vessel radius ranges of 120.1–140 µm, 140.1–160 µm, and 240.1–260 µm were present in only 1 out of 5 muscles (rat 3 and rat 5, respectively).

### 3.4. Nerve-Muscle-Junction and Myogenic Marker Expression

MHC staining revealed irregularly arranged myofibrils in the transplanted muscle constructs (Figure 10). Double staining for synaptophysin for nerve terminals and α-Bungarotoxin for acetylcholine receptors showed some scattering of neuromuscular junctions at the surface of the muscle near the epimysium (Figure 10). Synaptophysin expression dominated clearly over acetylcholine receptors, which only appeared scarcely at the muscle surface.

Table 4. Vessel distribution depicted from immunohistochemical analysis.

| Vessel Radius (µm) | Number of Vessel Lumen |
|---|---|
| 0.1–20 | 165.8 ± 109.5 |
| 20.1–40 | 17.4 ± 2.7 |
| 40.1–60 | 3.4 ± 1.5 |
| 60.1–80 | 1.8 ± 1.6 |
| 80.1–100 | 1.4 ± 0.9 |
| 100.1–120 | 0.4 ± 0.5 |
| 120.1–140 | 0.2 ± 0.4 |
| 140.1–160 | 0.2 ± 0.4 |
| 180.1–200 | 0.4 ± 0.5 |
| 220.1–240 | 0.4 ± 0.9 |
| 240.1–260 | 0.2 ± 0.4 |

All values are the mean ± SD.

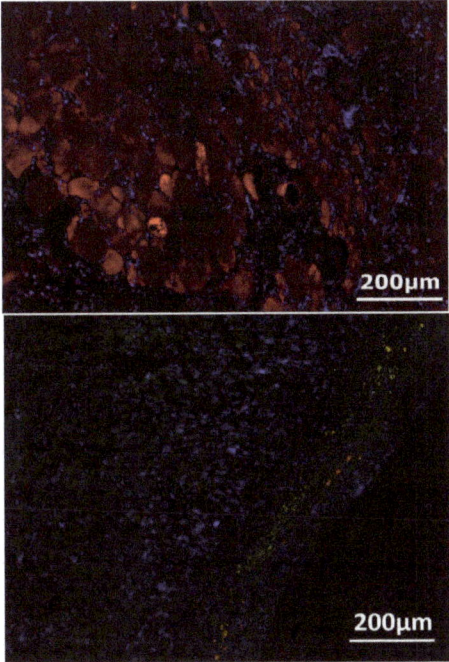

**Figure 10.** MHC staining (red) revealed irregularly arranged myofibrils in the transplanted muscle constructs (**top**). Double staining for synaptophysin (green) for nerve terminals and α-Bungarotoxin (red) for acetylcholine receptors showed neuromuscular junctions at the surface of the muscle near the epimysium after 2 weeks of transplantation and denervation (**bottom**).

*3.5. Myofiber Morphology and Macrophage Invasion*

HE staining showed partly well-preserved structures as well as partly inhomogenous and irregularly arrangement of the skeletal muscle similar to MHC staining (Figure 11). CD68 staining revealed invasion of macrophages, especially near the vessels (Figure 12).

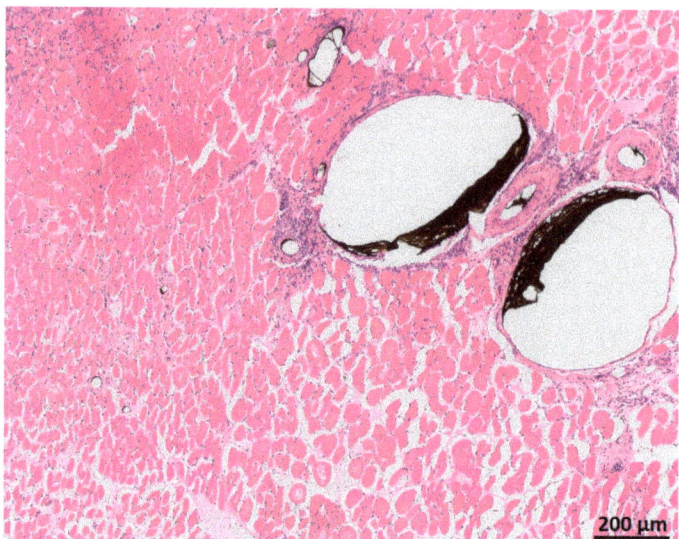

**Figure 11.** HE staining of the transplanted muscle showing partly well-preserved structures as well as partly inhomogenous and irregularly arrangement of the skeletal muscle.

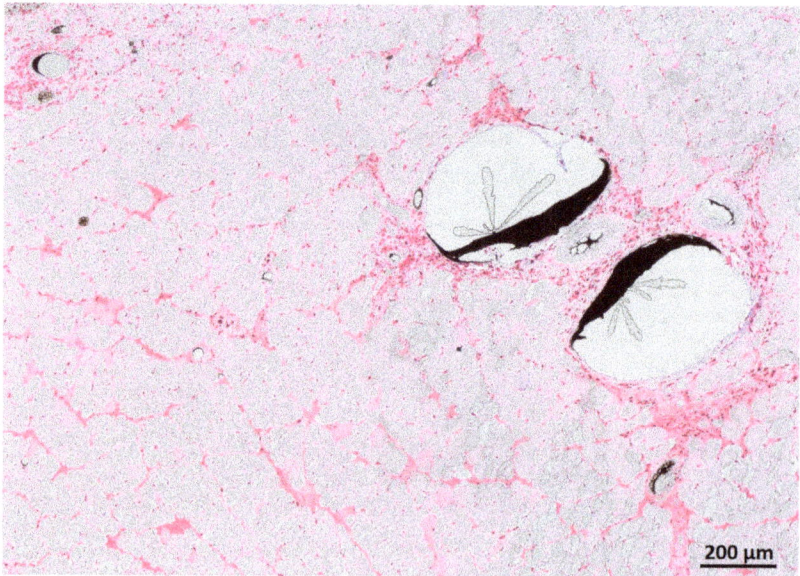

**Figure 12.** CD68 staining of transplanted muscle showing macrophages predominantly near the vessels filled with Microfil®.

## 4. Discussion

In the present study, a novel rat model of heterotopic muscle transplantation in an isolation chamber was proposed. In situ muscle contraction properties before and after transplantation and denervation of the muscle were assessed. Furthermore, vessel distribution after 2 weeks of transplantation was characterized with both µCT and immunohistochemical analysis.

Perfusion-decellularization of skeletal muscle has been successfully applied to the porcine rectus abdominis muscle [8]. Partial-thickness abdominal wall defects repaired with decellularized muscle scaffolds showed a higher amount of neo muscle tissue and neoangiogenesis compared to small intestinal submucosa, which showed the superiority of native tissue extracellular matrix for replacing muscle tissue [8]. Conconi et al. have shown the advantages of cell-seeded decellularized muscle matrices compared to matrices only, which were replaced by fibrous tissue shortly after implantation. However, after 60 days of implantation, even the cell–matrix constructs lost their full structural integrity, which could be explained by a missing axial vascularization [17]. The integration of a vascular axis results in prefabricated acellular matrices that can be transferred as flaps to repair defects [18]. Similarly, the goal of the present study was to set up a model which can be built on for whole muscle perfusion decellularization and subsequent recellularization and/or in vivo transplantation. For this purpose, a suitable muscle had to be chosen. There are various rodent models of muscle transplantation that have extensively described the anatomy and vascular supply of pectoralis major [19], gracilis [20], and quadriceps femoris muscles [21]. However, for the purposes of the present study, which is not solely a study of muscle transplantation, the medial head of the gastrocnemius muscle was chosen due to its single dominant vascular pedicle [22] and its spindle-like shape, which is beneficial for functional characterization and decellularization in a bioreactor as demonstrated recently [23]. In this study, gastrocnemius muscles were successfully perfusion-decellularized with their proximal tendinous parts being clamped in a bioreactor chamber, which enabled a continuous flow through the vascular system of the muscles while the muscles could be dynamically stretched [23]. As shown by others, repetitive stretching prevents denervation-induced muscle atrophy [24–26]. According to the aforementioned study, the mechanical stimulation in the reactor chamber preserved the effective decellularization [23]. Thus, this mechanism could be utilized for later recellularization of the constructs to preserve muscle functions. To set up baseline values for functionality and vascularization of such a de- and recellularized muscle construct, a native gastrocnemius muscle was transplanted within the present study. For minimizing external factors that could influence the transplanted muscle, e.g., extrinsic vascularization or fibrous tissue, an isolation chamber was designed that enclosed the muscle during the period of implantation. To enable tension-free closure of the wound, the size of the isolation chamber needed to be relatively small. This is also a reason for choosing the medial head of the gastrocnemius muscle of a smaller donor rat instead of a large muscle such as the quadriceps femoris muscle [21].

All force values decreased significantly after 2 weeks of transplantation. This finding is consistent with in vivo experiments that involved denervation of muscle, leading to muscle atrophy and a loss of isometric contraction force [27,28]. Microvascular flaps are denervated when transferred unless nerve coaptation is performed [29]. The effect of nerve coaptation (tibial nerve to a branch of the obturator nerve as described in the EPI-loop model [30]) would be the next step to analyze. Zhang et al. performed orthotopic transplantation of rat gracilis muscle with transection of the obturator nerve and subsequent neurorrhaphy of the nerve [31]. After 5–20 weeks after reinnervation, muscle function started to recover. Thus, it can be assumed that nerve coaptation would not have led to significant functional recovery in the present study where muscle transplantation was performed over a period of 2 weeks for establishing this novel model. Zhang et al. did not perform vessel anastomosis, which might have influenced the regeneration of nerve-muscle function. Cen et al. have shown that denervation impairs ischemic recovery of rat hindlimbs via impaired perfusion, lower capillary density, and narrower lumen of vessels, illustrating that angiogenesis depends on an intact peripheral nervous system [32]. In the present study, two different modalities were used to analyze vessel distribution. Both modalities showed that smaller vessels (0.1–20 µm in immunostains and 5–45 µm in µCT scans) were prevalent in the muscle constructs. While 2D immunosections only allowed for illustration of a few large vessels, 3D reconstruction of µCT scans enabled the quantification of cumulative lengths for different radius ranges. On the other hand, immunosections revealed smaller vessels more reliably since those vessels that were not filled with Microfil® were also counted. The density of the capillary network and capillary distribution is crucial for muscle oxygenation and function [33]. The vast presence of capillaries as shown by immunosections and μCT implies that blood flow through the vascular pedicle is sufficient for supplying the muscles in the present study, at least at the current duration of denervation. Thus, a longer period of muscle implantation with or without nerve coaptation and its impact on muscle transplant function would be the logical next step of investigation.

Unfortunately, muscle weight could not be determined after transplantation as explantation of the muscle took place after perfusion. This prohibited the normalization of peak force to muscle weight after transplantation. However, the significant decrease in absolute force values of more than 90% after transplantation shows that transplantation and denervation of the muscle lead to a loss of force, as would be expected. Fatigue index and passive stretch values did not change after transplantation which indicates that muscles remained vital after transplantation and did not develop a relevant amount of fibrosis after a period of 2 weeks.

Synaptophysin, which is a glycoprotein in neurons and an essential component of synaptic vesicles, has shown stable expression even after different periods of denervation of gastrocnemius rat muscles [34] while postsynaptic acetylcholine receptors are known to decline with increased duration of denervation [35]. Furthermore, denervated muscles have shown disorganized and atrophic myofibers with inhomogenous HE staining [32]. Peripheral nerve injury, associated with Wallerian degeneration, is associated with inflammation and macrophage invasion [36]. This feature is in conjunction with the results of immunohistochemical staining of the transplanted muscles in the present study. One limitation of this study includes a missing reference muscle, which has not undergone transplantation, during immunohistochemical analysis. However, the study design did not enable us to collect additional native gastrocnemius muscles for formalin fixation since the muscles from the contralateral legs of the sacrificed rats were used for decellularization experiments [23]. Another limitation is the sole method of immunohistochemistry for analyzing myogenic markers and neuromuscular junctions. Evaluation of gene expression by PCR was not possible because whole muscle constructs were fixed in formalin for μCT analysis and paraffin embedding. The use of five animals in the present study is another limitation that sometimes resulted in high standard deviations. However, it was possible to show obvious differences in force values before and after muscle transplantation and to establish this model of whole muscle transplantation as a preliminary step towards transplantation of perfusion-decellularized muscle constructs as the purpose of the present study.

The previously mentioned shortcomings of this study, including missing nerve coaption, short follow-up period, and missing control group, will determine the goals for future studies, which will specifically evaluate the influence of motoric innervation and of an extended time period of 6–12 weeks on the functional outcome and the vascularization of the muscle constructs.

## 5. Conclusions

A novel model of successful whole muscle construct transplantation in an isolation chamber was established. Force values were characterized for native and transplanted muscles and vascularization was determined for transplanted muscles with both μCT and immunohistochemical methods. The findings of this study serve as a base for transplantation of perfusion-decellularized muscle constructs, but they can also serve as a base for other models, e.g., transplantation of functional muscle constructs for replacing denervated muscle tissue and analysis of their regeneration.

**Author Contributions:** Conceptualization, A.C., T.F., J.P.B., B.F. and A.A.; methodology, A.C., Z.Z., J.B., B.F. and A.A.; validation, A.C., B.F., T.F.; formal analysis, A.C., T.F. and B.F.; investigation, A.C., Z.Z., W.M.-S., J.B. and B.F.; resources, A.C., T.F., R.E.H. and A.A.; data curation, A.C., T.F. and B.F.; supervision, A.C. and A.A.; visualization, A.C. and T.F.; writing—original draft preparation, A.C.; writing—review and editing, W.M.-S., T.F., J.P.B., B.F. and A.A.; project administration, A.C., R.E.H. and A.A.; funding acquisition, A.C., R.E.H. and A.A. All authors have read and agreed to the published version of the manuscript.

**Funding:** The research was funded by Manfred Roth Stiftung and Forschungsstiftung Medizin Universitätsklinikum Erlangen of the Friedrich-Alexander University Erlangen-Nürnberg (FAU). We acknowledge financial support by Deutsche Forschungsgemeinschaft and Friedrich-Alexander-Universität Erlangen-Nürnberg within the funding programme "Open Access Publication Funding".

**Institutional Review Board Statement:** The study was conducted according to the guidelines of the Declaration of Helsinki, and approved by the local Animal Care Committee of the University of Erlangen-Nürnberg (FAU) and the District Government of Lower Franconia (approval number RUF 55.2.2-2532.2-658-48).

**Informed Consent Statement:** Not applicable.

**Data Availability Statement:** The data represented in this study are available on request from the corresponding author.

**Acknowledgments:** The authors want to thank Andrea Beck and Stefan Fleischer for their excellent technical support.

**Conflicts of Interest:** The authors declare not conflict of interest.

# References

1. Lee, K.T.; Mun, G.H. A systematic review of functional donor-site morbidity after latissimus dorsi muscle transfer. *Plast. Reconstr. Surg.* **2014**, *134*, 303–314. [CrossRef]
2. Knox, A.D.C.; Ho, A.L.; Leung, L.; Tashakkor, A.Y.; Lennox, P.A.; Van Laeken, N.; Macadam, S.A. Comparison of Outcomes following Autologous Breast Reconstruction Using the DIEP and Pedicled TRAM Flaps: A 12-Year Clinical Retrospective Study and Literature Review. *Plast. Reconstr. Surg.* **2016**, *138*, 16–28. [CrossRef]
3. Cai, A.; Hardt, M.; Schneider, P.; Schmid, R.; Lange, C.; Dippold, D.; Schubert, D.W.; Boos, A.M.; Weigand, A.; Arkudas, A.; et al. Myogenic differentiation of primary myoblasts and mesenchymal stromal cells under serum-free conditions on PCL-collagen I-nanoscaffolds. *BMC Biotechnol.* **2018**, *18*, 75. [CrossRef]
4. Witt, R.; Weigand, A.; Boos, A.M.; Cai, A.; Dippold, D.; Boccaccini, A.R.; Schubert, D.W.; Hardt, M.; Lange, C.; Arkudas, A.; et al. Mesenchymal stem cells and myoblast differentiation under HGF and IGF-1 stimulation for 3D skeletal muscle tissue engineering. *BMC Cell Biol.* **2017**, *18*, 15. [CrossRef]
5. Dippold, D.; Cai, A.; Hardt, M.; Boccaccini, A.R.; Horch, R.; Beier, J.P.; Schubert, D.W. Novel approach towards aligned PCL-Collagen nanofibrous constructs from a benign solvent system. *Mater. Sci. Eng. C Mater. Biol. Appl.* **2017**, *72*, 278–283. [CrossRef]
6. Urciuolo, A.; Urbani, L.; Perin, S.; Maghsoudlou, P.; Scottoni, F.; Gjinovci, A.; Collins-Hooper, H.; Loukogeorgakis, S.; Tyraskis, A.; Torelli, S.; et al. Decellularised skeletal muscles allow functional muscle regeneration by promoting host cell migration. *Sci. Rep.* **2018**, *8*, 8398. [CrossRef]
7. Smoak, M.M.; Han, A.; Watson, E.; Kishan, A.; Grande-Allen, K.J.; Cosgriff-Hernandez, E.; Mikos, A.G. Fabrication and Characterization of Electrospun Decellularized Muscle-Derived Scaffolds. *Tissue Eng. Part C Methods* **2019**, *25*, 276–287. [CrossRef]
8. Zhang, J.; Hu, Z.Q.; Turner, N.J.; Teng, S.F.; Cheng, W.Y.; Zhou, H.Y.; Zhang, L.; Hu, H.W.; Wang, Q.; Badylak, S.F. Perfusion-decellularized skeletal muscle as a three-dimensional scaffold with a vascular network template. *Biomaterials* **2016**, *89*, 114–126. [CrossRef]
9. Masson-Meyers, D.S.; Tayebi, L. Vascularization strategies in tissue engineering approaches for soft tissue repair. *J. Tissue Eng. Regen. Med.* **2021**, *15*, 747–762. [CrossRef]
10. Weigand, A.; Beier, J.P.; Arkudas, A.; Al-Abboodi, M.; Polykandriotis, E.; Horch, R.E.; Boos, A.M. The Arteriovenous (AV) Loop in a Small Animal Model to Study Angiogenesis and Vascularized Tissue Engineering. *J. Vis. Exp.* **2016**, *117*, e54676. [CrossRef]
11. Tamayo, T.; Eno, E.; Madrigal, C.; Heydemann, A.; Garcia, K.; Garcia, J. Functional in situ assessment of muscle contraction in wild-type and mdx mice. *Muscle Nerve* **2016**, *53*, 260–268. [CrossRef]
12. Hayhurst, J.W.; O'Brien, B.M. An experimental study of microvascular technique, patency rates and related factors. *Br. J. Plast. Surg.* **1975**, *28*, 128–132. [CrossRef]
13. Arkudas, A.; Beier, J.P.; Pryymachuk, G.; Hoereth, T.; Bleiziffer, O.; Polykandriotis, E.; Hess, A.; Gulle, H.; Horch, R.E.; Kneser, U. Automatic quantitative micro-computed tomography evaluation of angiogenesis in an axially vascularized tissue-engineered bone construct. *Tissue Eng. Part C Methods* **2010**, *16*, 1503–1514. [CrossRef]

14. Steiner, D.; Winkler, S.; Heltmann-Meyer, S.; Trossmann, V.T.; Fey, T.; Scheibel, T.; Horch, R.E.; Arkudas, A. Enhanced vascularization andde novotissue formation in hydrogels made of engineered RGD-tagged spider silk proteins in the arteriovenous loop model. *Biofabrication* **2021**, *13*, 045003. [CrossRef]
15. Sarhaddi, D.; Poushanchi, B.; Merati, M.; Tchanque-Fossuo, C.; Donneys, A.; Baker, J.; Buchman, S.R. Validation of Histologic Bone Analysis Following Microfil Vessel Perfusion. *J. Histotechnol.* **2012**, *35*, 180–183. [CrossRef]
16. Winkler, S.; Mutschall, H.; Biggemann, J.; Fey, T.; Greil, P.; Korner, C.; Weisbach, V.; Meyer-Lindenberg, A.; Arkudas, A.; Horch, R.E.; et al. Human Umbilical Vein Endothelial Cell Support Bone Formation of Adipose-Derived Stem Cell-Loaded and 3D-Printed Osteogenic Matrices in the Arteriovenous Loop Model. *Tissue Eng. Part A* **2021**, *27*, 413–423. [CrossRef]
17. Conconi, M.T.; De Coppi, P.; Bellini, S.; Zara, G.; Sabatti, M.; Marzaro, M.; Zanon, G.F.; Gamba, P.G.; Parnigotto, P.P.; Nussdorfer, G.G. Homologous muscle acellular matrix seeded with autologous myoblasts as a tissue-engineering approach to abdominal wall-defect repair. *Biomaterials* **2005**, *26*, 2567–2574. [CrossRef]
18. Chung, S.; Hazen, A.; Levine, J.P.; Baux, G.; Olivier, W.A.; Yee, H.T.; Margiotta, M.S.; Karp, N.S.; Gurtner, G.C. Vascularized acellular dermal matrix island flaps for the repair of abdominal muscle defects. *Plast. Reconstr. Surg.* **2003**, *111*, 225–232. [CrossRef]
19. Zhang, F.; Kao, S.D.; Walker, R.; Lineaweaver, W.C. Pectoralis major muscle free flap in rat model. *Microsurgery* **1994**, *15*, 853–856. [CrossRef]
20. Atabay, K.; Hong, C.; Bentz, M.L.; Hrach, C.J.; Futrell, J.W. Variations in the vascular pedicle of the rat gracilis muscle flap. *J. Reconstr. Microsurg.* **1995**, *11*, 265–269. [CrossRef]
21. Dogan, T.; Kryger, Z.; Zhang, F.; Shi, D.Y.; Komorowska-Timek, E.; Lineaweaver, W.C.; Buncke, H.J. Quadriceps femoris muscle flap: Largest muscle flap model in the rat. *J. Reconstr. Microsurg.* **1999**, *15*, 433–437. [CrossRef]
22. Tetreault, M.W.; Della Valle, C.J.; Hellman, M.D.; Wysocki, R.W. Medial gastrocnemius flap in the course of treatment for an infection at the site of a total knee arthroplasty. *JBJS Essent Surg Tech.* **2017**, *7*, e14. [CrossRef]
23. Ritter, P.; Cai, A.; Reischl, B.; Fiedler, M.; Prol, G.; Frie, B.; Kretzschmar, E.; Michael, M.; Hartmann, K.; Lesko, C.; et al. MyoBio: An automated bioreactor system technology for standardized perfusion-decellularization of whole skeletal muscle. *IEEE Trans. Biomed. Eng.* **2022**, 1. [CrossRef]
24. Agata, N.; Sasai, N.; Inoue-Miyazu, M.; Kawakami, K.; Hayakawa, K.; Kobayashi, K.; Sokabe, M. Repetitive stretch suppresses denervation-induced atrophy of soleus muscle in rats. *Muscle Nerve* **2009**, *39*, 456–462. [CrossRef]
25. Sakakima, H.; Yoshida, Y. Effects of short duration static stretching on the denervated and reinnervated soleus muscle morphology in the rat. *Arch. Phys. Med. Rehabil.* **2003**, *84*, 1339–1342. [CrossRef]
26. Sakakima, H.; Yoshida, Y. The effect of short duration static stretching and reinnervation on the recovery of denervated soleus muscle in the rat. *J. Jpn. Phys. Ther. Assoc.* **2002**, *5*, 13–18. [CrossRef]
27. Finol, H.J.; Lewis, D.M. Proceedings: The effects of denervation on isometric contractions of rat skeletal muscle. *J. Physiol.* **1975**, *248*, 11P.
28. Billington, L. Reinnervation and regeneration of denervated rat soleus muscles. *Muscle Nerve* **1997**, *20*, 744–746. [CrossRef]
29. Kaariainen, M.; Kauhanen, S. Skeletal muscle injury and repair: The effect of disuse and denervation on muscle and clinical relevance in pedicled and free muscle flaps. *J. Reconstr. Microsurg.* **2012**, *28*, 581–587. [CrossRef]
30. Bitto, F.F.; Klumpp, D.; Lange, C.; Boos, A.M.; Arkudas, A.; Bleiziffer, O.; Horch, R.E.; Kneser, U.; Beier, J.P. Myogenic differentiation of mesenchymal stem cells in a newly developed neurotised AV-loop model. *Biomed. Res. Int.* **2013**, *2013*, 935046. [CrossRef]
31. Zhang, Y.; Liu, A.; Zhang, W.; Jiang, H.; Cai, Z. Correlation of contractile function recovery with acetylcholine receptor changes in a rat muscle flap model. *Microsurgery* **2010**, *30*, 307–313. [CrossRef]
32. Cen, Y.; Liu, J.; Qin, Y.; Liu, R.; Wang, H.; Zhou, Y.; Wang, S.; Hu, Z. Denervation in Femoral Artery-Ligated Hindlimbs Diminishes Ischemic Recovery Primarily via Impaired Arteriogenesis. *PLoS ONE* **2016**, *11*, e0154941. [CrossRef]
33. Hendrickse, P.; Degens, H. The role of the microcirculation in muscle function and plasticity. *J. Muscle Res. Cell Motil.* **2019**, *40*, 127–140. [CrossRef]
34. Ma, K.; Huang, Z.; Ma, J.; Shao, L.; Wang, H.; Wang, Y. Perlecan and synaptophysin changes in denervated skeletal muscle. *Neural Regen Res.* **2012**, *7*, 1293–1298. [CrossRef]
35. Miyamaru, S.; Kumai, Y.; Minoda, R.; Yumoto, E. Nerve-muscle pedicle implantation in the denervated thyroarytenoid muscle of aged rats. *Acta Otolaryngol.* **2012**, *132*, 210–217. [CrossRef]
36. Mueller, M.; Leonhard, C.; Wacker, K.; Ringelstein, E.B.; Okabe, M.; Hickey, W.F.; Kiefer, R. Macrophage response to peripheral nerve injury: The quantitative contribution of resident and hematogenous macrophages. *Lab. Investig.* **2003**, *83*, 175–185. [CrossRef]

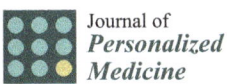

Article

# The Free Myocutaneous Tensor Fasciae Latae Flap—A Workhorse Flap for Sternal Defect Reconstruction: A Single-Center Experience

Amir Khosrow Bigdeli, Florian Falkner, Benjamin Thomas, Gabriel Hundeshagen, Simon Andreas Mayer, Eva-Maria Risse, Leila Harhaus, Emre Gazyakan, Ulrich Kneser and Christian Andreas Radu *

Department of Hand, Plastic and Reconstructive Surgery, Burn Center, BG Trauma Center Ludwigshafen, Plastic and Hand Surgery, University of Heidelberg, Ludwig-Guttmann-Str. 13, D-67071 Ludwigshafen, Germany; amir.bigdeli@bgu-ludwigshafen.de (A.K.B.); florian.falkner@bgu-ludwigshafen.de (F.F.); benjamin.thomas@bgu-ludwigshafen.de (B.T.); gabriel.hundeshagen@bgu-ludwigshafen.de (G.H.); simon.mayer@bgu-ludwigshafen.de (S.A.M.); eva-maria.risse@bgu-ludwigshafen.de (E.-M.R.); leila.harhaus@bgu-ludwigshafen.de (L.H.); emre.gazyakan@bgu-ludwigshafen.de (E.G.); ulrich.kneser@bgu-ludwigshafen.de (U.K.)
* Correspondence: christian.radu@bgu-ludwigshafen.de; Tel.: +49-151-2345-6112; Fax: +49-621-6810-2844

**Abstract:** Introduction: Deep sternal wound infections (DSWI) after cardiac surgery pose a significant challenge in reconstructive surgery. In this context, free flaps represent well-established options. The objective of this study was to investigate the clinical outcome after free myocutaneous tensor fasciae latae (TFL) flap reconstruction of sternal defects, with a special focus on surgical complications and donor-site morbidity. Methods: A retrospective chart review focused on patient demographics, operative details, and postoperative complications. Follow-up reexaminations included assessments of the range of motion and muscle strength at the donor-site. Patients completed the Quality of Life 36-item Short Form Health Survey (SF-36) as well as the Lower Extremity Functional Scale (LEFS) questionnaire and evaluated aesthetic and functional outcomes on a 6-point Likert scale. The Vancouver Scar Scale (VSS) and the Patient and Observer Scar Assessment Scales (POSAS) were used to rate scar appearance. Results: A total of 46 patients (mean age: 67 ± 11 years) underwent sternal defect reconstruction with free TFL flaps between January 2010 and March 2021. The mean defect size was 194 ± 43 cm$^2$. The mean operation time was 387 ± 120 min with a flap ischemia time of 63 ± 16 min. Acute microvascular complications due to flap pedicle thromboses occurred in three patients (7%). All flaps could be salvaged without complete flap loss. Partial flap loss of the distal TFL portion was observed in three patients (7%). All three patients required additional reconstruction with pedicled or local flaps. Upon follow-up, the range of motion (hip joint extension/flexion ($p = 0.73$), abduction/adduction ($p = 0.29$), and internal/external rotation ($p = 0.07$)) and muscle strength at the donor-sites did not differ from the contralateral sides ($p = 0.25$). Patient assessments of aesthetic and functional outcomes, as well as the median SF-36 (physical component summary (44, range of 33 to 57)) and LEFS (54, range if 35 to 65), showed good results with respect to patient comorbidities. The median VSS (3, range of 2 to 7) and POSAS (24, range of 18 to 34) showed satisfactory scar quality and scar appearance. Conclusion: The free TFL flap is a reliable, effective, and, therefore, valuable option for the reconstruction of extensive sternal defects in critically ill patients suffering from DSWIs. In addition, the TFL flap shows satisfactory functional and aesthetic results at the donor-site.

**Keywords:** sternal defect reconstruction; deep sternal wound infection; DSWI; reconstructive microsurgery; free flap; tensor fasciae latae flap; TFL flap

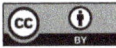

## 1. Introduction

Deep sternal wound infection (DSWI) after cardiac surgery is a severe complication that can result in devastating mortality rates between 10 and 47% [1,2]. Among these multimorbid patients, who often not only bear the burden of pre-existing coronary artery disease (CAD), but also chronic obstructive pulmonary disease (COPD) and diabetes mellitus (DM), reconstructive procedures are highly challenging [2]. The treatment of DSWIs requires radical surgical debridement of soft and bony tissue and, eventually, tension-free defect closure with well-perfused tissue [3]. For sternal defect reconstruction, microsurgeons have a vast armamentarium of pedicled and free flaps at their disposal: Common reconstructive options for sternal defect reconstruction are local flaps from the chest, abdomen, or the back, such as the vertical rectus abdominis musculocutaneous (VRAM) flap, the pectoralis major, and the latissimus dorsi (LD) flap [4,5]. When both internal mammary arteries (IMAs) have been harvested for coronary-artery bypass grafts (CABG) or after previous local flap failure, reconstruction can be difficult. This is partially due to the fact that the arc of rotation of pedicled flaps is limited [5,6] and closure of defects, which include the entirety of the sternum, can be critical, putting the most distal part of the pedicled flap at risk of impaired perfusion [7,8]. To offer these multimorbid patients the best possible care and optimal long-term outcomes, we are increasingly using the free myocutaneous tensor fasciae latae (TFL) flap for extended deep sternal defect reconstruction. With its voluminous muscle bulk and large skin paddle, it can be adapted to large and multilayered wounds, making it ideal for complex sternal reconstruction [9,10]. Here, we report our one-decade single-center experience of 46 free TFL flaps for deep sternal defect reconstruction following cardiac surgery. The study aimed at evaluating the feasibility of this free flap for sternal reconstruction by analyzing operative data, surgical complication rates, reconstructive outcomes, and donor-site morbidity.

## 2. Patients and Methods

The study has been performed in accordance with the guidelines and regulations of the Declaration of Helsinki and has been approved by the local ethics committee (Mainz, Germany, IRB approval reference number: 2021–15577). Retrospective clinical data were collected from our institutional database of patients undergoing free flap reconstruction from January 2010 until March 2021. A retrospective chart review for intraoperative details, surgical and medical complications, length of hospitalization, as well as outcome and mortality rates, was performed. The severity of DSWI was rated according to the El Oakley and Wright classification from I to V [11]. The ASA (American Society of Anesthesiologists) classification system was used to assess the perioperative risk for each patient. Postoperative surgical complications, which required additional surgical intervention, were considered as major. The primary outcomes studied were "re-explorations" because of acute vascular complications, such as pedicle thromboses, as well as flap necrosis, wound dehiscence, hematoma, and infection. Partial flap necrosis was considered as necrosis affecting >5% (maximum of 20%) of the flap surface area. In addition, any medical complications, such as respiratory failure or death throughout the postoperative hospital stay, were evaluated.

### 2.1. Pre-, Intra-, and Postoperative Treatment

All free TFL flap operations were performed in a two-team approach for the donor- and recipient-sites. Intraoperatively, 500 IU to 1500 IU (international units) of unfractionated heparin were applied prior to releasing the flap anastomosis or 2000 IU to 3000 IU in case of an arteriovenous loop (AVL). Intraoperative flap perfusion measurements were not performed regularly. However, since January 2017, indocyanine green angiography (ICG) has been performed occasionally, depending on the individual intraoperative decision of the senior surgeon. Primary closure of the TFL donor-site was performed in two layers. Closed suction drains were left in situ in all cases. No additional reconstruction of the fascia was performed. Postoperatively, all patients received 30 mg enoxaparin twice a day over a five-day period, followed by daily 40 mg doses for at least two weeks. Subsequently, the therapy was continued until adequate mobilization of the patient was achieved All free flaps were examined hourly by analyzing the capillary refill, skin temperature, and skin color for five days in order to detect any perfusion alterations.

*2.2. Follow-Up*

Follow-up was established from the date of surgery to the last outpatient visit at our department at least 3 months after discharge. Follow-up examinations included donor-site range of motion (ROM), with measurements in hip and knee joints, as well as strength measurements of the thigh muscles. Results were analyzed and compared to the contralateral healthy side. Muscle strength was assessed manually and scaled in six grades (0 = complete paralysis, 1 = contraction palpable, 2 = active movement with gravity eliminated, 3 = active movement against gravity, 4 = active movement against resistance, 5 = normal power) [12]. Additionally, each patient completed the Quality of Life 36-item Short Form Health Survey (SF-36) and the Lower Extremity Functional Scale (LEFS) questionnaire [13,14]. The subjective donor-site morbidity and satisfaction with the overall aesthetic and functional results were analyzed using a self-reported non-standardized 6-point Likert-questionnaire. Results were rated on a scale from 1 to 6 (1 = excellent, 6 = poor). The Vancouver Scar Scale (VSS) and the Patient and Observer Scar Assessment Scales (POSAS) were used to analyze scarring at the donor- and recipient-sites [15,16].

*2.3. Statistical Analysis*

Data were collected in excel sheets, and statistical analyses were performed using GraphPad Prism 7.0 (GraphPad Software, Inc., San Diego, CA, USA). For descriptive statistics of patients and flaps, the mean of continuous data accompanied by the standard deviation and the median or mode with interquartile ranges for ordinal data were reported. The paired two-sided Wilcoxon–Mann–Whitney-Test and the two-sided chi-square test were computed to assess differences in categorical and dichotomous variables, respectively. $p$-values of <0.05 were regarded statistically significant.

## 3. Results

Between January 2010 and March 2021, 46 patients underwent sternal defect reconstruction with free TFL flaps. Patients included 17 women (37%) and 29 men (63%), with a mean age of 67 ± 11 years (range: 38 to 85 years). Sternal osteomyelitis in all 46 patients was confirmed upon microbiology, clinical presentation, histology, and computed tomography. The defect etiologies were as follows: wound infection and sternum osteomyelitis after CABG with use of the left internal mammary artery (LIMA, $n$ = 35; 76%), CABG with use of both IMAs ($n$ = 1; 2%), valve replacement (VR, $n$ = 5; 11%), or combined valve replacement and LIMA-CABG ($n$ = 5, 11%). The median ASA classification was 3 (range: 2 to 4). Demographic data of patients, individual risk factors, chronic conditions, the El Oakley classification, as well as the results of microbiological examinations are summarized in Table 1.

**Table 1.** Patient demographics and comorbidities, El Oakley and Wright classification, and microbiological examination (SD = Standard Deviation).

| Patient Demographics | |
|---|---|
| Number of patients and flaps | 46 |
| Mean age (years) ± SD (range) | 67 ± 11 (38 to 85) |
| Median ASA class (range) | 3 (2 to 4) |
| Sex (female/male) | 17/29 |
| Comorbidities | $n$ (%) |
| Arterial hypertension (HTN) | 44 (96%) |
| Coronary artery disease (CAD) | 41 (89%) |
| Chronic heart failure (CHF) | 27 (59%) |
| Chronic obstructive pulmonary disease (COPD) | 20 (44%) |
| Chronic kidney disease (CKD) | 25 (54%) |
| Diabetes mellitus (DM) | 30 (65%) |
| Active smoker at time of surgery | 13 (28%) |

Table 1. *Cont.*

| Patient Demographics | |
|---|---|
| BMI (Body Mass Index) (kg/m$^2$) | 29 ± 6 |
| Obesity (BMI ≥ 30 kg/m$^2$) | 19 (41%) |
| El Oakley and Wright classification | |
| I | - |
| II | - |
| IIIA | 7 (15%) |
| IIIB | 11 (24%) |
| IVA | 2 (4%) |
| IVB | - |
| V | 26 (57%) |
| Microbiological examination of soft and bony tissue | |
| *Staphylococcus aureus* | 17 (37%) |
| Methicillin-resistant *Staphylococcus aureus* | 6 (13%) |
| *Staphylococcus epidermidis* | 14 (30%) |
| *Enterococcus faecalis* | 10 (22%) |
| *Escherichia coli* | 7 (15%) |
| Multiresistant Gram-negative bacteria | 9 (20%) |

A total of 16 patients (35%) underwent secondary reconstructions at our institution following failed prior attempts. Of these, 11 patients (*n* = 11; 24%) had previously undergone unsuccessful bilateral pedicled pectoralis major flaps at the referring cardiosurgical departments. Five patients, in detail, two VRAM and three bilateral pectoralis major flaps, developed partial flap losses requiring further free flap surgery at our institution (*n* = 5; 11%). These 16 patients underwent an average of 3 ± 2 debridements and negative pressure wound therapy cycles prior to free flap surgery. The mean operation time (OT) was 387 ± 120 min (range: 212 to 695 min), which included a mean flap ischemia time of 63 ± 16 min (range: 32 to 91 min). While the mean sternal defect size was 194 ± 43 cm$^2$, the mean skin paddle surface of the TFL flap was 205 ± 38 cm$^2$, with a mean flap length of 24 ± 3 cm and a mean flap width of 8 ± 1 cm. Single-stage AVLs were necessary in 22 cases to provide reliable recipient vessels (Figure 1). Operative characteristics are presented in Table 2.

**Table 2.** Operative characteristics (cm = centimeter, cm$^2$ = square-centimeter, min = minute, RIMA = Right Internal Mammary Artery, OT = Operation Time).

| Operative Characteristics | |
|---|---|
| Mean sternal defect size [cm$^2$] ± SD | 194 ± 43 (128 to 297) |
| Mean sternal defect length [cm] ± SD | 23 ± 3 (18 to 27) |
| Mean sternal defect width [cm] ± SD | 8 ± 1 (7 to 11) |
| Mean length of flap ischemia [min] ± SD | 63 ± 16 (32 to 91) |
| Mean skin paddle surface [cm$^2$] ± SD | 205 ± 38 (154 to 308) |
| Mean flap length [cm] ± SD | 24 ± 3 (19 to 28) |
| Mean flap width [cm] ± SD | 8 ± 1 (7 to 11) |
| Mean OT [min] ± SD (range) | 387 ± 120 (212 to 695) |
| Recipient vessel situation | |
| RIMA and concomitant vein | 9 (20%) |
| RIMA and cephalic vein | 15 (33%) |
| Cephalic vein-thoracoacromial artery arterio-venous loop | 3 (7%) |
| Cephalic vein-subclavian artery arterio-venous loop | 10 (22%) |
| Subclavian artery/vein arterio-venous loop using a greater saphenous vein graft | 9 (20%) |

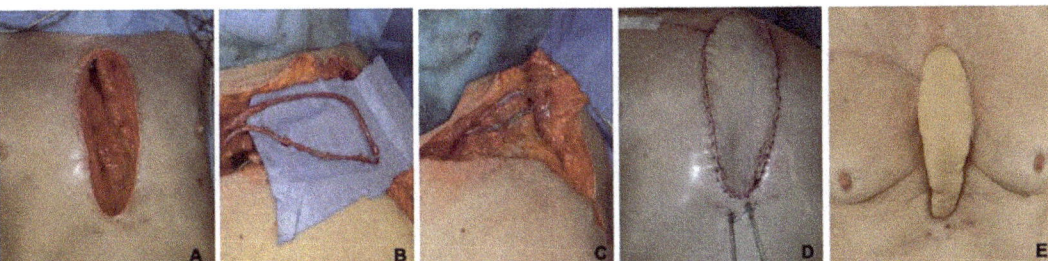

**Figure 1.** A 62-year-old male patient with DSWI and sternal osteomyelitis after a bilateral CABG procedure. The resulting defect measured 22 × 8 cm (**A**). Sternal reconstruction with a TFL flap and an AVL was planned. The AVL was created between the subclavian artery and vein in an end-to-side technique using a greater saphenous vein graft (**B**). Subsequently, arterial and venous end-to-end anastomoses with the TFL flap pedicle were performed (**C,D**). The patient's recovery was uneventful, and he was discharged 13 days postoperatively. Stable defect reconstruction without any sign of wound healing disorder or recurrent infection three month after surgery (**E**).

*3.1. Postoperative Complications*

The immediate postoperative course was uneventful in 38 of 46 patients (83%). Eight patients (17%) experienced acute microvascular complications or progredient hematoma at the recipient-site, which required emergency free flap re-exploration. In detail, acute microvascular compromise was observed during re-exploration in three cases (7%) in the form of acute arterial ($n = 2$; 4%) or venous thrombosis ($n = 1$; 2%). In this context, the use of single-stage AVLs did not increase the risk of microvascular thrombosis ($n = 1/21$ vs. $n = 2/22$; odds ratio: 0.50; 95% confidence interval: 0.03 to 4.6; $p = 0.9$). Postoperative hematoma evacuation was necessary in five patients (11%) within the first three days after flap surgery. All flaps could be salvaged. The further postoperative course was complicated in 6 patients (13%). In three patients, partial flap necroses of the most distal TFL parts were observed (7%). In these three patients, further secondary reconstructions with an intercostal anterior perforator flap ($n = 1$; 2%), a pedicled VRAM flap ($n = 1$; 2%), and two opposing local rotational flaps ($n = 2$; 4%) were performed. Wound dehiscence of the TFL flap with the need for debridement and secondary split-thickness skin-grafting (SSTG) was necessary in three patients (7%). Surgical donor-site complications occurred in five patients (11%), including three cases of impaired wound healing (7%), one case of donor-site infection (2%), and one case with the need for hematoma evacuation (2%). Of these patients, two received SSTG (4%) and three underwent successful secondary wound closure (7%). Eventually, all donor-sites healed satisfactorily. Table 3 shows the distribution of surgical complications. The average hospital stay was 34 ± 12 days, with a mean length of postoperative hospital stay of 23 ± 14 days. Postoperatively, 37 patients (80%) were monitored at the intensive care unit (ICU) for an average of 6 ± 9 days. Postoperative medical complications were seen in six patients (13%). These included: paralytic ileus ($n = 1$; 2%), postoperative delirium ($n = 1$; 2%), and cardiovascular instability with severe hypotension ($n = 2$; 4%). Two patients (4%) died due to respiratory failure and cardiovascular instability within the first 30 days post-surgery. The 1-year mortality rate was 17% ($n = 8$), but these deaths were not related to flap surgery. At the time of discharge, all successfully treated patients presented with stable soft-tissue conditions and without a sign of recurrent sternal infection.

*3.2. Follow-Up Examinations*

Follow-up donor-site examinations were performed 34 ± 19 months after free flap surgery, including a total of 28 patients (61% follow-up rate). From the initial cohort of 46 patients, 8 patients (17%) had died, and 10 patients (22%) could not be reached. At the TFL donor-sites, the ROM of hip and knee joints revealed no restrictions when compared to the contralateral healthy sides (Table 4). Three patients subjectively described a weakness in knee extension ($n = 3$; 11%); however, muscle strength was not notably impaired in any patient (donor-site: median of 5, range of 4 to 5 vs. healthy-site: median of 5, range of 4 to 5; $p = 0.25$). Herniation of the quadriceps muscle was not seen in any patient at follow-up. The patient-reported satisfaction showed an overall good result for both functional and aesthetic outcomes at the donor-site (function: median of 2, range of 1 to 4; aesthetic: median of 2, range of 1 to 4). With respect to general health and satisfaction, the SF-36 questionnaire (physical component summary, median of 44, range: 33 to 57; mental component summary, median of 29, range: 19 to 40) as well as the LEFS (median of 54, range: 35 to 65) revealed satisfactory results. The mean donor-site scar length was $24.8 \pm 3.3$ cm. Scar examinations revealed a median VSS score of 3 (range: 2 to 7) at the donor-site and a median of 3 (range: 2 to 5) at the corresponding recipient-site. In accordance, the POSAS showed an overall good satisfaction with scar quality and scar appearance at the donor-site (median: 24, range: 18 to 34) and recipient-site (median: 23, range: 19 to 31) with comparable results for the patients' and observers' scale (Table 4).

Table 3. Postoperative complications.

| Surgical Complications | n (%) |
|---|---|
| **Flap Complications** | |
| Arterial thrombosis | 2 (4%) |
| Venous thrombosis | 1 (2%) |
| Hematoma | 5 (11%) |
| Wound dehiscence | 3 (7%) |
| Partial flap necrosis (>5% of the skin paddle) | 3 (7%) |
| **Donor-site complications** | |
| Impaired wound healing | 3 (7%) |
| Wound infection | 1 (2%) |
| Hematoma | 1 (2%) |

Table 4. Follow-up examination (VSS = Vancouver Scar Scale, POSAS = Patient and Observer Scar Assessment Scale, SD = Standard Deviation).

| Follow-Up Examinations | | | |
|---|---|---|---|
| Range of Motion | Donor-Site | Healthy Side | p-Value |
| Mean knee joint extension/flexion (mean ± SD) | 110° ± 9° | 114° ± 9° | $p = 0.08$ |
| Mean hip joint extension/flexion (mean ± SD) | 118° ± 10° | 122° ± 8° | $p = 0.73$ |
| Mean hip joint abduction/adduction (mean ± SD) | 69° ± 5° | 71° ± 6° | $p = 0.29$ |
| Mean hip internal-/external rotation (mean ± SD) | 58° ± 7° | 62° ± 7° | $p = 0.07$ |
| Scarring | Donor-Site | Recipient-Site | |
| Median VSS (range) | 3 (2 to 7) | 3 (2 to 5) | - |
| Median POSAS (range) | 24 (18 to 34) | 23 (19 to 31) | - |
| Median patients' scar assessment (range) | 12 (9 to 21) | 12 (10 to 16) | - |
| Median observers' scar assessment (range) | 11 (9 to 17) | 11 (9 to 15) | - |

## 4. Discussion

In the present study, we report on our treatment of a selective group of patients with DSWI and sternal osteomyelitis after cardiac surgery resulting in large sternal defects. The patients in this study had multiple previous surgeries (El Oakley III to V), with their overall morbidity leading to a median ASA score of 3. Nowadays, microsurgical free flap transfer is a safe and reliable procedure, with failure rates ranging between 1 and 6% [17–19]. However, it is technically complex, time-consuming, and often debilitating on multimorbid patients due to their diminished physical reserves [20–22]. A particularly challenging situation arises when free flaps become the only remaining reconstructive option because defects cannot be closed with local or pedicled flaps. Nevertheless, a persisting disfiguring, painful, and infected defect is hardly ever an alternative for the patient's remaining life span. In order to avoid additional complications, any reconstructive procedure in these patients needs to be as safe and reliable as possible. Hereby, operative time should be kept as short as possible, with the designated flap being "easily accessible". Pursuing the objective of optimizing the treatment of these critically ill patients, we have increasingly been choosing the free TFL flap with its large skin paddle, which makes it ideal for the reconstruction of extensive three-dimensional sternal defects.

The TFL muscle is a weak flexor and lateral rotator of the thigh. The muscle is dispensable, and its absence usually causes no remarkable functional deficit or donor-site morbidity [9]. This was confirmed by the results of our clinical follow-up examinations. Hereby, muscle strength and range of motion were not considerably impaired. However, our method of muscle strength assessment may not have been precise enough to discriminate between the donor-site and uninjured side. The LEFS, a well-established and sensitive tool to measure lower extremity functional impairment [14], also did not reveal considerable impairment in any patient (median LEFS = 54) when compared to normative median values (LEFS = 66) for patients older than 65 [23]. Donor-site morbidity in this study was negligible when compared to other flaps, such as the rectus abdominis muscle flap, for example [24,25]. The TFL flap can comprise a maximal skin paddle three times the size of the muscle [26]. Therefore, it combines the freedom of abundant skin coverage and a strong fascial layer with the versatility of a microvascular pedicle. The fascia is a highly vascularized semirigid layer, which provides additional structural support to cover large defects [9,27]. The TFL flap is easily accessible and can be harvested in a supine position, thus eliminating the need for lengthy intraoperative repositioning, when compared to flaps from the thoracodorsal system. The operating time can be kept short by working in a two-team approach. Another advantage of the large muscular TFL flap is its suitability for anastomoses to AVLs, as opposed to fasciocutaneous perforator flaps, such as the anterior lateral thigh (ALT) flap. In this context, Henn and colleagues stated that ALT flaps in combination with AVLs might be prone to microvascular complications due to an elevated flow resistance of the small-caliber perforator in comparison to the low-resistance conditions of the vein graft used in AVLs [28]. Because of these findings, we refrain from using fasciocutaneous perforator flaps in combination with AVLs and only use muscle-based flaps in these scenarios. In line with this notion, the combination of TFL flaps with AVLs showed no increased risk of microvascular thrombosis in this study.

Certainly, we want to point out that, in general, the full armamentarium of reconstructive procedures is required to cover sternal defects. Hereby, the most prevalent reconstructive options usually comprise pedicled muscle flaps, as they provide well-vascularized tissue with enough bulk to fill the defect cavity. The pedicled VRAM flap, LD flap, and bilateral pectoralis major flap have been the method of choice for decades [5,6,8]. In this context, it is recommended to cover cranial sternal wounds with pectoralis major flaps, whereas VRAM flaps are of better use to cover caudal sternal wounds. Davison and colleagues compared the outcome of 41 modified pectoralis major flaps against 56 pedicled VRAM flaps and reported equal wound dehiscence rates (VRAM: 14.2% vs. PM: 14.6%) [4]. However, it has to be considered that in the majority of patients developing DSWI after cardiovascular surgery, the LIMA is harvested for CABG. Therefore only the RIMA can be used for a cranially pedicled VRAM flap [8]. Furthermore, the most distal part of the pedicled flap, which is of paramount importance to the reconstructive outcome, especially in larger defects, is at risk of impaired perfusion, with a higher risk for wound dehiscence and infection [29]. We agree with Davison and colleagues that both pedicled flaps are straight forward and easy to harvest; nevertheless, the free TFL flap showed lower rates of wound dehiscence and partial flap necrosis in this study.

The latissimus dorsi muscle is the largest human muscle and is ideal to cover larger sternal defects. Even when the insertion to the humeral bone is detached, the maximum arc of rotation of a pedicled LD flap is an important limitation, particularly when a midline exceeding defect must be reconstructed [29]. This can put the most distal part of the flap at risk of impaired perfusion. Spindler and colleagues published a study of 106 patients undergoing sternal reconstruction with a pedicled myocutaneous LD flap. Besides no total flap loss, they reported 35% revision surgeries because of wound healing disorders, hematoma, or persistent infection [30]. In comparison to their results, the number of revision surgeries for partial flap necrosis ($n = 3$), wound healing disorders ($n = 3$), and hematomas ($n = 5$) was lower in our cohort (24%). According to the current literature, the free LD transfer can show reliable results, with encouragingly low rates of revision surgeries or serious complications [31]. However, raising a free LD flap to cover sternal defects has some disadvantages that need to be considered. First, patients must be repositioned intraoperatively, and the flap must be banked in the axilla. Second, the latissimus dorsi muscle, as the rectus abdominis muscle, is an auxiliary breathing muscle; thus, sacrificing this muscle can affect breathing mechanisms in these already multimorbid patients [30]. While some authors state that the greater omentum (OM) flap is a valuable alternative to muscle flaps, we do not consider the OM flap as a first line procedure [32]. Kolbenschlag and colleagues presented a study of 50 patients undergoing sternal defect reconstruction with a pedicled OM flap and reported high surgical complication rates and high donor-site morbidity, with one patient even developing acute intestinal incarceration [33]. Therefore, the OM flap should be considered a last resort backup option rather than a first-line treatment. Furthermore it should be considered than an increasing defect size can be related to a higher incidence of partial flap necrosis of pedicled flaps, leading to a higher rate of revisional surgeries and impaired postoperative recovery [34]. In this context we can recommend the myocutaneous TFL flap as a workhorse flap for extensive sternal defect reconstruction.

Despite the promising nature of our data, which highlight the feasibility of the free TFL flap for the reconstruction of large sternal defects in a one-stage procedure, our study has important limitations that need to be discussed. First, our study is limited by its retrospective nature and involvement of several different surgeons and their various flap planning routines. Second, the study comprises a relatively small number of patients. Therefore, we conclude that a larger cohort of patients and a longer follow-up period are necessary to gain more reliable data regarding the choice of the reconstructive approach in this context. Third, the follow-up response rate was low, and follow-up times varied greatly, which may have resulted in different stages of rehabilitation, wound healing, and scarring assessed.

## 5. Conclusions

In conclusion, the free TFL flap represents a valuable option for sternal reconstruction in critically ill patients with large defects and a history of previously failed reconstructive procedures. It is associated with an encouragingly low morbidity at the corresponding donor-site. We therefore regard the free TFL flap, in combination with AVLs if needed, as a workhorse flap for sternal reconstruction, rather than merely a backup option.

**Author Contributions:** A.K.B., F.F., B.T. and C.A.R. designed the study. F.F. carried out data acquisition, performed the statistical analysis and data interpretation, and drafted the first version of the manuscript. G.H., S.A.M. and E.-M.R. supported the manuscript writing. L.H., E.G., U.K. and C.A.R. helped in data interpretation and manuscript revision. A.K.B. and C.A.R. further participated in the conception of the study, interpretation of data, as well as manuscript preparation. All authors have read and agreed to the published version of the manuscript.

**Funding:** No funding was received for this article. None of the authors has a financial interest in any of the products, devices, or drugs mentioned in this manuscript.

**Institutional Review Board Statement:** This study was approved by the local ethics committee (Mainz, Germany) under the IRB approval reference number 2021-15577. The need for consent was deemed unnecessary according to German national regulations (ethical committee of Rhineland palatinate, Germany). The study has been performed in accordance with the guidelines and regulations of the Declaration of Helsinki.

**Informed Consent Statement:** Not applicable.

**Data Availability Statement:** The datasets used and/or analyzed during the current study are available from the corresponding author on reasonable request.

**Conflicts of Interest:** The authors declare no conflict of interest.

## References

1. Strecker, T.; Rösch, J.; Horch, R.E.; Weyand, M.; Kneser, U. Sternal wound infections following cardiac surgery: Risk factor analysis and interdisciplinary treatment. *Heart Surg. Forum.* **2007**, *10*. [CrossRef] [PubMed]
2. Yusuf, E.; Chan, M.; Renz, N.; Trampuz, A. Current perspectives on diagnosis and management of sternal wound infections. *Infect. Drug Resist.* **2018**, *11*, 961–968. [CrossRef]
3. Cabbabe, E.B.; Cabbabe, S.W. Surgical management of the symptomatic unstable sternum with pectoralis major muscle flaps. *Plast. Reconstr. Surg.* **2009**, *123*, 1495–1498. [CrossRef] [PubMed]
4. Davison, S.P.; Clemens, M.W.; Armstrong, D.; Newton, E.D.; Swartz, W. Sternotomy wounds: Rectus flap versus modified pectoral reconstruction. *Plast. Reconstr. Surg.* **2007**, *120*, 929–934. [CrossRef] [PubMed]
5. Daigeler, A.; Falkenstein, A.; Pennekamp, W.; Duchna, H.W.; Birger Jettkant, D.; Goertz, O.; Homann, H.-H.; Steinau, H.-U.; Lehnhardt, M. Sternal osteomyelitis: Long-term results after pectoralis muscle flap reconstruction. *Plast. Reconstr. Surg.* **2009**, *123*, 910–917. [CrossRef] [PubMed]
6. Baumann, D.P.; Butler, C.E. Component separation improves outcomes in VRAM flap donor sites with excessive fascial tension. *Plast. Reconstr. Surg.* **2010**, *126*, 1573–1580. [CrossRef]
7. Taeger, C.D.; Horch, R.E.; Arkudas, A.; Schmitz, M.; Stübinger, A.; Lang, W.; Meyer, A.; Seitz, T.; Weyand, M.; Beier, J.P. Combined free flaps with arteriovenous loops for reconstruction of extensive thoracic defects after sternal osteomyelitis. *Microsurgery* **2016**, *36*, 121–127. [CrossRef]
8. Li, Y.H.; Zheng, Z.; Yang, J.; Su, L.L.; Liu, Y.; Han, F.; Liu, J.-Q.; Hu, D.-H. Management of the extensive thoracic defects after deep sternal wound infection with the rectus abdominis myocutaneous flap: A retrospective case series. *Medicine* **2017**, *96*, e6391. [CrossRef]
9. O'Hare, P.M.; Leonard, A.G.; Brennen, M.D. Experience with the tensor fasciae latae free flap. *Br. J. Plast. Surg.* **1983**, *36*, 98–104. [CrossRef]
10. Engel, H.; Pelzer, M.; Sauerbier, M.; Germann, G.; Heitmann, C. An innovative treatment concept for free flap reconstruction of complex central chest wall defects—The cephalic-thoraco-acromial (CTA) loop. *Microsurgery* **2007**, *27*, 481–486. [CrossRef]
11. El Oakley, R.M.; Wright, J.E. Postoperative mediastinitis: Classification and management. *Ann. Thorac. Surg.* **1996**, *61*, 1030–1036. [CrossRef]
12. Medical Research Council. *Aids to the Investigation of Peripheral Nerve Injuries*, 2nd ed.; Her Majesty's Stationery Office: London, UK, 1943.
13. Ware, J.E.; Sherbourne, C.D. The MOS 36-item short-form health survey (Sf-36): I. conceptual framework and item selection. *Med. Care* **1992**, *30*, 473–483. [CrossRef] [PubMed]
14. Binkley, J.M.; Stratford, P.W.; Lott, S.A.; Riddle, D.L. The Lower Extremity Functional Scale (LEFS): Scale development, measurement properties, and clinical application. *Phys. Ther.* **1999**, *79*, 371–383. [CrossRef] [PubMed]
15. Tyack, Z.; Simons, M.; Spinks, A.; Wasiak, J. A systematic review of the quality of burn scar rating scales for clinical and research use. *Burns* **2012**, *38*, 6–18. [CrossRef] [PubMed]
16. Draaijers, L.J.; Tempelman, F.R.; Botman, Y.A.M.; Tuinebreijer, W.E.; Middelkoop, E.; Kreis, R.W.; Van Zuijlen, P.P. The Patient and Observer Scar Assessment Scale: A Reliable and Feasible Tool for Scar Evaluation. *Plast. Reconstr. Surg.* **2004**, *113*, 1960–1965. [CrossRef]
17. Xiong, L.; Gazyakan, E.; Kremer, T.; Hernekamp, F.J.; Harhaus, L.; Saint-Cyr, M.; Knesser, U.; Hirche, C. Free flaps for reconstruction of soft tissue defects in lower extremity: A meta-analysis on microsurgical outcome and safety. *Microsurgery* **2016**, *36*, 511–524. [CrossRef]
18. Mirzabeigi, M.N.; Wang, T.; Kovach, S.J.; Taylor, J.A.; Serletti, J.M.; Wu, L.C. Free flap take-back following postoperative microvascular compromise: Predicting salvage versus failure. *Plast. Reconstr. Surg.* **2012**, *130*, 579–589. [CrossRef]
19. Serletti, J.M.; Higgins, J.P.; Moran, S.; Orlando, G.S. Factors Affecting Outcome in Free-Tissue Transfer in the Elderly. *Plast. Reconstr. Surg.* **2000**, *106*, 66–70. [CrossRef]
20. Makary, M.A.; Segev, D.L.; Pronovost, P.J.; Syin, D.; Bandeen-Roche, K.; Patel, P.; Takenaga, R.; Devgan, L.; Holzmueller, C.G.; Tian, J.; et al. Frailty as a Predictor of Surgical Outcomes in Older Patients. *J. Am. Coll. Surg.* **2010**, *210*, 901–908. [CrossRef]
21. Wong, A.K.; Nguyen, J.; Peric, M.; Shahabi, A.; Vidar, E.N.; Hwang, B.H.; Niknam Leilabadi, S.; Chan, L.S.; Urata, M.M. Analysis of risk factors associated with microvascular free flap failure using a multi-institutional Database. *Microsurgery* **2015**, *35*, 6–12. [CrossRef]
22. Wähmann, M.; Wähmann, M.; Henn, D.; Xiong, L.; Hirche, C.; Harhaus, L.; Knesser, U.; Kremer, T. Geriatric Patients with Free Flap Reconstruction: A Comparative Clinical Analysis of 256 Cases. *J. Reconstr. Microsurg.* **2020**, *36*, 127–135. [CrossRef] [PubMed]
23. Dingemans, S.A.; Kleipool, S.C.; Mulders, M.A.M.; Winkelhagen, J.; Schep, N.W.; Goslings, J.C.; Schepers, T. Normative data for the lower extremity functional scale (LEFS). *Acta Orthop.* **2017**, *88*, 422–426. [CrossRef] [PubMed]

24. Rao, V.K.; Baertsch, A. Microvascular reconstruction of the upper extremity with the rectus abdominis muscle. *Microsurgery* **1994**, *15*, 746–750. [CrossRef] [PubMed]
25. Galli, A.; Raposio, E.; Santi, P. Reconstruction of full-thickness defects of the thoracic wall by myocutaneous flap transfer: Latissimus dorsi compared with transverse rectus abdominis. *Scand. J. Plast. Reconstr. Surg. Hand. Surg.* **1995**, *29*, 39–43. [CrossRef]
26. Nahai, F.; Hill, L.H.; Hester, R.T. Experiences with the tensor fascia lata flap. *Plast. Reconstr. Surg.* **1979**, *63*, 788–799. [CrossRef]
27. Gruen, L.; Morrison, W.A.; Vellar, I.V.D. Surgical Technique The Tensor Fasciae Latae myocutaneous Flap Closue Of Major Chest And Abdominal Wall Defects. *Aust. N. Z. J. Surg.* **1998**, *68*, 666–669. [CrossRef]
28. Henn, D.; Wähmann, M.S.T.; Horsch, M.; Hetjens, S.; Kremer, T.; Gazyakan, E.; Hirche, C.; Schmidt, V.J.; German, G.; Knesser, U. One-Stage versus Two-Stage Arteriovenous Loop Reconstructions: An Experience on 103 Cases from a Single Center. *Plast. Reconstr. Surg.* **2019**, *143*, 912–924. [CrossRef]
29. Beier, J.P.; Arkudas, A.; Lang, W.; Weyand, M.; Horch, R.E. Sternumosteomyelitis—Chirurgische Behandlungskonzepte Sternal osteomyelitis—Surgical treatment concepts. *Der Chir.* **2016**, *87*, 537–550. [CrossRef]
30. Spindler, N.; Kade, S.; Spiegl, U.; Misfeld, M.; Josten, C.; Mohr, F.W.; Borger, M.; Langer, S. Deep sternal wound infection—Latissimus dorsi flap is a reliable option for reconstruction of the thoracic wall. *BMC Surg.* **2019**, *19*, 173. [CrossRef]
31. Wettstein, R.; Erni, D.; Berdat, P.; Rothenfluh, D.; Banic, A. Radical sternectomy and primary musculocutaneous flap reconstruction to control sternal osteitis. *J. Thorac. Cardiovasc. Surg.* **2002**, *123*, 1185–1190. [CrossRef]
32. López-Monjardin, H.; De-la-Peña-Salcedo, A.; Mendoza-Muñoz, M.; López-Yáñez-de-la-Peña, A.; Palacio-López, E.; López-García, A. Omentum flap versus pectoralis major flap in the treatment of mediastinitis. *Plast. Reconstr. Surg.* **1998**, *101*, 1481–1485. [CrossRef] [PubMed]
33. Kolbenschlag, J.; Hörner, C.; Sogorski, A.; Goertz, O.; Ring, A.; Harati, K.; Lehnhardt, M.; Diageler, A. Sternal Reconstruction with the Omental Flap—Acute and Late Complications, Predictors of Mortality, and Quality of Life. *J. Reconstr. Microsurg.* **2018**, *34*, 376–382. [PubMed]
34. Falkner, F.; Thomas, B.; Haug, V.; Nagel, S.S.; Vollbach, F.H.; Kneser, U.; Bigdeli, A.K. Comparison of pedicled versus free flaps for reconstruction of extensive deep sternal wound defects following cardiac surgery. *Microsurgery* **2021**, *41*, 309–318. [CrossRef] [PubMed]

# Article

# Intra- and Early Postoperative Evaluation of Malperfused Areas in an Irradiated Random Pattern Skin Flap Model Using Indocyanine Green Angiography and Near-Infrared Reflectance-Based Imaging and Infrared Thermography

Wibke Müller-Seubert [1,*], Patrick Ostermaier [1], Raymund E. Horch [1], Luitpold Distel [2], Benjamin Frey [3], Aijia Cai [1] and Andreas Arkudas [1]

1. Laboratory for Tissue Engineering and Regenerative Medicine, Department of Plastic and Hand Surgery, University Hospital Erlangen, Friedrich Alexander University Erlangen-Nuremberg FAU, 91054 Erlangen, Germany; patrickostermaier@yahoo.com (P.O.); raymund.horch@uk-erlangen.de (R.E.H.); aijia.cai@uk-erlangen.de (A.C.); andreas.arkudas@uk-erlangen.de (A.A.)
2. Department of Radiation Oncology, University Hospital Erlangen, Friedrich Alexander University Erlangen-Nuremberg FAU, 91054 Erlangen, Germany; luitpold.distel@uk-erlangen.de
3. Translational Radiobiology, Department of Radiation Oncology, University Hospital Erlangen, Friedrich Alexander University Erlangen-Nuremberg FAU, 91054 Erlangen, Germany; benjamin.frey@uk-erlangen.de
* Correspondence: wibke.mueller-seubert@uk-erlangen.de; Tel.: +49-9131-85-33296; Fax: +49-9131-85-39327

**Abstract:** Background: Assessment of tissue perfusion after irradiation of random pattern flaps still remains a challenge. Methods: Twenty-five rats received harvesting of bilateral random pattern fasciocutaneous flaps. Group 1 served as nonirradiated control group. The right flaps of the groups 2–5 were irradiated with 20 Gy postoperatively (group 2), 3 × 12 Gy postoperatively (group 3), 20 Gy preoperatively (group 4) and 3 × 12 Gy preoperatively (group 5). Imaging with infrared thermography, indocyanine green angiography and near-infrared reflectance-based imaging were performed to detect necrotic areas of the flaps. Results: Analysis of the percentage of the necrotic area of the irradiated flaps showed a statistically significant increase from day 1 to 14 only in group 5 ($p < 0.05$). Indocyanine green angiography showed no differences ($p > 0.05$) of the percentage of the nonperfused area between all days in group 1 and 3, but a decrease in group 2 in both the left and the right flaps. Infrared thermography and near-infrared reflectance-based imaging did not show evaluable differences. Conclusion: Indocyanine green angiography is more precise in prediction of necrotic areas in random pattern skin flaps when compared to hyperspectral imaging, thermography or clinical impression. Preoperative fractional irradiation with a lower individual dose but a higher total dose has a more negative impact on flap perfusion compared to higher single stage irradiation.

**Keywords:** irradiation; imaging; malperfusion

## 1. Introduction

Defect reconstruction still remains one of the main fields of interest in plastic surgery. Assessment of flap viability has been shown to be effective using the correct length-to-width ratio in the case of random pattern flaps for clinical evaluation [1,2].

When multimorbid oncological patients who might have undergone irradiation preoperatively or should undergo irradiation postoperatively, further reliable assessment of flap perfusion is necessary to avoid complications such as wound healing disorders and partial or complete flap loss [1]. Therefore, the correct intraoperative detection of malperfused areas is one of the points of interest [1,3]. Skin is especially one of the common areas for collateral injury caused by radiotherapy and increasingly in diagnostic radiology by the use of fast multislice CT scanners and fluoroscopically guided interventions [4]. Skin tolerance has often been the limiting factor in radiotherapy [5]. Currently, skin injuries lead to long-lasting burdens for the patients being treated.

Irradiation of tissue leads to ischemia and finally results in tissue fibrosis [6]. Briefly, irradiation induces DNA damage and the generation of reactive oxygen species leading to activation of the immune system and the recruitment of inflammatory cells. These neutrophils release additional inflammatory mediators. Furthermore, lymphocytes and monocytes migrate to the irradiated tissue. Monocytes differentiate into macrophages, which—together with other cells such as fibroblasts—release the transforming growth factor-beta (TGF-β), which stimulates fibroblasts to differentiate into myofibroblasts. In the end, myofibroblasts secrete extracellular matrix proteins and lead to increased tissue stiffness [7]. Besides these factors, vascular injury and changes in microvascular function are a primary pathogenetic signal for the procedure of fibrosis [8]. Early inflammatory vascular changes such as an increase in leukocyte adhesion due to irradiation can be seen within one hour after irradiation [9]. The developed tissue fibrosis itself reduces the perfusion of the irradiated tissue [7,10]. Furthermore, irradiation seems to have a negative impact on flap dimension [11].

To determine tissue perfusion, different imaging modalities have been tested, such as laser Doppler flowmetry for cutaneous circulation [12], infrared thermography [13], indocyanine green angiography [1,14] and near-infrared reflectance-based imaging [15]. While these devices may eventually predict the malperfusion accurately, there might be differences in their features such as application handling and invasivity.

This study evaluates the different imaging modalities—infrared thermography, indocyanine green angiography and near-infrared reflectance-based imaging [16,17]—to predict malperfused areas in an irradiated random pattern fasciocutaneous flap model.

## 2. Materials and Methods

Twenty-five male Lewis rats (age $14 \pm 2.5$ weeks (range 10–19 weeks)) weighing $336 \pm 22.4$ g (range 283–390 g) were operated in 5 different treatment groups. The study was approved by the ethic committee of the government of Middle Franconia (RUF-55.2.2-2532-2-1275-15).

### 2.1. Surgical Procedure

Anesthesia was performed using isofluran. For analgesia, the animals received butorphanol (0.5–2 mg per kg) and meloxicam (1 mg per kg). Two modified caudally based McFarlane flaps were harvested at the rat's back with a length of 6 cm and a width of 1 cm. The flaps were located parallel and 1 cm lateral to the spine (Figure 1). The flaps were harvested by incision along their medial, lateral and cranial side so that their caudal base was 1 cm cranial of the spina iliaca posterior superior. The dissection was deep to the panniculus carnosus and superficial to the deep fascia. After raising the flap, it was reinserted to its bed and sutured using monofilament sutures. Postoperative analgesia was performed using meloxicam. The rats received an antibiotic treatment with enrofloxacin (7.5 mg per kg) for 5 days.

### 2.2. Irradiation Procedure

An orthovoltage X-ray device performed the irradiation with a current of 20 mA and a voltage of 150 kV. For the irradiation, the rats received intramuscular anesthesia using ketamine (100 mg per kg) and medetomidine (0.2 mg per kg). Rats were positioned on the belly and transferred to the irradiation unit in a closed isolation cage to protect the rats from pathogens. An area of $7 \times 2$ cm$^2$ including the right flap or the area of the prospective right flap in case of preoperative irradiation was irradiated (Figure 2). The rest of the body of the rat was covered with lead shields as protection from irradiation. The left flap served as nonirradiated internal control. Postoperative irradiation was performed on the first day after the operation. Postoperative fractional irradiation was performed on the first, second and third day after the operation. Single stage preoperative irradiation was performed

4 weeks before the operation and fractional preoperative irradiation on the three following days starting 4 weeks preoperatively (Figure 3).

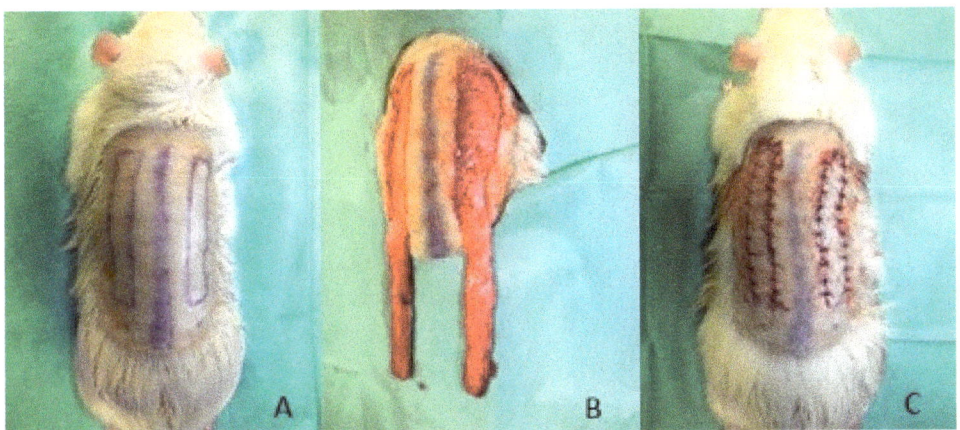

**Figure 1.** Harvest of two modified McFarlane flaps: (**A**) preoperative markings parallel and 1 cm lateral to the spine; (**B**) two flaps harvested; (**C**) reinsertion of the flaps.

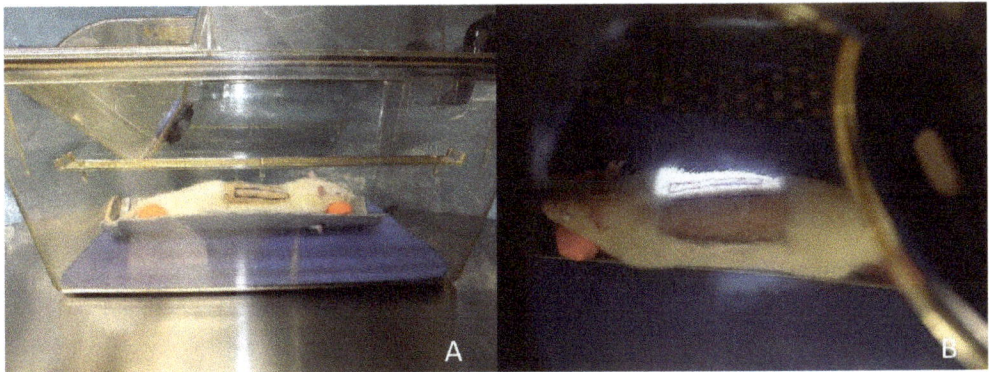

**Figure 2.** Irradiation procedure: (**A**) rat positioned for irradiation; (**B**) irradiated area.

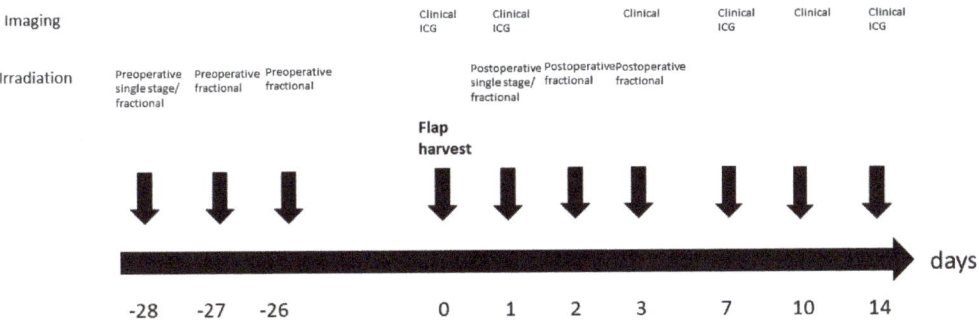

**Figure 3.** Study protocol.

## 2.3. Groups

Animals were divided in 5 groups ($n = 5$). Group 1 included the control group without irradiation. The rats of group 2 received postoperative irradiation with 20 Gy. The rats of group 3 had postoperative irradiation with $3 \times 12$ Gy. Rats of group 4 received preoperative irradiation with 20 Gy and rats of group 5 fractional preoperative irradiation with $3 \times 12$ Gy (Table 1).

**Table 1.** Groups.

| Group. | Irradiation Regimen |
| --- | --- |
| Group 1 | None = control |
| Group 2 | Single stage postoperative irradiation 20 Gy 1 day after flap harvest |
| Group 3 | Fractional postoperative irradiation 12 Gy each day 1, 2 and 3 after flap harvest |
| Group 4 | Single stage preoperative irradiation 20 Gy 28 days before flap harvest |
| Group 5 | Fractional preoperative irradiation 12 Gy each day 28, 27 and 26 before flap harvest |

## 2.4. Imaging

Indocyanine green angiography using an IC-Flow™ Imaging System (Diagnostic Green, Farmington Hills, MI, USA) was performed directly after flap harvest and on day 1, 7 and 14 after the operation in groups 1, 2 and 3 (Figure 4). Therefore, indocyanine green was injected via the tail vein (1 mg per kg). An intensity of less than 20% of the maximum intensity was defined as malperfused area.

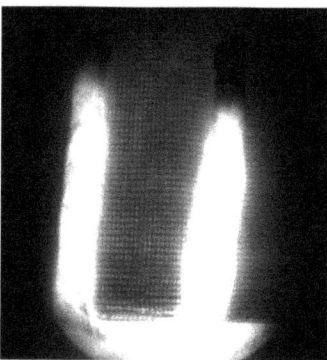

**Figure 4.** Indocyanine green angiography after flap harvest in group 2.

Standard clinical imaging was performed directly after the operation and on day 1, 3, 7, 10 and 14 after the operation. The animals were sacrificed 14 days after the operation. As previously described [16], near-infrared reflectance-based imaging was performed on the same days using Snapshot NIR® (Kent Imaging Inc.; Calgary, AB, Canada) to measure tissue oxygenation in superficial tissue. Near-infrared light is transmitted onto the skin surface and reflected off the blood within the tissue [16]. There is a difference of oxygenated and deoxygenated light absorption of hemoglobin that depends on the wavelength. In conclusion, the ratio from oxygenated to deoxygenated blood and therefore the viability can be determined by this method. Poorly perfused skin has a lower percentage of oxygenated hemoglobin than well-perfused skin [16,18]. Infrared thermography images were obtained on the same days by a smartphone-compatible thermographic camera (FLIR ONE Pro, FLIR Systems, Inc.; Wilsonville, OR, USA). The camera uses a long-wave infrared sensor. It has an effective temperature range from $-20$ to $400\ °C$ with a resolution of $0.1\ °C$ with a sensitivity that detects temperature differences as low as 70 mK. Image processing is used to merge the photo with a thermal image and thus measure the temperature [16].

## 2.5. Blood Samples

Blood samples were taken 30 min after irradiation in the postoperative irradiation groups for staining of DNA double-strand breaks in lymphocytes as previously described [19]. Briefly, lymphocytes were isolated using Pancoll Separating Solution (Pan Biotech, Aidenbach, Germany). After separation, the lymphocytes were incubated overnight with the antibody detecting the phosphorylated variant of the histone H2AX ($\gamma$-H2AX) (Purified anti-H2A.X Phospho (Ser139); BioLegend, San Diego, CA, USA).

## 2.6. Statistical Analysis

Flap size and malperfused/necrotic areas were calculated using Image J (U.S. National Institutes of Health, Bethesda, MD, USA). The statistical analysis was performed using Microsoft Excel (Microsoft, Redmond, WA, USA) and Prism 8 (GraphPad Software, San Diego, CA, USA). The normal distribution was identified graphically using QQ plots. For the comparison of the medians of the same group at different timepoints and the comparison of different groups at the same timepoint, mixed effect models with the Geisser–Greenhouse correction following the Tukey test were used. The level for statistical significance was set at $p < 0.05$.

## 3. Results

All animals tolerated the operative procedure without complications. Postoperative irradiation resulted in weight loss of approximately 10% (group 2, weight day at 0: 322 ± 20.3 g, weight at day 14: 297 ± 17.2 g; group 3 weight at day 0: 329 ± 17.8 g, weight at day 14: 296 ± 14.2 g). The weight of the rats in groups 1, 4 and 5 remained stable.

### 3.1. Flap Size

Mean flap size (including all well- and mal- or nonperfused areas) was slightly reduced ($p > 0.05$) 14 days after the operation in all groups (Figure 5).

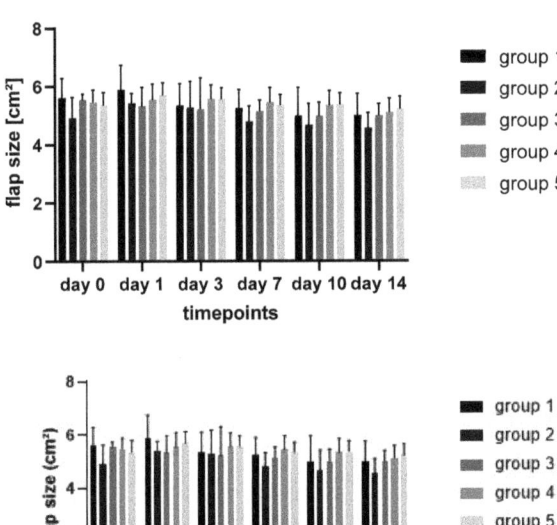

**Figure 5.** Flap size over time in the different treatment groups.

## 3.2. Necrotic Areas of Flaps

There was no difference ($p > 0.05$) in the percentage of the necrotic area of the flaps between days 1 and 14 in the control group (comparison day 1 to 7: $p = 0.04$; day 1 to 10: $p = 0.01$). Furthermore, there was no difference between the control group and the treatment groups or between the right and left flaps within each group.

Comparison of the percentage of the necrotic area of the irradiated flaps showed an increase in all groups from day 1 to 14 (Figure 6). The difference between day 1 and 14 was statistically significant only in group 5 (comparison day 1 to 7: $p = 0.03$; day 1 to day 10: $p = 0.01$; day 1 to 14: $p = 0.02$).

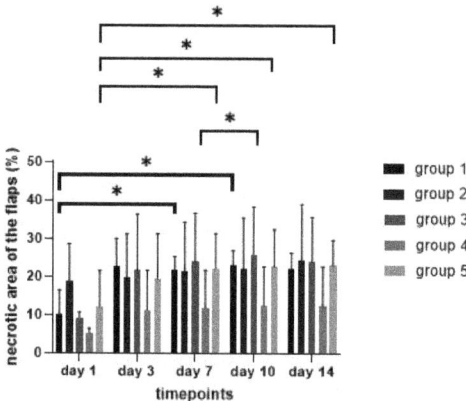

**Figure 6.** Necrotic area of the flaps over time in the different treatment groups. * showing statiscally significant differences ($p \leq 0.05$).

## 3.3. Nonperfused Areas of the Flaps in the Indocyanine Green Angiography

The indocyaningreen angiography during the operation showed no differences ($p > 0.05$) of the mean percentage of the nonperfused area between all groups or between the left and the right flaps within each group (Figure 7). On days 1, 7 and 14, no difference ($p > 0.05$) of the percentage of the nonperfused area of the flaps in group 1 and 3 was measured. The percentage of the nonperfused area of the flaps in group 2 decreased between day 1 and 7 ($p < 0.01$) and between day 1 and 14 ($p = 0.01$). However, as the percentage of the nonperfused area in the intraindividual control group in group 2 decreased as well, there was no difference between the left and the right flap of group 2 on the days 1, 7 and 14.

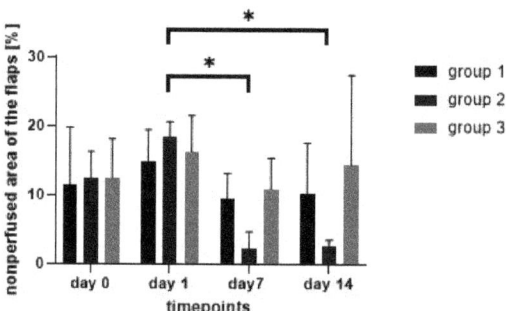

**Figure 7.** Nonperfused areas of the flaps in the indocyanine green angiography over time in the different treatment groups. * showing statiscally significant differences ($p \leq 0.05$).

*3.4. Staining of Double-Strand Breaks*

Staining of the lymphocytes, which were extracted from the blood samples taken 30 min after the end of the irradiation procedure, showed double-strand breaks in all groups with a lower number in group 2 and a higher number in group 3 (Figure 8). These double-strand breaks show that all irradiation regimens had an influence on the rat's organism and that the irradiation was not just applied locally on the flaps.

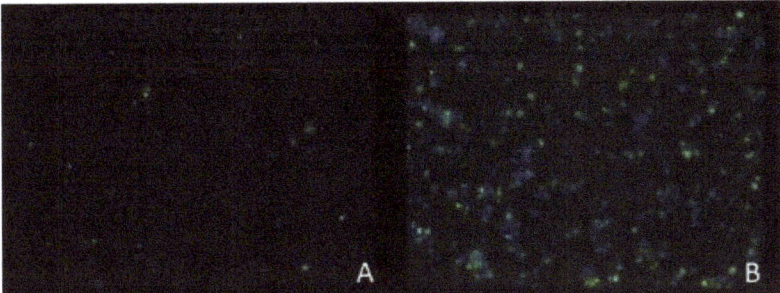

**Figure 8.** Staining of DNA double-strand breaks (green) in lymphocytes (blue) showing an increase in double-strand breaks after higher total dose irradiation: (**A**) group 2; (**B**) group 3.

*3.5. Near-Infrared Reflectance-Based Imaging and Infrared Thermography*

Near-infrared reflectance-based imaging did not produce valuable data in our study. As seen in Figure 9, the sutures and the wound scab at the sides did not allow for capturing the oxygen levels in these areas, thus making precise evaluation impossible.

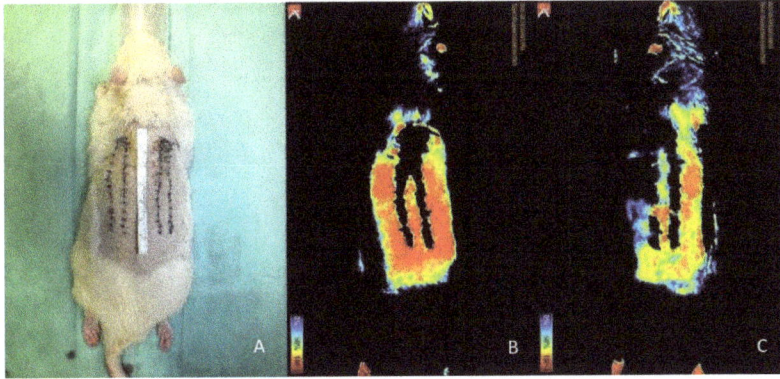

**Figure 9.** Group 2 comparison of clinical imaging (**A**) and near-infrared reflectance-based imaging at day 14: (**B**) right flap; (**C**): left flap.

Evaluation of the images of the infrared thermography did not show evaluable differences of the temperature. Due to the previous shaving and the hair loss after irradiation, the measured temperature was generally high without specific differences between the flaps, the surrounding tissue or between the different areas of the flap itself (Figure 10).

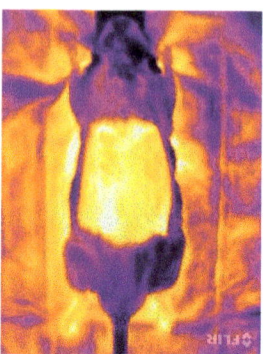

**Figure 10.** Infrared thermography on day 14 in group 2.

## 4. Discussion

In times of multimorbid patients undergoing complicated reconstructive procedures including reconstructive flap surgery [20], predictable complications such as partial flap necrosis due to malperfusion should be avoided. Replacing irradiated tissue with unirradiated flaps is one way to circumvent such surgical site sequelae [21–23]. To assess the viability and perfusion of flaps properly, different imaging modalities have been evaluated in this study in the setting of pre- and postoperative irradiation of random pattern skin flaps.

From the three imaging methods tested, the indocyanine green angiography was shown to be the most precise. The advantages of the infrared thermography such as its noninvasive use have been already shown in other studies [13]. In contrast to the study of Li et al.; infrared thermography was shown not to reproduce evaluable results in our study. One reason might be that the areas of interest—the flaps—were hairless during the total period of observation. Repetitive shaving was not possible due to the developed desquamation and necrosis. Hairless areas might be a necessary condition for infrared thermography [24].

While Chin et al. stated that prediction of region-of-flap necrosis might be possible due to the detection of early changes in deoxygenated hemoglobin seen by near-infrared reflectance-based imaging [15], we could not produce evaluable data. The reason for this might be similar to those of the limitations of the infrared thermography.

Indocyanine green angiography has been proven to predict flap survival area on the first postoperative day more accurately than other imaging modalities such as laser Doppler [1]. Especially, the early detection of malperfused areas of flaps is important to adapt the flap design at best intraoperatively, for example, by resection of the malperfused parts to prevent partial flap loss. Indocyanine green angiography supports the intraoperative decision-making process of flap design in daily clinical practice [3]. Giunta et al. stated that a perfusion index of less than 25% of the reference skin could be considered as a sign of developing flap necrosis [14], which is similar to the 20% we chose for our study. While the percentage of the necrotic area of the flaps increased in all groups, when evaluated clinically, the percentage of the nonperfused areas of the flaps—seen in the indocyanine green angiography—remained at least constant. These data support the assumption that indocyanine green angiography reliably foresees the well- and nonperfused areas of random pattern flaps. Interestingly, we measured a reduction of the nonperfused areas in group 2 after 20 Gy irradiation on days 7 and 14 compared to day 1. One reason might be that single irradiation with 20 Gy does not lead to harmful effects on flap perfusion. The improved perfusion might be due to the mechanism of flap delay, where linking or so-called choke vessels dilatate and reorientate due to increased blood flow because of opening of arteriovenous anastomoses and result in an enlarged perfused area [25,26]. As we measured the decrease in both the irradiated and the nonirradiated flaps without difference between these two groups, it might be possible that the animals in these groups were more susceptible to the changes of the delay phenomenon.

When comparing clinical evaluation of the necrotic area of the flaps to evaluation by indocyanine green angiography, the percentage generally turns out to be higher when compared to indocyanine green angiography. One reason for this difference might be that the indocyanine green angiography is able to evaluate the flap in its total thickness. In contrast, the clinical impression just assesses the visible superficial layers of the flap. It might be that the necrotic tissue, which was seen, does not affect all layers of the flap and is just necrotic scab as a sign of partial flap necrosis.

In addition to the imaging used in this study, duplex sonography may provide additional evidence of changes in flap perfusion. For example, Heitland et al. measured an increase in blood flow after anastomosis in musculocutaneous and perforator flaps compared to the donor vessel that indicates flap hyperperfusion [27]. Duplex sonography was not indicated in this model due to the random pattern perfusion. The irradiation had a systemic impact on the rats. This could be seen as DNA double-strand breaks were visible in all groups as proof of the systemic influence. Previous tests in our laboratory have shown that postoperative irradiation with 30 Gy was the lethal dose in our setting with a weight loss of more than 20% over several weeks. A reason might be that shorter, more intense irradiation treatments can increase acute effects because they do not allow sufficient time for regeneration [28].

Irradiation of the flaps resulted in a shrinking of the flaps in all groups, but the difference was not statistically significant. This might be explained by the fact that irradiation reduces the elasticity of the affected skin [5]. It is well known that tissue fibrosis is one of the hallmarks of chronic damage due to irradiation and changes the form, function and the appearance of the irradiated tissue [7]. In general, tissue fibrosis is a dynamic process with constant remodeling and long-term fibroblast activation. Initiation of these processes, however, could be seen 24 h after irradiation [29]. Especially early microvascular changes are seen within hours after irradiation [9]. As microvascular depletion leads to tissue ischemia, tissue hypoxia might be relevant for early fibrogenesis [8]. Skin reactions on irradiation such as desquamation were first visible at day 7 after irradiation with a peak at day 14 in a mouse model after 50 Gy irradiation [30]. The clinical sign of alopecia [5] or reduced hair growth due to irrradiation was seen in all flaps. High dose irradiation has been shown to cause dermal thickening [5], which unfortunately was not measured in our study. The shrinkage of the flap, however, is seen as sign of the developed fibrosis. Lin et al. performed fractioned irradiation with fractions up to 400 cGy and in total up to 40 Gy four weeks postoperatively [11]. The animals were killed six weeks after the end of irradiation. Greater tissue damage in both skin and muscle tissue of rat rectus muscle flaps with histological changes such as fibrosis and vascular damages were seen after irradiation with greater dose per fraction and less total dose compared to lower dose fraction groups and higher total dose. In our study, we did not see a statistically significant difference in all groups.

We did not see statistically significant differences in the size of the necrotic area between the treatment groups and the control group. However, we did see an increase of the necrotic area in all irradiated groups with a statistically significant increase in group 5. This could indicate that the damage of irradiation on tissue perfusion was not completely detected in our study setting. Similarly, postoperative irradiation of free skin flaps in rats one week after transplantation did not show statistical significant differences in the mechanical strength of the healing interface or the biochemical markers compared to the control group [31]. The irradiated flaps just showed minimal histomorphological changes compared to the nonirradiated flaps. Additionally, the irradiation with 20 Gy did not affect flap survival.

Furthermore, our study examines the acute phase after irradiation. It might be possible that the late harmful effects of irradiation are not included. As the study of Sumi et al. suggested, however, postoperative irradiation of skin flaps in rats that begins 3–4 weeks postoperatively should not affect flap survival negatively [32]. In this study, the postoperative irradiation begins at the first day after the operation. Therefore, one might expect that this study captures the majority of the negative side effects of irradiation.

In contrast to the harmful influence of irradiation observed in our study, low dose irradiation of ischemic pedicled skin flaps in mice with 5 Gy upregulates angiogenic chemokines and resulted in an increase of the vascularity of the flaps measured by laser Doppler. In addition, the irradiated flaps did not show an increase in flap ischemia or in flap necrosis compared to controls. Thus, it is suggested that neovascularization after ischemic injury is a multifactorial process [33]. Furthermore, low dose irradiation of ischemic legs in mice with 2 Gy promoted neovascularization by release of vascular endothelial growth factor (VEGF) [34]. Besides neovascularization, low dose fractionated irradiation with four fractions of 0.3 Gy in murine ischemic limbs improved capillary density and stimulated collateral vessel formation [35]. In conclusion, it can be assumed that the harmful effects of irradiation are directly related to the applied dose. For example, human endothelial cells have been shown to be viable up to an irradiation dose of 10 Gy [36]. However, it has been shown that irradiation with 40 Gy one month before harvesting an axial fasciocutaneous flaps resulted in an increased flap necrosis and a decrease in vascular density compared to the nonirradiated control group [37].

Limitations of this study include the small number of animals per group, which might be a reason for the results that showed just a few statistically significant differences. The irradiation regimen that was chosen in this study can only be transferred to clinical daily routine to a limited extent, since, for example, postoperative irradiation is usually only carried out after wound healing has been completed and not, as in this study, on the first postoperative day. The timing in this study was chosen so that the possible influence of the delay phenomenon could be kept as low as possible. Histopathological examinations or examinations on the molecular level, which could provide an indication of a possible neoangiogenesis, were not performed. This study deliberately wanted to focus on the use and comparison of imaging as it is also practiced in routine clinical practice. To distinguish necrotic areas in all layers from superficial necrosis more precisely, histopathological staining could be performed in future studies. In addition, the influence of irradiation could then also be studied at the molecular level. There is a wide range of different diagnostic procedures to measure tissue perfusion. For example, the measurement of transcutaneous oxygen pressure has been proven useful for the evaluation of free flap viability [38]. Skin perfusion pressure seems to be an accurate predictor of wound healing potential, especially in patients with limb ischemia [39]. In this study, we focused on three different imaging modalities that assessed the entire flap. Future studies could compare the indocyaningreen angiography, which in this study has been shown to be more precise, with other procedures.

## 5. Conclusions

This study shows that indocyanine green angiography is more precise in the prediction of necrotic areas in random pattern skin flaps when compared to hyperspectral imaging, thermography or clinical impression, since infrared thermography and near-infrared reflectance-based imaging did not produce reliable data in this setting. The impact of pre- and postoperative irradiation on flap perfusion seems to be the same. Furthermore, preoperative fractional irradiation with a lower individual dose but a higher total dose has a more negative impact on flap perfusion compared to higher single stage irradiation.

**Author Contributions:** Conceptualization, A.A.; methodology, A.A.; formal analysis, P.O.; investigation, W.M.-S.; data curation, W.M.-S.; P.O.; writing—original draft preparation, W.M.-S.; writing—review and editing, P.O.; R.E.H.; L.D.; A.C.; A.A.; B.F.; supervision, R.E.H.; L.D.; A.A.; B.F.; project administration, W.M.-S. All authors have read and agreed to the published version of the manuscript.

**Funding:** We acknowledge financial support by Deutsche Forschungsgemeinschaft and Friedrich-Alexander-Universität Erlangen-Nürnberg within the funding programme "Open Access Publication Funding".

**Institutional Review Board Statement:** The animal study protocol was approved by the Institutional Ethics Committee of the government of Middle Franconia (RUF-55.2.2-2532-2-1275; 29 October 2020).

**Informed Consent Statement:** Not applicable.

**Data Availability Statement:** Data sharing is not applicable to this article.

**Conflicts of Interest:** The authors declare no conflict of interest.

## References

1. Fourman, M.S.; Gersch, R.P.; Phillips, B.T.; Nasser, A.; Rivara, A.; Verma, R.; Dagum, A.B.; Rosengart, T.K.; Bui, D.T. Comparison of laser doppler and laser-assisted indocyanine green angiography prediction of flap survival in a novel modification of the mcfarlane flap. *Ann. Plast. Surg.* **2015**, *75*, 102–107. [CrossRef]
2. Wei, J.W.; Dong, Z.G.; Ni, J.D.; Liu, L.H.; Luo, S.H.; Luo, Z.B.; Zheng, L.; He, A.Y. Influence of flap factors on partial necrosis of reverse sural artery flap: A study of 179 consecutive flaps. *J. Trauma Acute Care Surg.* **2012**, *72*, 744–750. [CrossRef] [PubMed]
3. Moyer, H.R.; Losken, A. Predicting mastectomy skin flap necrosis with indocyanine green angiography: The gray area defined. *Plast. Reconstr. Surg.* **2012**, *129*, 1043–1048. [CrossRef] [PubMed]
4. Jaschke, W.; Schmuth, M.; Trianni, A.; Bartal, G. Radiation-induced skin injuries to patients: What the interventional radiologist needs to know. *Cardiovasc. Intervent. Radiol.* **2017**, *40*, 1131–1140. [CrossRef]
5. Thanik, V.D.; Chang, C.C.; Zoumalan, R.A.; Lerman, O.Z.; Allen, R.J., Jr.; Nguyen, P.D.; Warren, S.M.; Coleman, S.R.; Hazen, A. A novel mouse model of cutaneous radiation injury. *Plast. Reconstr. Surg.* **2011**, *127*, 560–568. [CrossRef] [PubMed]
6. Yoshida, S.; Yoshimoto, H.; Hirano, A.; Akita, S. Wound healing and angiogenesis through combined use of a vascularized tissue flap and adipose-derived stem cells in a rat hindlimb irradiated ischemia model. *Plast. Reconstr. Surg.* **2016**, *137*, 1486–1497. [CrossRef]
7. Borrelli, M.R.; Shen, A.H.; Lee, G.K.; Momeni, A.; Longaker, M.T.; Wan, D.C. Radiation-induced skin fibrosis: Pathogenesis, current treatment options, and emerging therapeutics. *Ann. Plast. Surg.* **2019**, *83*, S59–S64. [CrossRef]
8. Yarnold, J.; Brotons, M.C. Pathogenetic mechanisms in radiation fibrosis. *Radiother. Oncol.* **2010**, *97*, 149–161. [CrossRef]
9. Kimura, H.; Wu, N.Z.; Dodge, R.; Spencer, D.P.; Klitzman, B.M.; McIntyre, T.M.; Dewhirst, M.W. Inhibition of radiation-induced up-regulation of leukocyte adhesion to endothelial cells with the platelet-activating factor inhibitor, BN52021. *Int. J. Radiat. Oncol. Biol. Phys.* **1995**, *33*, 627–633. [CrossRef]
10. Phulpin, B.; Gangloff, P.; Tran, N.; Bravetti, P.; Merlin, J.L.; Dolivet, G. Rehabilitation of irradiated head and neck tissues by autologous fat transplantation. *Plast. Reconstr. Surg.* **2009**, *123*, 1187–1197. [CrossRef]
11. Lin, K.Y.; Patterson, J.W.; Simmons, J.; Long, M.D.; Schultz, R.O.; Amiss, L.R.; Molloy, J.A.; Kelly, M.D. Effects of external beam irradiation on the TRAM flap: An experimental model. *Plast. Reconstr. Surg.* **2001**, *107*, 1190–1197, discussion 1198–1200. [CrossRef]
12. Özyazgan, İ.; Baykan, H. The effect of TENS on random pattern flap survival in nicotinized rats. *Ann. Plast. Surg.* **2015**, *74*, 365–370. [CrossRef] [PubMed]
13. Li, X.; Chen, M.; Jiang, Z.; Liu, Y.; Lu, L.; Gong, X. Visualized identification of the maximal surgical delay effect in a rat flap model. *Wound Repair Regen.* **2019**, *27*, 39–48. [CrossRef]
14. Giunta, R.E.; Holzbach, T.; Taskov, C.; Holm, P.S.; Brill, T.; Busch, R.; Gansbacher, B.; Biemer, E. Prediction of flap necrosis with laser induced indocyanine green fluorescence in a rat model. *Br. J. Plast. Surg.* **2005**, *58*, 695–701. [CrossRef]
15. Chin, M.S.; Chappell, A.G.; Giatsidis, G.; Perry, D.J.; Lujan-Hernandez, J.; Haddad, A.; Matsumine, H.; Orgill, D.P.; Lalikos, J.F. Hyperspectral imaging provides early prediction of random axial flap necrosis in a preclinical model. *Plast. Reconstr. Surg.* **2017**, *139*, 1285e–1290e. [CrossRef] [PubMed]
16. Müller-Seubert, W.; Roth, S.; Hauck, T.; Arkudas, A.; Horch, R.E.; Ludolph, I. Novel imaging methods reveal positive impact of topical negative pressure application on tissue perfusion in an in vivo skin model. *Int. Wound J.* **2021**, *18*, 932–939. [CrossRef] [PubMed]
17. Schmauss, D.; Beier, J.P.; Eisenhardt, S.U.; Horch, R.E.; Momeni, A.; Rab, M.; Rieck, B.; Rieger, U.; Schaefer, D.J.; Schmidt, V.J.; et al. The "safe" flap—Preoperative perforator-mapping and intraoperative perfusion assessment to reduce flap-associated morbidity—Consensus statement of the German speaking working group for microsurgery of the peripheral nerves and vessels. *Handchir. Mikrochir. Plast. Chir.* **2019**, *51*, 410–417. [PubMed]
18. Landsman, A.S.; Barnhart, D.; Sowa, M. Near-infrared spectroscopy imaging for assessing skin and wound oxygen perfusion. *Clin. Podiatr. Med. Surg.* **2018**, *35*, 343–355. [CrossRef]
19. Kuefner, M.A.; Grudzenski, S.; Schwab, S.A.; Wiederseiner, M.; Heckmann, M.; Bautz, W.; Lobrich, M.; Uder, M. DNA double-strand breaks and their repair in blood lymphocytes of patients undergoing angiographic procedures. *Investig. Radiol.* **2009**, *44*, 440–446. [CrossRef]

20. Müller-Seubert, W.; Horch, R.E.; Schmidt, V.F.; Ludolph, I.; Schmitz, M.; Arkudas, A. Retrospective analysis of free temporoparietal fascial flap for defect reconstruction of the hand and the distal upper extremity. *Arch. Orthop. Trauma Surg.* **2021**, *141*, 165–171. [CrossRef]
21. Horch, R.E.; Ludolph, I.; Arkudas, A. Reconstruction of oncological defects of the perianal region. *Chirurg* **2021**, *92*, 1159–1170. [CrossRef] [PubMed]
22. Horch, R.E.; Ludolph, I.; Cai, A.; Weber, K.; Grützmann, R.; Arkudas, A. Interdisciplinary surgical approaches in vaginal and perineal reconstruction of advanced rectal and anal female cancer patients. *Front. Oncol.* **2020**, *10*, 719. [CrossRef]
23. Schellerer, V.S.; Bartholomé, L.; Langheinrich, M.C.; Grützmann, R.; Horch, R.E.; Merkel, S.; Weber, K. Donor site morbidity of patients receiving vertical rectus abdominis myocutaneous flap for perineal, vaginal or inguinal reconstruction. *World J. Surg.* **2021**, *45*, 132–140. [CrossRef] [PubMed]
24. Lahiri, B.B.; Bagavathiappan, S.; Jayakumar, T.; Philip, J. Medical applications of infrared thermography: A review. *Infrared Phys. Technol.* **2012**, *55*, 221–235. [CrossRef] [PubMed]
25. Reinisch, J.F. The pathophysiology of skin flap circulation. The delay phenomenon. *Plast. Reconstr. Surg.* **1974**, *54*, 585–598. [CrossRef] [PubMed]
26. Dhar, S.C.; Taylor, G.I. The delay phenomenon: The story unfolds. *Plast. Reconstr. Surg.* **1999**, *104*, 2079–2091. [CrossRef]
27. Heitland, A.S.; Markowicz, M.; Koellensperger, E.; Schoth, F.; Feller, A.M.; Pallua, N. Duplex ultrasound imaging in free transverse rectus abdominis muscle, deep inferior epigastric artery perforator, and superior gluteal artery perforator flaps: Early and long-term comparison of perfusion changes in free flaps following breast reconstruction. *Ann. Plast. Surg.* **2005**, *55*, 117–121.
28. McBride, W.H.; Schaue, D. Radiation-induced tissue damage and response. *J. Pathol.* **2020**, *250*, 647–655. [CrossRef]
29. Martin, M.; Lefaix, J.; Delanian, S. TGF-beta1 and radiation fibrosis: A master switch and a specific therapeutic target? *Int. J. Radiat. Oncol. Biol. Phys.* **2000**, *47*, 277–290. [CrossRef]
30. Chin, M.S.; Freniere, B.B.; Lo, Y.C.; Saleeby, J.H.; Baker, S.P.; Strom, H.M.; Ignotz, R.A.; Lalikos, J.F.; Fitzgerald, T.J. Hyperspectral imaging for early detection of oxygenation and perfusion changes in irradiated skin. *J. Biomed. Opt.* **2012**, *17*, 026010. [CrossRef]
31. Virolainen, P.; Aitasalo, K. Effect of postoperative irradiation on free skin flaps: An experimental study in rats. *Scand J. Plast. Reconstr. Surg. Hand Surg.* **2002**, *36*, 257–261. [CrossRef] [PubMed]
32. Sumi, Y.; Ueda, M.; Oka, T.; Torii, S. Effects of irradiation of skin flaps. *J. Oral Maxillofac. Surg.* **1984**, *42*, 447–452. [CrossRef]
33. Thanik, V.D.; Hang, C.C.; Lerman, O.Z.; Greives, M.R.; Le, H.; Warren, S.M.; Schneider, R.J.; Formenti, S.C.; Saadeh, P.B.; Levine, J.P. Cutaneous low-dose radiation increases tissue vascularity through upregulation of angiogenic and vasculogenic pathways. *J. Vasc. Res.* **2010**, *47*, 472–480. [CrossRef] [PubMed]
34. Heissig, B.; Rafii, S.; Akiyama, H.; Ohki, Y.; Sato, Y.; Rafael, T.; Zhu, Z.; Hicklin, D.J.; Okumura, K.; Ogawa, H.; et al. Low-dose irradiation promotes tissue revascularization through VEGF release from mast cells and MMP-9-mediated progenitor cell mobilization. *J. Exp. Med.* **2005**, *202*, 739–750. [CrossRef]
35. Ministro, A.; de Oliveira, P.; Nunes, R.J.; Dos Santos Rocha, A.; Correia, A.; Carvalho, T.; Rino, J.; Faísca, P.; Becker, J.D.; Goyri-O'Neill, J.; et al. Low-dose ionizing radiation induces therapeutic neovascularization in a pre-clinical model of hindlimb ischemia. *Cardiovasc. Res.* **2017**, *113*, 783–794. [CrossRef] [PubMed]
36. Kermani, P.; Leclerc, G.; Martel, R.; Fareh, J. Effect of ionizing radiation on thymidine uptake, differentiation, and VEGFR2 receptor expression in endothelial cells: The role of VEGF(165). *Int. J. Radiat. Oncol. Biol. Phys.* **2001**, *50*, 213–220. [CrossRef]
37. Luginbuhl, A.; Modest, M.; Yan, K.; Curry, J.; Heffelfinger, R. Novel irradiated axial rotational flap model in the rodent. *JAMA Facial Plast. Surg.* **2013**, *15*, 344–348. [CrossRef]
38. Geis, S.; Schreml, S.; Lamby, P.; Obed, A.; Jung, E.M.; Nerlich, M.; Babilas, P.; Szeimies, R.M.; Prantl, L. Postoperative assessment of free skin flap viability by transcutaneous $pO_2$ measurement using dynamic phosphorescence imaging. *Clin. Hemorheol. Microcirc.* **2009**, *43*, 11–18. [CrossRef]
39. Pan, X.; Chen, G.; Wu, P.; Han, C.; Ho, J.K. Skin perfusion pressure as a predictor of ischemic wound healing potential. *Biomed. Rep.* **2018**, *8*, 330–334. [CrossRef]

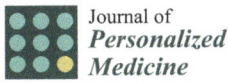 

Article

# Combined versus Single Perforator Propeller Flaps for Reconstruction of Large Soft Tissue Defects: A Retrospective Clinical Study

Amir K. Bigdeli [1,2,*,†], Oliver Didzun [1,2,†], Benjamin Thomas [1,2], Leila Harhaus [1,2], Emre Gazyakan [1,2], Raymund E. Horch [3] and Ulrich Kneser [1,2]

1. Department of Hand, Plastic and Reconstructive Surgery, Burn Center, BG Trauma Center Ludwigshafen, Ludwig-Guttmann-Strasse 13, 67071 Ludwigshafen, Germany; oliver.didzun@googlemail.com (O.D.); benjamin.thomas@bgu-ludwigshafen.de (B.T.); leila.harhaus@bgu-ludwigshafen.de (L.H.); emre.gazyakan@bgu-ludwigshafen.de (E.G.); ulrich.kneser@bgu-ludwigshafen.de (U.K.)
2. Department of Hand and Plastic Surgery, University of Heidelberg, 69117 Heidelberg, Germany
3. Department of Plastic and Hand Surgery, Friedrich-Alexander-University Erlangen-Nuremberg, Krankenhausstrasse 12, 91054 Erlangen, Germany; Raymund.Horch@uk-erlangen.de
* Correspondence: amir.bigdeli@bgu-ludwigshafen.de; Tel.: +49-621-6810-8926; Fax: +49-0621-6810-2844
† These authors contributed equally.

**Abstract:** Sufficient wound closure of large soft tissue defects remains a challenge for reconstructive surgeons. We aimed to investigate whether combined perforator propeller flaps (PPFs) are suitable to expand reconstructive options. Patients undergoing PPF reconstruction surgery between 2008 and 2021 were screened and evaluated retrospectively. Of 86 identified patients, 69 patients received one perforator propeller flap, while 17 patients underwent combined PPF reconstruction with multiple flaps. We chose major complications as our primary outcome and defined those as complications that required additional surgery. Postoperatively, 27 patients (31.4%) suffered major complications. The propeller flap size, the type of intervention as well as the operation time were not associated with a higher risk of major complications. A defect size larger than 100 cm$^2$, however, was identified as a significant risk factor for major complications among single PPFs but not among combined PPFs (OR: 2.82, 95% CI: 1.01−8.36; $p$ = 0.05 vs. OR: 0.30, 95% CI: 0.02−3.37; $p$ = 0.32). In conclusion, combined PPFs proved to be a reliable technique and should be preferred over single PPFs in the reconstruction of large soft tissue defects at the trunk and proximal lower extremity.

**Keywords:** perforator propeller flap; combined perforator propeller flap; microsurgery; soft tissue reconstruction; propeller flap; perforator flap

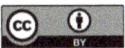

## 1. Introduction

Modern reconstructive surgery offers a vast variety of surgical techniques for the reconstruction of soft tissue defects [1,2]. Although free flaps have been established as the standard procedure in the reconstruction of soft tissue defects, regional flaps might be used depending on the size and characteristics of a defect [3]. However, large defects often require complex solutions with multiple flaps or tissue expansion to ensure sufficient wound closure [4,5]. Frequently used combinations consist of muscle flaps, sliding flaps as well as rotation flaps, which are either combined with one another or with a free flap [6,7]. Nevertheless, limitations of regional flaps are due to arc of flap rotation, flap size to defect size ratio, wound infections, and donor-site morbidity while free flaps are limited whenever vessels for anastomosis are insufficient [8]. Furthermore, prior surgeries often lead to significant scarring and, hence, may impede the use of conventional regional flaps.

Since the introduction of perforator propeller flaps (PPFs), they have gained increasing popularity [9,10]. By the definition of the "Tokyo consensus" on propeller flaps, propeller flaps are "island flaps that reach the recipient-site through an axial rotation" [11]. As a combination of a reliable pedicled flap along with low donor-site morbidity, PPFs offer high flexibility and, therefore, have led to versatile use. First employed in the reconstruction of the upper and lower extremity, PPFs have also become an established technique in the reconstruction of soft tissue defects of the trunk [12]. Even though PPFs have shown to be a reliable reconstructive option, there is a gap in the literature regarding the potential advantages associated with using combined PPFs instead of single PPFs (Table 1). This study aims to compare the outcome of single and combined PPFs, to determine the prevalence of complications among both techniques, and to assess the potential use of combined PPFs in the reconstruction of large soft tissue defects.

Table 1. Articles [1] reporting the use of combined perforator propeller flaps.

| Title | Author | Year | No. of Patients | Body Region |
|---|---|---|---|---|
| Dual Reconstruction of Lumbar and Gluteal Defects with Freestyle Propeller Flap and Muscle Flap | Ellabban et al. [13] | 2021 | 18 | Trunk/Gluteal |
| Lumbar Perforator Flaps for Coverage of Extensive Defects With Osteomyelitis | Schaffer et al. [14] | 2021 | 7 | Trunk |
| Perforator-Based Flaps for Defect Reconstruction of the Posterior Trunk | Hernekamp et al. [9] | 2021 | 36 | Trunk |
| Use of the Propeller Lumbar Perforator Flap: A Series of 32 Cases | Falinower et al. [15] | 2020 | 31 | Trunk |
| The SCIP propeller flap: Versatility for reconstruction of locoregional defect | Boissière et al. [16] | 2019 | 56 | Trunk |
| Freestyle multiple propeller flap reconstruction (jigsaw puzzle approach) for complicated back defects | Park et al. [17] | 2015 | 18 | Trunk |

[1] Case reports as well as articles that did not include combined perforator propeller flaps were excluded.

## 2. Materials and Methods

### 2.1. Patients

Medical records of all patients who received a PPF reconstruction surgery between 2008 and 2021 at the University Clinic of Erlangen Nuremberg and the BG Trauma Center Ludwigshafen were identified and evaluated retrospectively. All surgeries were performed under the senior author's direct supervision. This study was approved by the ethics board of the Friedrich Alexander University of Erlangen Nuremberg (registration number: 21-433-Br) and the local ethic committee of Rhineland-Palatinate (registration number: 2021-16096). Patients who either received single or combined PPF reconstruction with a minimum rotation arc of 45 degrees were included in the study. Combined PPFs were defined as "double PPF" if two perforator propeller flaps were used whereas those combined with any kind of regional flap were assigned to the group of "PPF plus regional flap".

We utilized patients' digital charts to collect data on individual characteristics, flap surgery, risk factors as well as postoperative complications. Risk factors considered were diabetes, arterial hypertension, peripheral artery disease, coronary heart disease, coagulation disorders, prior thrombotic events, obesity (BMI > 30 kg/m$^2$), radiation therapy, chemotherapy, and smoking. All risk factors as well as postoperative complications were assessed separately before creating a dichotomous variable. Furthermore, postoperative complications requiring surgical treatment were considered as a "major complication" whereas those manageable by conservative therapy were considered as a "minor complication". Partial flap loss was defined as a flap necrosis of at least five percent, which did not result in a total flap removal, while "total flap loss" was defined as a flap loss of more than 50 percent leading to reconstructive failure and, thus, total removal of the flap. Additionally, we recorded the total time of hospitalization as well as the total amount of surgeries related to the specific type of PPF reconstruction surgery (single or combined PPF). We chose "major complication" as the primary outcome variable since, by definition, all kinds of major complications resulted in additional surgeries and, hence, a more complex course of disease.

*2.2. Methods*

Flap Harvesting

Prior to surgery, relevant perforating vessels were identified by either using a handheld Doppler device (2008–2014) or duplex ultrasound (2015–2021) [18,19]. Preoperative planning of flap design, flap dimensions as well as flap orientation were adapted to the size, location, and vascular territory of the defect. If appropriate, combined PPF designs were considered to ensure tension-free donor-site closure. Flap dissection was performed with subsequent localization and preservation of significant perforators. It was conducted in a manner for which the chance of converting to a conventional random pattern flap was preserved. This procedure was intended as a rescue strategy if suitable perforators were absent or turned out to be insufficient. However, conversion to random pattern skin flaps was not necessary. Since the vascular pedicle represents the central axis of rotation and its length is inversely proportional to the critical angle of twisting, we aimed, whenever possible, for a minimum pedicle length of 3 to 5 centimeters to ensure adequate flap perfusion (Figure 1a) [20–22]. To verify sufficient blood flow, we intraoperatively clamped all preserved perforators except for the dominant one prior to complete flap harvest. Evaluation of the dominant perforator followed in terms of caliber size, pulsatility, and morphology. The flap was then rotated into the defect either in a clockwise or counterclockwise direction, depending on which method led to lower twisting of the pedicle. Flap perfusion was assessed clinically. In addition to clinical flap assessment, indocyanine green fluorescence angiography was performed for objective flap perfusion assessment in selected cases [23]. Figure 1 visualizes the principle of flap harvesting in further detail.

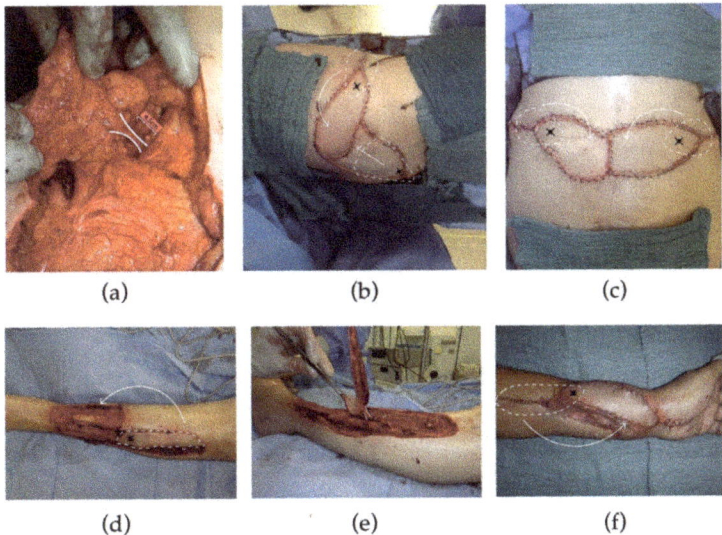

**Figure 1.** Principle of flap harvesting. (**a–c**) demonstrates PPF reconstruction on the trunk. (**a**) Meticulous dissection of the perforator. We aimed for a minimum length of 3 to 5 centimeters to avoid vascular complications; (**b**) PPF plus perforator-based VY advancement flap. Black crosses indicate perforators of the flaps. After skin incision and dissection of surrounding tissue, the PPF was rotated (curved arrow) into the defect, while the VY advancement flap was transposed (straight arrow) into the defect; (**c**) Double PPF: Black crosses indicate pivot points given by the perforators. Those were marked together with the regions of flap harvesting (white dashed lines) prior to surgery. After skin incision and dissection of surrounding tissue, flaps were rotated into the defect (white dashed lines); (**d**,**e**) Demonstrates PPF reconstruction of the lower extremity; (**f**) Demonstrates PPF reconstruction of the upper extremity (Abbreviations: PPF, perforator propeller flap).

## 2.3. Statistical Analysis

Separately for single PPF and combined PPF reconstruction surgery, we estimated the prevalence of major complications. To identify whether characteristics among the approaches differ, we conducted Wilcoxon–Mann–Whitney tests on continuous variables of defect size, PPF size, total days of hospitalization, age, total number of surgeries, and operation time against a patients' type of perforator propeller reconstruction surgery as well as Fisher's exact tests on categorical variables of sex, major complications, and existing risk factors. Furthermore, separately for the groups of (I) all PPFs, (II) single PPFs, and (III) combined PPFs, we regressed major complications onto individuals' defect size, propeller flap size, and operation time. Those analyses were applied to assess the effect an independent variable had on the outcome depending on the type of surgical intervention. Finally, we regressed the type of reconstructive flap surgery on major complications. All regression models were performed by employing univariable binary logistic regression analyses. We considered an error probability of $p \leq 0.05$ as statistically significant. Statistical analyses were conducted using R (version 3.6.1, open source). Visualization was performed wherever necessary using RStudio (version 1.1.456, RStudio PBC, Boston, MA, USA) and Adobe Illustrator CS6 (Adobe Systems Incorporated, Mountain View, San Jose, CA, USA).

## 3. Results

### 3.1. Overall Sample Characteristics

Of 86 patients (38 female, 48 male) that underwent PPF reconstruction surgery between 2008 and 2021, 69 patients received single PPFs (69 flaps) whereas 17 patients received combined PPF reconstruction (28 PPFs). Mean age of patients was 56.7 years ranging from 4 years to 88 years. Twenty-nine patients (33.7%) presented with risk factors for postoperative complications prior to surgery (Table 2). Tumor and pressure ulcer were the most common indications for PPF reconstruction and accounted for more than 66.3% of all indications. A total of 62 (72.1%) reconstructions were performed on the trunk, 18 (20.9%) on the lower extremity, and 6 (7.0%) on the upper extremity. Of all single PPF reconstructions performed, 47 (68.1%) were performed on the trunk, 16 (23.2%) on the lower extremity and 6 (8.7%) on the upper extremity. Among combined PPF reconstructions 15 (88.2%) were performed on the trunk and 2 (11.8%) on the lower extremity. Mean operation time was 178 minutes, ranging from 80 to 480 minutes. Mean defect size was $117.8 \pm 88.6$ cm$^2$ ranging from 12 to 504 cm$^2$, while mean PPF size was $137.3 \pm 85.1$ cm$^2$ ranging from 24 to 532 cm$^2$. Overall, major complications occurred in 27 patients (31.4%). Partial flap loss occurred in 5 patients (7.2%) and total flap loss in 5 patients (5.8%). In summary, primary reconstruction was successful in 60 out of 69 patients (87.0%) with single PPFs and in 16 out of 17 patients (94.1%) with combined PPFs by the time of discharge from our department. Patient and flap characteristics are shown in detail in Table 2.

**Table 2.** Patient characteristics.

| Characteristic | Total | Single PPF | Combined PPF | p-Value |
|---|---|---|---|---|
| No. of patients (%) | 86 | 69 (80.2) | 17 (19.8) | |
| Combined PPF, No. (%) | 17 (19.8) | | | |
| Double PPF | | | 11 (64.7) | |
| PPF plus regional flap | | | 6 (35.3) | |
| Sex, No. (%) | | | | 0.79 |
| Female | 38 (44.2) | 30 (43.5) | 8 (47.1) | |
| Male | 48 (55.8) | 39 (56.5) | 9 (52.9) | |
| Mean age [years] (SD, range) | 56.7 (19.7, 4–88) | 55.7 (20.0, 4–86) | 60.8 (18.6, 21–88) | 0.34 |

**Table 2.** *Cont.*

| Characteristic | Total | Single PPF | Combined PPF | *p*-Value |
|---|---|---|---|---|
| Risk factors [1] present, No. (%) | 29 (33.7) | 19 (27.5) | 10 (58.8) | 0.02 |
| Defect etiology (%) | | | | |
| Burn injury | 1 (1.2) | 1 (1.4) | 0 (0.0) | 0.36 |
| Pressure ulcer | 13 (15.1) | 10 (14.5) | 3 (17.6) | 0.72 |
| Infection | 8 (9.3) | 6 (8.7) | 2 (11.8) | 0.65 |
| Trauma | 6 (7.0) | 4 (5.8) | 2 (11.8) | 0.39 |
| Tumor | 44 (51.2) | 34 (49.3) | 10 (58.8) | 0.59 |
| Other | 14 (16.3) | 14 (20.3) | 0 (0.0) | |
| Defect size in [$cm^2$] (SD, range) | 117.8 (88.6, 12–504) | 103.0 (73.5, 12–450) | 178.2 (73.8, 25–504) | <0.01 |
| PPF size [$cm^2$] (SD, range) | 137.3 (85.1, 24–532) | 132.8 (88.0, 24–532) | 155.2 (71.6, 32–341) | 0.10 |
| Flap location (%) | | | | |
| Trunk | 62 (72.1) | 47 (68.1) | 15 (88.2) | 0.13 |
| Lower limb | 18 (20.9) | 16 (23.2) | 2 (11.8) | 0.50 |
| Upper limb | 6 (7.0) | 6 (8.7) | 0 (0.0) | 0.34 |
| Operation time [min] (SD, range) | 177.6 (68.0, 80–480) | 164.0 (59.0, 80–440) | 232.9 (75.6, 127–480) | <0.01 |
| Flap rotation [degree] (SD, range) | 149.9 (35.0, 50–180) | 147.1 (37.1, 50–180) | 156.4 (29.8, 90–180) | 0.53 |
| Number of surgeries [2] (SD, range) | 1.7 (1.4, 1–8) | 1.5 (1.1, 1–7) | 2.3 (2.0, 1–8) | 0.16 |
| Major complications [3] (%) | 27 (31.4) | 22 (31.9) | 5 (29.4) | 0.32 |
| Flap loss (%) | | | | |
| Partial | 5 (7.2) | 5 (7.2) | 0 (0.0) | 0.56 |
| Complete | 5 (5.8) | 4 (5.8) | 1 (5.9) | 0.99 |
| Total hospitalization [days] (SD, range) | 34.7 (15.7, 14–84) | 32.5 (13.6, 15–61) | 39.7 (19.7, 14–84) | 0.31 |

Abbreviations: PPF, perforator propeller flap; [1] includes risk factors of diabetes, arterial hypertension, peripheral artery disease, coronary heart disease, coagulation disorders, prior thrombotic events, obesity (BMI > 30 kg/m$^2$), radiation therapy, chemotherapy, and smoking; [2] with PPF surgery being the first surgery counted; [3] includes postoperative complications that required surgical revision during the time of hospitalization.

*3.2. Comparison of Single PPFs and Combined PPFs*

Both groups had similar characteristics in terms of age ($p$ = 0.34), sex ($p$ = 0.79), PPF size ($p$ = 0.10), flap rotation ($p$ = 0.53), total number of surgeries associated with flap surgery ($p$ = 0.16), and days of hospitalization ($p$ = 0.31) (Table 2, Figure 2). Risk factors were more frequent among patients undergoing combined PPF reconstruction (58.8% vs. 27.5%; $p$ = 0.02). Furthermore, tumors and pressure ulcers were the main causes for PPFs in both groups with a shared proportion of 63.8% among single PPFs and 76.4% among combined PPFs, respectively (Table 2). While most reconstructions were performed on the trunk, this proportion was 88.2% among combined PPFs and 68.1% among single PPFs. Lumbar artery perforator flaps (14.5% of single PPFs vs. 28.6% of combined PPFs), inferior gluteal artery perforator flaps (13.0% of single PPFs vs. 21.4% of combined PPFs), and superior gluteal artery perforator flaps (11.6% of single PPFs vs. 21.4% of combined PPFs) were the most common flaps used among both groups (Table 3). Defect sizes of combined PPFs were significantly larger than they were among single PPFs (178.2 ± 73.8 cm$^2$ vs. 103.0 ± 73.5 cm$^2$, $p < 0.01$) and mean operation time was significantly longer among combined PPFs than those among single PPFs (164 ± 59 vs. 233 ± 76 minutes, $p < 0.01$) (Figure 2). However, there were no significant differences in the occurrence of major complications (31.9% (single PPFs) vs. 29.4% (combined PPFs), $p = 0.32$) as well as complete flap losses (5.8% (single PPFs) vs. 5.9% (combined PPFs), $p = 0.99$). Table 2 provides a detailed summary of the results.

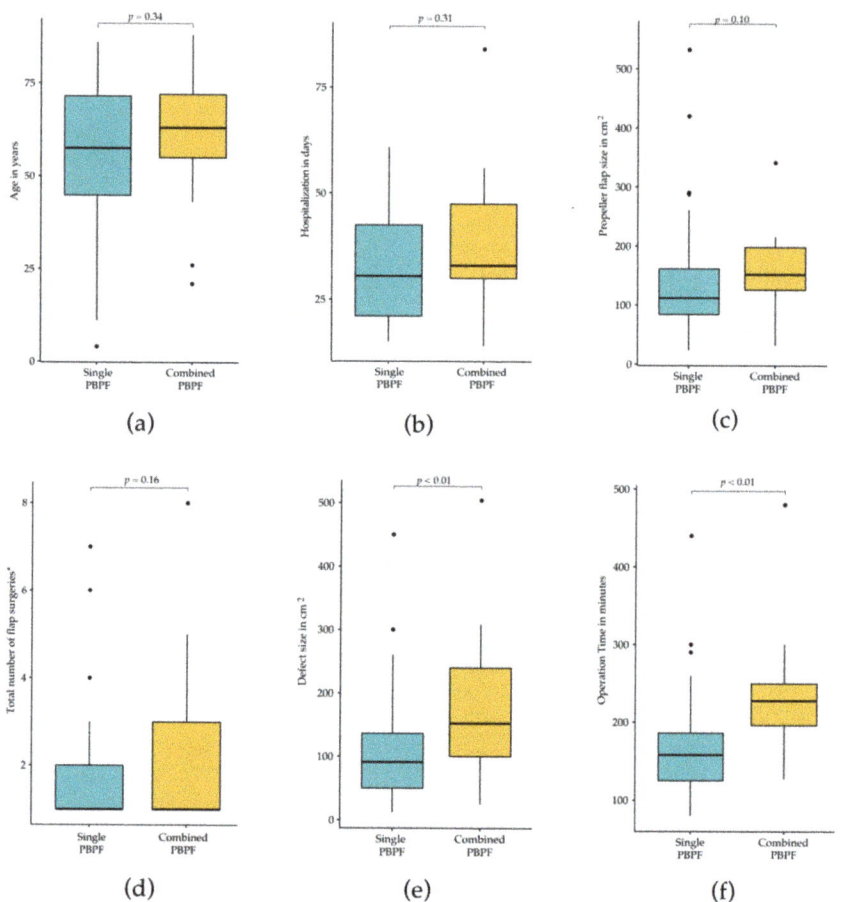

**Figure 2.** Wilcoxon–Mann–Whitney test on continuous variables. (**a**) Age in years; (**b**) Total hospitalization in days; (**c**) Perforator propeller flap size in cm$^2$; (**d**) Total number of surgeries starting with PPF surgery; (**e**) Defect size in cm$^2$; (**f**) Operation time in minutes (Abbreviations: PPF, perforator propeller flap).

**Table 3.** Flap distribution.

| Characteristics | Total | Single PPF | Combined PPF |
|---|---|---|---|
| No. of PPFs (%) | 97 | 69 (71.1) | 28 (28.9) |
| PPF type, No. (%) | | | |
| Adductor perforator | 5 (5.2) | 3 (4.3) | 2 (7.1) |
| ALT | 5 (5.2) | 4 (5.8) | 1 (3.6) |
| ATA | 3 (3.0) | 3 (4.3) | 0 (0.0) |
| AIA | 3 (3.0) | 3 (4.3) | 0 (0.0) |
| PTA | 5 (5.2) | 5 (7.2) | 0 (0.0) |
| Brachial artery | 4 (4.1) | 4 (5.8) | 0 (0.0) |
| DICAP | 7 (7.3) | 4 (5.8) | 3 (10.7) |
| IGAP | 15 (15.5) | 9 (13.0) | 6 (21.4) |
| LICAP | 3 (3.0) | 2 (2.9) | 1 (3.6) |
| Radial artery | 3 (3.0) | 3 (4.3) | 0 (0.0) |
| SGAP | 14 (14.4) | 8 (11.6) | 6 (21.4) |
| Lateral genicular artery | 1 (1.0) | 1 (1.4) | 0 (0.0) |
| LAP | 18 (18.6) | 10 (14.5) | 8 (28.6) |
| Posterior thigh perforator | 2 (2.0) | 2 (2.9) | 0 (0.0) |
| Profound femoral artery | 3 (3.0) | 3 (4.3) | 0 (0.0) |
| Pudendal artery | 2 (2.0) | 1 (1.4) | 1 (3.6) |
| Thoracoacromial artery | 2 (2.0) | 2 (2.9) | 0 (0.0) |
| Trapezius perforator | 2 (2.0) | 2 (2.9) | 0 (0.0) |

Abbreviations: PPF, perforator propeller flap; ALT, anterior lateral thigh; ATA, anterior tibial artery; AIA, anterior intercostal artery; PTA, posterior tibial artery; DICAP, dorsal intercostal artery perforator; IGAP, inferior gluteal artery perforator; LICAP, lateral intercostal artery perforator; SGAP, superior gluteal artery perforator; LAP, lumbar artery perforator.

*3.3. Univariable Binary Logistic Regression*

We included independent variables we thought could be used for clinical decision-making due to the prediction of major complications and that could be relatively easy to be ascertained by clinicians without needing to undertake complex imaging or laboratory measurements. We included independent variables of operation time, type of intervention, PPF size, and defect size. Defect size was included in our analysis as broad categories (<50 cm$^2$ [reference], 50–99 cm$^2$, 100–149 cm$^2$, 150–199 cm$^2$, and >200 cm$^2$) under the rationale that defect sizes are rather approximations than precise measurements due to complex geometry and the unclear extent of many defects. Regression analyses revealed that the type of intervention (OR: 0.95, 95% CI: 0.27–2.93; $p = 0.29$), the operation time (OR: 1.00, 95% CI: 1.00–1.01; $p = 0.25$) and the PPF size (OR: 1.00, 95% CI: 0.99–1.01; $p = 0.15$) had no significant impact on the occurrence of major complications (Table 4). However, we found a substantial higher probability of having major complications among defects larger than 200 cm$^2$ (OR: 8.50, 95% CI: 1.51–70.24; $p < 0.01$). To find out whether this was true for both groups, we conducted subgroup analyses separately for single PPFs and combined PPFs. Subgroup analyses revealed that there was a significant increase of major complications in defects larger than 100 cm$^2$ only in the group of single PPFs. However due to little data, confidence intervals of the subgroup analyses were disproportionately large. Consequently, we conducted an additional univariable binary logistic regression analysis, which only considered defect sizes larger than 100 cm$^2$. This analysis verified prior results. Defects larger than 100 cm$^2$ were significantly associated with an increased risk of having major complications among single PPFs (OR: 2.82, 95% CI: 1.01–8.36; $p = 0.05$). In contrast, there was no increased risk among combined PPFs (OR: 0.30, 95% CI: 0.02–3.37; $p = 0.32$). In fact, defects larger than 100 cm$^2$ only proved to be a significant predictor of major complications among single PPFs. Results of the regression analyses are shown in detail in Table 4.

**Table 4.** Univariable binary logistic regressions of major complications among 86 patients.

| Characteristics | Total PPF ($n = 86$) Odds Ratio (95% CI) | $p$-Value | Single PPF ($n = 69$) Odds Ratio (95% CI) | $p$-Value | Combined PPF ($n = 17$) Odds Ratio (95% CI) | $p$-Value |
|---|---|---|---|---|---|---|
| Intervention | | | | | | |
| Single PPF | 1 [Reference] | | | | | |
| Combined PPF | 0.95 (0.27–2.93) | 0.29 | | | | |
| Operation time (min) | 1.00 (1.00–1.01) | 0.25 | 1.00 (0.99–1.01) | 0.80 | 1.01 (1.00–1.04) | 0.33 |
| PPF size (cm$^2$) | 1.00 (0.99–1.01) | 0.15 | 1.00 (1.00–1.01) | 0.50 | 1.01 (1.00–1.03) | 0.11 |
| Defect size (cm$^2$) | | | | | | |
| <50 | 1 [Reference] | | 1 [Reference] | | 1 [Reference] | |
| 50–99 | 3.97 (0.80–29.48) | 0.17 | 6.85 (1.00–137.99) | 0.13 | 1.00 (0.01–69.47) | 0.99 |
| 100–199 | 4.25 (0.97–29.89) | 0.08 | 10.00 (1.63–194.65) | 0.05 | 0.17 (0.01–6.53) | 0.58 |
| >200 | 8.50 (1.51–70.24) | <0.01 | 32.00 (3.05–850.50) | 0.01 | 0.50 (0.01–17.47) | 0.99 |
| Defect size (cm$^2$) | | | | | | |
| <100 | 1 [Reference] | | 1 [Reference] | | 1 [Reference] | |
| >100 | 1.88 (0.74–4.91) | 0.18 | 2.82 (1.01–8.36) | 0.05 | 0.30 (0.02–3.37) | 0.32 |

Abbreviations: PPF = perforator propeller flap.

## 4. Discussion

While complete flap losses were rare events, we found a considerable prevalence of major complications of 31.9% among patients that received single PPFs and 29.4% among patients that received combined PPFs. Individual characteristics of sex, age, flap location, flap size, arc of flap rotation, total number of surgeries, and total flap loss were similar among the groups. Notably, defect sizes of combined PPF reconstructions were substantially larger than they were among single PPF reconstructions. While the operation time, the type of flap surgery, and the PPF size were not associated with the probability of having an increase in major complications, the defect size was. Interestingly, this was true for defects larger than 100 cm$^2$ among single PPFs but not among combined PPFs. Our findings have several important implications.

First, with a total flap loss of less than six percent, we have shown that combined PPFs were a reliable and promising reconstructive approach in the reconstruction of large soft tissue defects, which has thus far received little attention from a research perspective.

Second, the propeller flap size, the operation time as well as the type of flap surgery were not associated with a higher risk of having major complications among perforator propeller flaps. This, however, is interesting since flap size and operation time are known predictors for postoperative complications in free and regional flap surgery [24,25]. One possible explanation why we did not observe more major complications among larger flaps might be because most PPFs were performed on the trunk where perforasomes are usually quite large and, thus, may guarantee adequate flap perfusion. Another explanation could be the use of indocyanine green fluorescence angiography additional to clinical flap perfusion assessment in critical cases. Prior research implies that this method can reduce the rate of partial flap necrosis and improves flap survival through detection of insufficiently perfused flap areas [23,26,27]. However, further studies are needed to understand the underlaying factors of our findings. Additionally, our results showed that combined PPFs were as safe as single PPFs regardless of the significantly larger defect size among combined PPFs.

Third, a defect size of more than 100 cm$^2$ was a significant predictor of major complications only among single PPFs, suggesting that surgeons should prefer combined PPFs for the reconstruction of large soft tissue defects. This is an important finding since free flap surgery constitutes the alternative approach that might require complex surgical procedures, such as arteriovenous loops in order to provide adequate recipient vessels [28].

Fourth, the prevalence of major complications among combined PPF surgery is comparable to that reported among free flap surgery indicating that both options should be weighed carefully against each other when it comes to the reconstruction of large soft tissue defects [29–31]. For instance, due to microvascular anastomosis, free flaps require a longer operation time as well as longer postoperative immobilization than PPFs. Thus, the use of PPFs might decrease morbidity and mortality in selected patients [32–34].

Despite PPFs gaining popularity in recent years, research has mainly focused on single PPFs which, however, have proven to be a reliable method with a low complication rate [35,36]. Combined PPFs may allow reconstruction of extended defects and therefore, extent reconstructive possibilities [37]. For instance, Scaglioni and colleagues reported successful reconstruction of a large gluteal defect by a combination of two PPFs and a VY advancement flap [38]. This supports our experience as we could demonstrate sufficient reconstruction of the posterior trunk by a combination of two PPFs. Due to scarcity of recipient vessels, this body region is often unsuited for free flap reconstruction [8]. However, the combined PPF technique still is considered as a rescue strategy whenever established reconstructive approaches were not suitable. Given that, we suggest further prospective studies to specifically investigate the safety of combined PPFs in the reconstruction of large soft tissue defects and to assess the implementation of combined PPFs in the daily routine of reconstructive surgeons.

Although our results are promising, this study has several limitations. First, due to the retrospective design and small number of cases, this study might be underpowered. Second, we could only collect data documented in a patient's digital chart. Third, we used major complication rates of free flaps that were reported in the literature for comparison. Patients included in those studies might not reflect our patients, which is why further studies should aim for a prospective approach that include both, PPF and free flap surgery, to avoid possible bias. Fourth, most of the patients included in our study received PPF reconstructions on the trunk, which is why our results mainly account for this region of the body. Even though it is likely that our results can be applied to any region of the body, we strongly recommend further studies that specifically focus on the comparison of single and combined PPFs on the upper and lower extremity.

## 5. Conclusions

Our study is the first to compare single and combined perforator propeller flaps in terms of major postoperative complications. We could show that combined PPFs are not just a reliable reconstructive option, but eventually presented fewer major complications than single PPFs in the reconstruction of large soft tissue defects. Furthermore, major complication rates of combined PPFs were comparable to those among free flap surgery. Consequently, combined PPFs should be considered as a first line technique in the reconstruction of large soft tissue defects of the trunk. However, since combined PPFs require a flexible surgical strategy and intraoperative decision-making is sometimes challenging, we recommend proper training before implementing combined PPFs in a daily routine to achieve reliable results.

**Author Contributions:** Conceptualization: A.K.B. and U.K.; data curation, O.D.; formal analysis, O.D. and B.T.; investigation, O.D.; methodology, O.D. and B.T.; project administration, A.K.B. and R.E.H.; supervision, A.K.B. and R.E.H.; visualization, O.D. and B.T.; writing–original draft, A.K.B., O.D., and U.K.; writing–review and editing, A.K.B., B.T., L.H., E.G., R.E.H., and U.K. All authors have read and agreed to the published version of the manuscript.

**Funding:** This research received no external funding.

**Institutional Review Board Statement:** The study was conducted according to the guidelines of the Declaration of Helsinki, and approved by the Ethics board of the Friedrich Alexander University of Erlangen Nuremberg (registration number: 21-433-Br) and the local ethic committee of Rhineland-Palatinate (registration number: 2021-16096).

**Informed Consent Statement:** Informed consent was obtained from all subjects involved in the study.

**Data Availability Statement:** Data sharing is not applicable to this article.

**Conflicts of Interest:** The authors declare no conflict of interest.

## References

1. Baumann, D.P.; Butler, C.E. Soft tissue coverage in abdominal wall reconstruction. *Surg. Clin. N. Am.* **2013**, *93*, 1199–1209. [CrossRef] [PubMed]
2. Falkner, F.; Thomas, B.; Haug, V.; Nagel, S.S.; Vollbach, F.H.; Kneser, U.; Bigdeli, A.K. Comparison of pedicled versus free flaps for reconstruction of extensive deep sternal wound defects following cardiac surgery: A retrospective study. *Microsurgery* **2021**, *41*, 309–318. [CrossRef]
3. Xiong, L.; Gazyakan, E.; Kremer, T.; Hernekamp, F.J.; Harhaus, L.; Saint-Cyr, M.; Kneser, U.; Hirche, C. Free flaps for reconstruction of soft tissue defects in lower extremity: A meta-analysis on microsurgical outcome and safety. *Microsurgery* **2016**, *36*, 511–524. [CrossRef] [PubMed]
4. Bigdeli, A.K.; Thomas, B.; Falkner, F.; Radu, C.A.; Gazyakan, E.; Kneser, U. Microsurgical reconstruction of extensive lower extremity defects with the conjoined parascapular and latissimus dorsi free flap. *Microsurgery* **2020**, *40*, 639–648. [CrossRef]
5. Beier, J.P.; Horch, R.E.; Kneser, U. Bilateral pre-expanded free TFL flaps for reconstruction of severe thoracic scar contractures in an 8-year-old girl. *J. Plast. Reconstr. Aesthetic Surg.* **2013**, *66*, 1766–1769. [CrossRef] [PubMed]
6. Wanjala, N.F.; Dan, K. Local/regional flaps for extensive abdominal wall defects: Case series. *Int. J. Surg. Case Rep.* **2020**, *74*, 10–14. [CrossRef]
7. Ebehr, B.; Wagner, J.M.; Ewallner, C.; Eharati, K.; Elehnhardt, M.; Daigeler, A. Reconstructive Options for Oncologic Posterior Trunk Defects: A Review. *Front. Oncol.* **2016**, *6*, 51. [CrossRef]
8. Hernekamp, J.-F.; Cordts, T.; Kremer, T.; Kneser, U. Perforator-Based Flaps for Defect Reconstruction of the Posterior Trunk. *Ann. Plast. Surg.* **2020**, *86*, 72–77. [CrossRef]
9. Hallock, G.G. The Propeller Flap Version of the Adductor Muscle Perforator Flap for Coverage of Ischial or Trochanteric Pressure Sores. *Ann. Plast. Surg.* **2006**, *56*, 540–542. [CrossRef]
10. Yang, C.-H.; Kuo, Y.-R.; Jeng, S.-F.; Lin, P.-Y. An Ideal Method for Pressure Sore Reconstruction: A freestyle perforator-based flap. *Ann. Plast. Surg.* **2011**, *66*, 179–184. [CrossRef]
11. Pignatti, M.; Ogawa, R.; Hallock, G.G.; Mateev, M.; Georgescu, A.V.; Balakrishnan, G.; Ono, S.; Cubison, T.C.S.; D'arpa, S.; Koshima, I.; et al. The "Tokyo" Consensus on Propeller Flaps. *Plast. Reconstr. Surg.* **2011**, *127*, 716–722. [CrossRef]
12. Yu, S.; Zang, M.; Xu, L.; Zhao, Z.; Zhang, X.; Zhu, S.; Chen, B.; Ding, Q.; Liu, Y. Perforator Propeller Flap for Oncologic Reconstruction of Soft Tissue Defects in Trunk and Extremities. *Ann. Plast. Surg.* **2016**, *77*, 456–463. [CrossRef]
13. Ellabban, M.A.; Wyckman, A.; Abdelrahman, I.; Steinvall, I.; Elmasry, M. Dual Reconstruction of Lumbar and Gluteal Defects with Freestyle Propeller Flap and Muscle Flap. *Plast. Reconstr. Surg. Glob. Open* **2021**, *9*, e3376. [CrossRef]
14. Schaffer, C.; Guillier, D.; Raffoul, W.; di Summa, P.G. Lumbar Perforator Flaps for Coverage of Extensive Defects With Osteomyelitis. *Ann. Plast. Surg.* **2021**, *86*, 67–71. [CrossRef]
15. Falinower, H.; Herlin, C.; Laloze, J.; Bodin, F.; Kerfant, N.; Chaput, B. Use of the Propeller Lumbar Perforator Flap: A Series of 32 Cases. *Plast. Reconstr. Surg. Glob. Open* **2020**, *8*, e2522. [CrossRef]
16. Boissière, F.; Luca-Pozner, V.; Vaysse, C.; Kerfant, N.; Herlin, P.C.; Chaput, P.B. The SCIP propeller flap: Versatility for reconstruction of locoregional defect. *J. Plast. Reconstr. Aesthetic Surg.* **2019**, *72*, 1121–1128. [CrossRef]

17. Park, S.W.; Oh, T.S.; Eom, J.S.; Sun, Y.C.; Suh, H.S.; Hong, J.P. Freestyle Multiple Propeller Flap Reconstruction (Jigsaw Puzzle Approach) for Complicated Back Defects. *J. Reconstr. Microsurg.* **2015**, *31*, 261–267. [CrossRef] [PubMed]
18. Thomas, B.; Haug, V.; Falkner, F.; Arras, C.; Nagel, S.S.; Boecker, A.; Schmidt, V.J.; Kneser, U.; Bigdeli, A.K. A single-center retrospective comparison of Duplex ultrasonography versus audible Doppler regarding anterolateral thigh perforator flap harvest and operative times. *Microsurgery*, 2021; *published online ahead of print*. [CrossRef]
19. Daigeler, A.; Schubert, C.; Hirsch, T.; Behr, B.; Lehnhardt, M. Colour duplex sonography and "Power-Duplex" in Perforator Surgery—Improvement of patients safety by efficient planning. *Handchir. Mikrochir. Plast. Chir.* **2018**, *50*, 101–110. [CrossRef]
20. Wong, C.-H.; Cui, F.; Tan, B.-K.; Liu, Z.; Lee, H.-P.; Lu, C.; Foo, C.-L.; Song, C. Nonlinear Finite Element Simulations to Elucidate the Determinants of Perforator Patency in Propeller Flaps. *Ann. Plast. Surg.* **2007**, *59*, 672–678. [CrossRef] [PubMed]
21. Selvaggi, G.; Anicic, S.; Formaggia, L. Mathematical explanation of the buckling of the vessels after twisting of the microanastomosis. *Microsurgery* **2006**, *26*, 524–528. [CrossRef] [PubMed]
22. Topalan, M.; Bilgin, S.S.; Ip, W.; Chow, S. Effect of torsion on microarterial anastomosis patency. *Microsurgery* **2003**, *23*, 56–59. [CrossRef]
23. Bigdeli, A.K.; Thomas, B.; Falkner, F.; Gazyakan, E.; Hirche, C.; Kneser, U. The Impact of Indocyanine-Green Fluorescence Angiography on Intraoperative Decision-Making and Postoperative Outcome in Free Flap Surgery. *J. Reconstr. Microsurg.* **2020**, *36*, 556–566. [CrossRef] [PubMed]
24. Lin, P.; Kuo, P.; Kuo, S.C.H.; Chien, P.; Hsieh, C. Risk factors associated with postoperative complications of free anterolateral thigh flap placement in patients with head and neck cancer: Analysis of propensity score-matched cohorts. *Microsurgery* **2020**, *40*, 538–544. [CrossRef]
25. Peng, P.; Dong, Z.; Wei, J.; Liu, L.; Luo, Z.; Zheng, L. Risk factors related to the partial necrosis of the posterior tibial artery perforator-plus fasciocutaneous flap. *Eur. J. Trauma Emerg. Surg.* **2021**. published online ahead of print. [CrossRef] [PubMed]
26. Jakubietz, R.G.; Schmidt, K.; Bernuth, S.; Meffert, R.H.; Jakubietz, M.G. Evaluation of the Intraoperative Blood Flow of Pedicled Perforator Flaps Using Indocyanine Green-fluorescence Angiography. *Plast. Reconstr. Surg. Glob. Open* **2019**, *7*, e2462. [CrossRef]
27. Kneser, U.; Beier, J.P.; Schmitz, M.; Arkudas, A.; Dragu, A.; Schmidt, V.J.; Kremer, T.; Horch, R.E. Zonal perfusion patterns in pedicled free-style perforator flaps. *J. Plast. Reconstr. Aesthetic Surg.* **2013**, *67*, e9–e17. [CrossRef] [PubMed]
28. Henn, D.; Wähmann, M.S.T.; Horsch, M.; Hetjens, S.; Kremer, T.; Gazyakan, E.; Hirche, C.; Schmidt, V.J.; Germann, G.; Kneser, U. One-Stage versus Two-Stage Arteriovenous Loop Reconstructions: An Experience on 103 Cases from a Single Center. *Plast. Reconstr. Surg.* **2019**, *143*, 912–924. [CrossRef]
29. Farquhar, D.R.; Masood, M.M.; Pappa, A.K.; Patel, S.N.; Hackman, A.T.G. Predictors of Adverse Outcomes in Free Flap Reconstruction: A Single-Institution Experience. *Otolaryngol. Neck Surg.* **2018**, *159*, 973–980. [CrossRef]
30. Le Nobel, G.J.; Higgins, K.M.; Enepekides, D.J. Predictors of complications of free flap reconstruction in head and neck surgery: Analysis of 304 free flap reconstruction procedures. *Laryngoscope* **2012**, *122*, 1014–1019. [CrossRef]
31. Classen, D.A.; Ward, H. Complications in a Consecutive Series of 250 Free Flap Operations. *Ann. Plast. Surg.* **2006**, *56*, 557–561. [CrossRef]
32. Guo, F.; Shashikiran, T.; Chen, X.; Yang, L.; Liu, X.; Song, L. Clinical features and risk factor analysis for lower extremity deep venous thrombosis in Chinese neurosurgical patients. *J. Neurosci. Rural. Pract.* **2015**, *6*, 471–476. [CrossRef] [PubMed]
33. Brogan, E.; Langdon, C.; Brookes, K.; Budgeon, C.; Blacker, D. Respiratory Infections in Acute Stroke: Nasogastric Tubes and Immobility are Stronger Predictors than Dysphagia. *Dysphagia* **2014**, *29*, 340–345. [CrossRef] [PubMed]
34. Chou, C.-L.; Lee, W.-R.; Yeh, C.-C.; Shih, C.-C.; Chen, T.-L.; Liao, C.-C. Adverse Outcomes after Major Surgery in Patients with Pressure Ulcer: A Nationwide Population-Based Retrospective Cohort Study. *PLoS ONE* **2015**, *10*, e0127731. [CrossRef] [PubMed]
35. Vitse, J.; Bekara, F.; Bertheuil, N.; Sinna, R.; Chaput, B.; Herlin, C. Perforator-based propeller flaps reliability in upper extremity soft tissue reconstruction: A systematic review. *J. Hand Surg. Eur. Vol.* **2016**, *42*, 157–164. [CrossRef] [PubMed]
36. Iida, T.; Yoshimatsu, H.; Koshima, I. Reconstruction of Anterolateral Thigh Defects Using Perforator-Based Propeller Flaps. *Ann. Plast. Surg.* **2017**, *79*, 385–389. [CrossRef]
37. Arco, G.; Horch, R.E.; Arkudas, A.; Dragu, A.; Bach, A.D.; Kneser, U. Double pedicled perforator flap to close flank defects: An alternative for closure of a large lumbar defect after basalioma excision—A case report and review of the literature. *Ann. Plast. Surg.* **2009**, *63*, 422–424. [CrossRef]
38. Scaglioni, M.F.; Grufman, V.; Meroni, M.; Fritsche, E. Soft tissue coverage of a total gluteal defect with a combination of perforator-based flaps: A case report. *Microsurgery* **2020**, *40*, 797–801. [CrossRef]

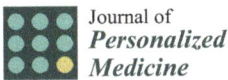 

Article

# Non-Invasive and Surgical Modalities for Scar Management: A Clinical Algorithm

Khaled Dastagir *,†, Doha Obed †, Florian Bucher, Thurid Hofmann, Katharina I. Koyro and Peter M. Vogt

Department of Plastic, Aesthetic, Hand and Reconstructive Surgery, Medical School Hannover, 30625 Hannover, Germany; Obed.doha@mh-hannover.de (D.O.); Bucher.florian@mh-hannover.de (F.B.); Hofmann.Thurid@mh-hannover.de (T.H.); Koyro.Katharina@mh-hannover.de (K.I.K.); Vogt.Peter@mh-hannover.de (P.M.V.)
* Correspondence: Khaleddastagir@hotmail.com
† Equally contributed as first author.

**Abstract:** Scars can lead to aesthetic and functional impairments. The treatment of scars requires meticulous planning and an individually adapted therapeutic strategy. A conceptual algorithm for scar treatment makes everyday clinical work easier for the practitioner and offers more safety for the patient. Based on a retrospective analysis of 1427 patients who presented for treatment of a variety of scars, we developed an algorithm for scar management and treatment. The treatments are presented using case descriptions. Additionally, an electronic search of MEDLINE, EMBASE, and ClinicalTrials.gov databases was performed utilizing combinations of relevant medical subject headings for "scar treatment", "hypertrophic scar treatment" and "keloid treatment". Reference lists of relevant articles and reviews were hand-searched for additional reports. Observed outcomes included: conservative scar therapy, minimally invasive scar therapy, and surgical scar therapy using local, regional and free flaps. With this work, we provide an algorithm for safe scar treatment. For better understanding, we have described a clinical case for each algorithm modality.

**Keywords:** scar; scar therapy; algorithm; free flap; tissue transfer

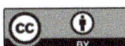

## 1. Introduction

Despite preventative efforts made after trauma or surgical procedures, dermal wounds will mostly heal by scarring with potentially devastating consequences e.g., emotional distress, deformity, and impaired quality of life. Patients suffering from scar tissue frequently experience stigmatization and social distress, which marks the importance of the search for efficient treatment in order to ameliorate scar tissue towards vital skin. An extensive number of techniques and treatment options exist for the management of scars. Nonetheless, the increasing prevalence of scar tissue formation and its functional and aesthetic impact remains a financial burden for the health care system. The global scar treatment market magnitude is estimated to value approximately $32 billion by 2027 [1], highlighting that scar management in the health care system will remain a significant challenge.

The concept of scar treatment ranges from simple conservative treatment options to highly complex operations that must be planned individually for each patient. The most important aim for scar treatment is the improvement of functional and aesthetical deformities [2,3]. Additionally, in order to achieve aesthetically pleasing results, homogeneous skin texture and pigmentation are essential, as well as soft tissue pliability for adequate functionality e.g., of adjacent joints [4]. Despite the efforts of clinicians and researchers, identifying successful scar treatments has remained elusive.

Currently, there is no evidence-based gold-standard treatment algorithm for the treatment of functionally and aesthetically disruptive scars. This unsatisfactory knowledge of scar treatment is based on the complex pathophysiology, lack of suitable model systems for the evaluation of therapeutic outcomes, difficulties in quantifying changes in scar appearance, and the limited prospective, randomized controlled clinical trials of scar treatment options. Thus, patient management has been driven by clinical experience rather than adherence to a professional consensus. The last recommended algorithm was described by Gold et al. in 2014 [5]. Mostly, conservative treatment algorithms were described here without the incorporation of complex surgical scar treatment options.

We hereby present an algorithm for scar management in the clinical setting. Each step of the algorithm is described using representative cases with simple to complex scar therapy strategies. In this article, the concepts, the algorithm for scar management, and an original catalog of indications that apply to treatments from conservative to complex operative therapies are provided based on the German and international scar management guidelines [6,7].

## 2. Patients and Methods

Based on retrospective data analysis of 1427 patients we developed an algorithm for scar management and treatment. Furthermore, an electronic search of MEDLINE, EMBASE, and ClinicalTrials.gov databases was performed utilizing combinations of relevant medical subject headings for "scar treatment", "hypertrophic scar treatment" and "keloid treatment". Reference lists of relevant articles and reviews were hand-searched for additional reports. Observed outcomes included: conservative scar therapy, minimally invasive scar therapy, surgical scar therapy using local flaps, and surgical scar therapy using regional- and free flaps. The treatments are presented using case descriptions.

## 3. Results

### 3.1. Conservative Treatment Options

Conservative treatment procedures such as scar massage and compression therapy using compression dressings or scar plasters containing silicone are gold standard therapies to obtain flat, soft, and aesthetically acceptable scars [8]. Furthermore, for functional rehabilitation, physiotherapy and occupational therapy remain integral treatment pillars [4]. Naturally, scar tissue shows spontaneous improvement whilst maturing. Therefore, scar revision usually will be performed after 6 to 12 months upon formation. However, conservative treatment modalities frequently will not yield satisfactory results and are often limited with regard to sustainability in complex and extensive cases, leaving surgical treatment alternatives necessary. Whether and when to perform surgical procedures is the patient's and doctor's joint decision upon extensive medical education about treatment alternatives and risks. The selection of an adequate surgical procedure itself remains a highly individualized concept since it is in fact dependent on a variety of factors such as the size of the scar, the texture of the skin, the anatomical region, and its pigmentation. Prior to surgery, it remains crucial to evaluate the resolution of acute tissue inflammation.

### 3.2. Laser Therapy

Laser therapy depicts a safe and effective first-line therapy in the management of traumatic scars and contractures. Early laser treatment may aid in minimizing pathological scar formation and associated disability [9]. In the treatment of hypertrophic scars, ablative lasers (10,600-nm), $CO_2$ lasers, and the 2940-Er:YAG lasers, are frequently used [10]. The main goal of this treatment option is to destroy collagen and promote new collagen growth. However, treatment with ablative lasers can lead to prolonged downtime, edema, persistent erythema, keloid formation, and pigment disorders [11]. Non-ablative lasers, which also cause collagen remodeling, have fewer side effects compared to ablative lasers. Due to the superior degree of extracellular remodeling, ablative lasers generally achieve superior outcomes than non-ablative lasers. The introduction of fractional $CO_2$ lasers has facilitated reduced ablative resurfacing that allows for corrections of scar surface irregularities and pliability, as well as dermal collagen reorientation in all skin types. Unlike non-ablative lasers, these $CO_2$ lasers rely on a filtering system that produces microfractioned laser beams, that allow for local tissue damage with resulting ablation of the epidermis. The damaged tissue areas show spontaneous healing within 48 hours and subsequent tissue remodelling leads to flattening of scars and surface irregularities and collagen reorganization [12].

### 3.3. Triamcinolone Injections

Hypertrophic scars and keloids depict a special challenge in scar treatment. Triamcinolone acetate injections have been demonstrated to be effective short-term. Their intralesional application remains one of the most widely used treatments. Causing a reduction of collagen synthesis through fibroblast hypoactivity and a reduction in fibroblast density presumably derives their efficacy. Apart from this, triamcinolone seems to cause a decrease in endothelial bud formation from blood vessels [13]. Still, recent studies have shown, that up to 50% of keloids show no response to triamcinolone injections and may show significant relapse upon initial response [14,15]. Besides, an array of side-effects e.g., telangiectasia and tissue atrophy have been described which should not be underestimated [16]. Alternatively, the incorporation of verapamil and 5-Fluorouracil may produce superior results for medium- and long-term treatments with a reduction of given side-effects [17]. Recent clinical studies have shown that in comparison with intralesional triamcinolone treatment, combination treatment with triamcinolone and 5-fluorouracil was more effective in keloid and hypertrophic scar treatment and allowed for more significant improvement in erythema, scar height, observer assessment, and patient self-assessment. Additionally, the combination therapy offered easy administration, greater patient safety, and a reduced rate of recurrence [18]. Further studies have assessed the efficacy of oral medication on scar tissue treatment. A recent experimental study investigating the effectiveness of enalapril, candesartan, and intralesional steroid therapies in rabbits has shown that all treatment modalities were effective in the reduction of scar tissue development, whilst the best macroscopic results were obtained by triamcinolone treatment and the best microscopic results were obtained by enalapril and triamcinolone [19].

Case Report

A 25-year-old female patient presented with a hypertrophic scar in the area of the décolleté, which had occurred after a scratch injury sustained during her childhood. External keloid excision was performed at the age of 15 years, whereupon a scar keloid formed again. We performed triamcinolone injections in three sessions and applied silicone patches, after which the scar texture improved significantly (Figure 1).

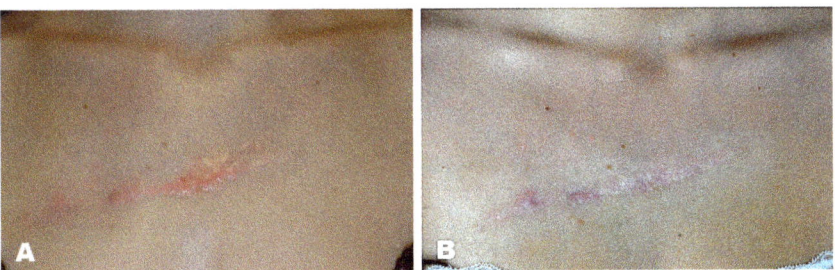

**Figure 1.** (**A**) Preoperative hypertrophic scar, (**B**) 3 months postoperative outcome after triamcinolone treatment.

### 3.4. Lipofilling

Autologous fat grafting as a treatment for scars includes lipofilling procedures. These are particularly indicated for patients with painful, hypertrophic, or retracted scars. The technique is usually performed under general anesthesia and is based on autologous fat extraction (i.e., abdominal fat). Upon fat processing, the injection of the remaining adipose tissue occurs in the hypodermis under the scar. In general, lipofilling procedures can be regarded as minimally invasive procedures that can contribute to a reduction of tension in scar tissue. Besides, the cosmetic appearance of a scar can be improved [20]. A disadvantage of the free fat transfer is the physiological reabsorption ranging from 10–70% of the initially injected fat grafting. Therefore, multiple sessions of fat transfer might be necessary, and permanently stable outcomes cannot be guaranteed. The technique cannot be performed in malnourished patients as fatty areas are needed for liposuction [21].

Case Report

This 46-year-old patient had breast ablation on the left side after breast cancer. After an unsuccessful attempt to reconstruct the breast using a deep inferior epigastric perforator (DIEP) flap, the patient's left breast was reconstructed using a superior gluteal artery perforator (S-GAP) flap. The patient developed a retracted scar at the donor site which was painful and visible (Figure 2A). We proposed a lipofilling procedure and explained that multiple lipofilling might be necessary for a satisfactory aesthetic outcome. We performed the first lipofilling procedure (application of 337 mL, thigh liposuction). The patient was satisfied after the first complected procedure (Figure 2B). Therefore, no further lipofilling procedures were required.

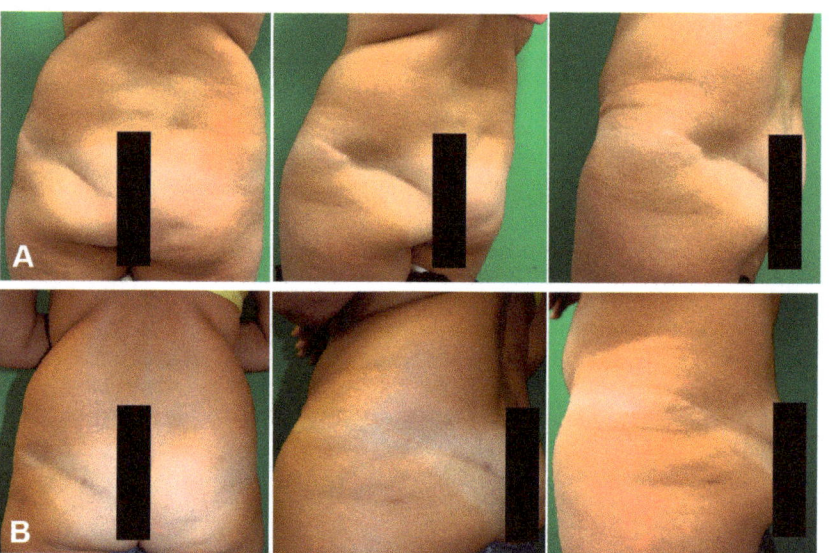

**Figure 2.** (**A**) Preoperative donor site scar after S-GAP flap harvest for breast reconstruction, (**B**) 3 month postoperative outcome after lipofilling.

*3.5. Medical Needling*

Based on the principle of percutaneous collagen induction, medical needling consists of applying needle rollers with pressure on the target area, causing an array of microwounds in the dermal layer. The procedure that can be performed under local or general anesthesia is supposed to trigger a posttraumatic inflammatory cascade whilst preserving the epidermal structures and thereby allowing skin regeneration and collagen formation [22]. Particularly the increased expression of growth factors, e.g., vascular endothelial growth factor (VEGF) and tissue growth and transforming factor (TGF-ß) is a key component of the treatment's effect. Besides, the proliferation of dermal cells, which are crucial for skin remodeling, is initiated [23]. Apart from this, by triggering the reorganization of the extracellular matrix, the thickness of the epidermis can be shaped [24]. As an effective treatment modality for rejuvenation procedures and the treatment of wrinkles, it has advanced to a reliable method for larger scar tissue areas, which unlike laser and topically ablative treatments does not damage the epidermis. Therefore, medical needling sessions can be performed multiple times to yield optimal results.

Case Report

An 18-year-old patient suffered a car accident, sustaining 2b-3° burns to the left side of her face and décolleté. During the course of intensive medical therapy at our burn center, multiple necrectomies and split-thickness skin grafts were performed to reconstruct the burned areas. During the process, hypertrophic scarring occurred in the area of the left eye, face, and décolleté, which was associated with pain and limitation of the facial field. Initially, we performed three medical needling sessions in a row in 2017, which resulted in an improvement of the scar appearance due to collagen induction. Subsequently, in 2019, we were able to treat the visual field restriction using canthotomy and canthopexy on the left eye, as well as scar transection and full-thickness skin grafting. In the area of the décolleté, thoracic scar resection could be performed by means of expander treatment in 2019 and the reduction of the scar could be achieved (Figure 3).

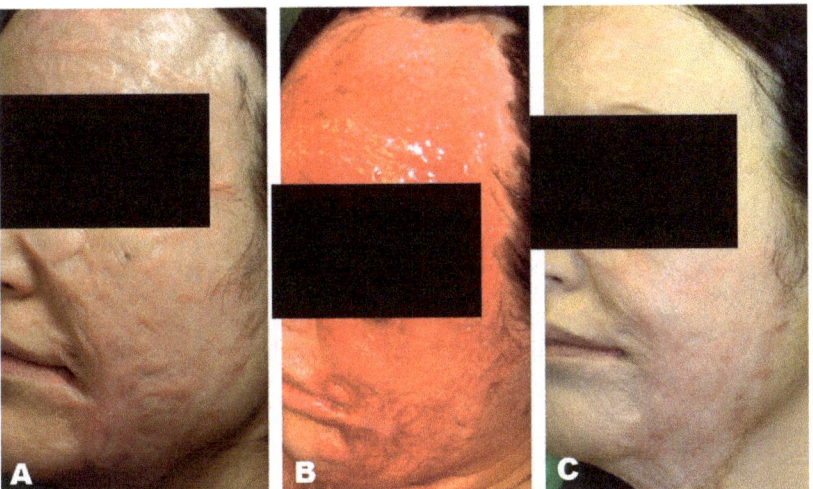

**Figure 3.** (**A**) Preoperative hypertrophic scar, (**B**) Intraoperative picture after Medical Needling, (**C**) Postoperative outcome after 3 medical needling treatments.

*3.6. Skin Grafting*

Skin grafts provide many functional and aesthetic benefits when it comes to tissue repair. Paramount in skin grafting is the choice of split- or full-thickness grafts and choosing a sufficient texture and pigmentation match for the recipient site [25]. Whilst full-thickness grafts are particularly beneficial for covering facial defects after scar excision due to minimal skin contraction, split-thickness grafts are preferred when large defects need coverage and in areas in which skin contraction is favorable to some degree for defect size reduction [26].

The meshing of skin grafts additionally may be beneficial for instance by allowing a reduction of donor-site morbidity, by the expansion of the skin graft, and by avoiding fluid retention in infected recipient-sites [27].

*3.7. Dermal Regeneration Templates (DRT)*

Dermal templates are used when split-thickness skin grafts are not sufficient for the reconstruction of tissue defects. They provide a scaffold, which promotes tissue regeneration, immediate wound closure and depicts a physical barrier to prevent wound infections [28]. Advantages include the restoration of the skin's pliability and mobility whilst providing sufficient sturdiness [28,29]. Types of DRTs include products derived from animal and human sources as well as scaffolds that have been artificially constructed of highly purified biomaterial or entirely synthetic polymers. For scars developing following large burn injuries, synthetic polyurethane dermal templates such as Integra (Life Sciences Corp., Princeton, NJ, USA) or NovoSorb Biodegradable Temporising Matrix (Polymedics, Denkendorf, Germany) have been established to address the lack of autologous skin to graft and to restore the dermal skin layer [30]. Integra presents a decellularized dermal template derived from animal sources and consists of purified collagen from bovine tendons crosslinked with glycosaminoglycan obtained from shark cartilage and may be supplied with a removable silicone layer that functions as a temporary epidermis [30]. In contrast, BTM is a fully synthetic dermal template which consists of biodegradable polyurethane foam with a temporary non-biodegradable polyurethane seal [31]. Compared to Integra, BTM evades the risk of cross-species immune rejection or disease transmission, as well as circumvents ethical and cultural objections to using animal-derived products [28].

BTM application has shown to be successful in improving scar quality upon application and limiting wound contraction significantly [32,33]. Its reconstructive possibilities can be used for a variable range of tissue defects that are not responsive to instant skin grafting. Key advantages are the vascularization and integration of the template even in the presence of infection, thereby allowing an application in patients with an array of comorbidities [34].

Case Report

A 79-year-old woman with a deep burn injury scar on the right lateral thigh was referred to our center. She had suffered from a scalding injury in her early childhood. The initial injury was treated conservatively. In 2017, the patient underwent surgical excision of keloids in the formerly burned area. Subsequently, she developed a wound-healing deficit and wound dehiscence. The following treatment comprised of wound debridement, scar excision, and primary wound closure shortly after. Three-months postoperatively, the patient had presented with a recurrent wound dehiscence that was surgically revised by wound debridement and skin advancement flap. After 14 days, the wound had healed sufficiently. The representation of the patient occurred three years later with a flap skin dehiscence. Sufficient healing could not be achieved by conservative treatment with disinfecting topicals. Additionally, the patient described an uncomfortable and painful feeling of tension in the formerly burned areas. Physical examination showed a predominantly non-irritated extensive scar area of approximately 20 × 10 cm on the lateral aspect of the right thigh with scar tissue extending into the gluteal and trochanter region. On the latero-proximal border of the scar was an approximately 3 × 1 cm sized wound dehiscence. We performed another wound debridement and opted for extensive scar excision and application of Novosorb BTM. Efforts were made in order to ensure sufficiently vascularized subcutaneous tissue. The wound was sealed by vacuum-assisted closure (VAC) dressing. On days 8 and 16 the patient was taken back to theater for BTM evaluation and VAC dressing change. On day 21 we performed the surgical delamination of the BTM. It showed full adhesion to the underlying wound bed. We went on to perform split-thickness grafting over the delaminated BTM. At 1-month follow-up, the reconstructed area presented with a natural appearance with flexible skin and minimal skin contraction. The uncomfortable feeling of tension was fully regressive, and the patient's mobility was fully preserved. Post-dressing removal, we initiated physiotherapeutic rehabilitation for flexibility and endurance (Figure 4).

*3.8. Local Flaps*

Local flaps, such as Z-plasties, can be performed in order to achieve reorientation of scar tissue and to position it further into relaxed skin tension lines. Surgically it is accomplished by performing a double transposition local flap, positioning the central limb of the Z-platy perpendicularly to the former scar [35]. Advantages also include the breaking up of scar tissue resulting in an irregularization, which renders scar perception less conspicuous. Presumably, the Z-plasty's variety of tension vectors may aid in the prevention of scar contraction and hypertrophy.

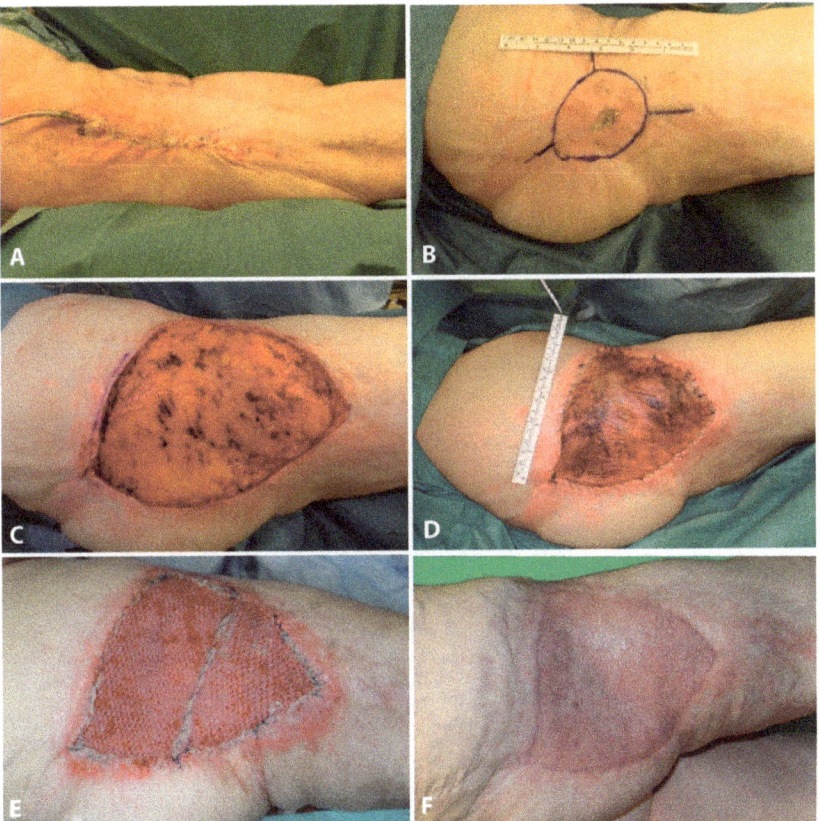

**Figure 4.** (**A**) Postoperative picture after scar excision and primary wound closure, (**B**) Postoperative development of a wound healing disorder, (**C**) Another scar excision, (**D**) Application of BTM, (**E**) Split-skin graft 3 weeks after BTM application, (**F**) Final outcome.

For extensive scars, Z-plasties can be performed with multiple and continuous incisions. Disadvantages that go in hand with performing Z-plasties include the increase of the scar's lengths as well as the addition of scar lines, which partially cannot be positioned within relaxed skin lines.

Case Report

The patient suffered a severe childhood burn affecting the trunk, thighs, and right upper arm including the axilla (30% total body surface). The initial therapy consisted of necrosectomy with skin grafting. Further, three sessions of medical needling were performed to improve the scar pattern. The patient presented to our special consultation hour complaining about a hypertrophic scar with local contracture in the right axilla.

During clinical examination the patient was unable to abduct his right shoulder >90° due to contracture of a hypertrophic scar measuring approximately 30 cm. Operative resection of hypertrophic scar tissue was performed under general anesthesia. Wound closure was performed using Z-plasties in order to achieve a free range of motion of the right shoulder. Postoperatively the patient received a Gilchrist sling for seven days and was discharged after four days.

The patient returned to our consultation hour three months postoperatively. The scar healing was smooth with no hypertrophic areas. Range of motion for the right shoulder was without any restriction in all planes (Figure 5).

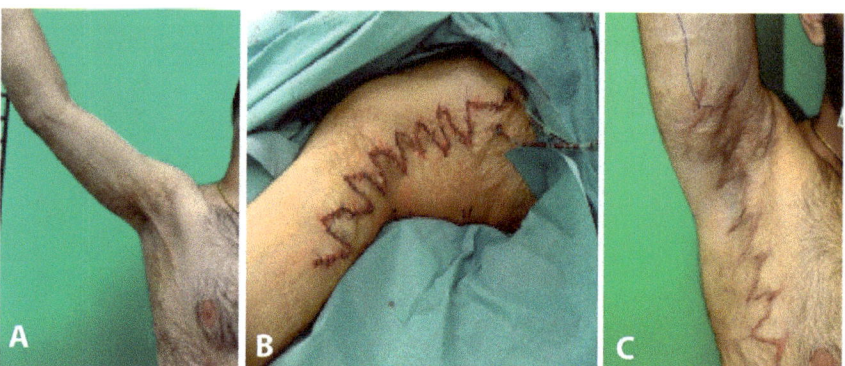

**Figure 5.** (**A**)Preoperative hypertrophic scar with functional limitation of the arm, (**B**) Intraoperative picture after Z-plasty, (**C**) Postoperative outcome.

*3.9. Expander*

Advantages of gaining skin and soft tissue using expanders include suitable aesthetic results due to the superior skin quality and color match and no donor-site morbidity.

They are usually used for reconstruction in the area of the scalp, face, chest, and extremities. The soft tissue obtained by expanders can also be used as a pedicled flap to cover defects of the head, neck, or face area. For this purpose, pre-expanded supraclavicular flaps or super thin posterior thorax flaps can be used, too [36]. However, the practitioner should be aware that the expander can severely limit the functioning of the patient, cause pain, and cannot be tolerated by all patients. In case that all above-mentioned options are not applicable, free flaps are indicated to cover the tissue defect after scar excision [37].

Case Report

The patient suffered a scalding injury by boiling water affecting the chest with contracture of the upper pole of both breasts 20 years ago. Previously, multiple sessions of medical needling were performed in our clinic. However, the patient complained about a persisting hypertrophic scar contracture. An area of hypertrophic scar tissue measuring $10 \times 12$ cm was identified. Due to scar contracture, the upper breast poles were drawn upwards.

In order to achieve distension of fibrous scar tissue, two subcutaneous expanders (55 mL each) were placed presternally using a horizontal incision. The expanders were explanted two months postoperatively. During the same surgery, the hypertrophic scar area was resected completely, and wound closure was achieved using a V-shaped advancement flap.

The patient was satisfied with the functional and aesthetic result. Further on, a local lipofilling was performed to improve the local scar condition (Figure 6).

*3.10. Vascularized Flaps*

Regional flaps such as vascularized pedicled fasciocutaneous or myocutaneous flaps are applied if there is a lack of adjacent tissue to cover the defect after scar excision [38,39]. Due to the complexity of these operations and the risk of donor-site morbidity, regional flaps are only indicated in cases of severe functional or aesthetic impairment. The most commonly used pedicled flaps include groin flaps for covering defects in the hand area or transverse rectus abdominis myocutaneous (TRAM) flaps for covering tissue defects in the lumbar and hip areas. In the case of the inguinal flap, it should be noted that a two-stage surgical treatment is necessary. Multistage treatment strategies e.g., serial scar excisions tissue expander are indicated if the expanded soft tissue has better quality compared to other options and the patient does not mind undergoing multiple interventions [36].

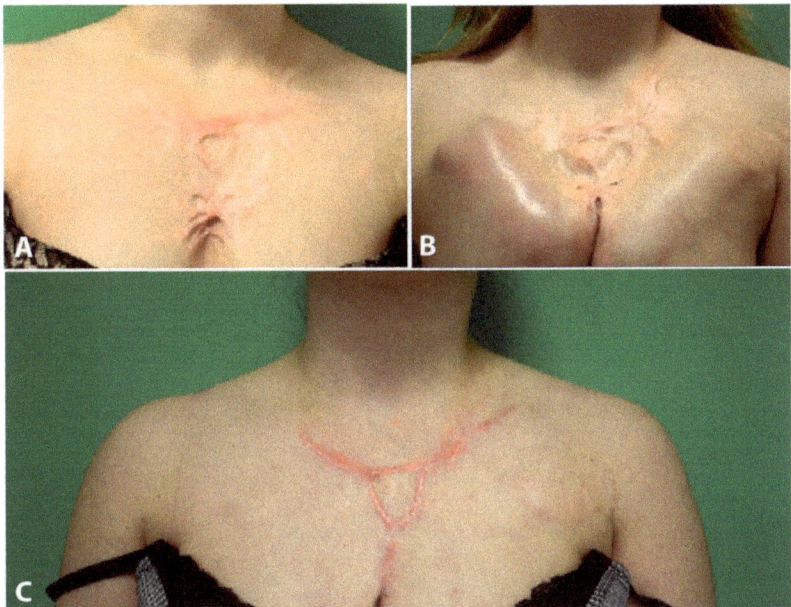

**Figure 6.** (**A**) Hypertrophic scar in the chest area, (**B**) After expander implantation, (**C**) Outcome after 6 month.

Case Report

The patient had breast cancer (right side) in 2011. She got neoadjuvant chemotherapy (Epirubicin) via a port catheter. During the first cycle of chemotherapy, the patient suffered from an extravasate. However, no surgical therapy was needed, and the tissue was healing. After completion of all chemotherapy cycles, the patient got a breast-conserving surgical treatment, an axillary lymph node dissection (level 1 and 2) and radiation. Subsequently, the port got removed and the patient suffered from a wound-healing disorder. Multiple surgical wound debridements were performed including VAC-therapy and the application of a split-skin graft. However, the patient developed a massive and painful scar contracture in the chest area. The scar was excised and a musculus latissimus dorsi pedicle flap was performed. As the pedicel flap was prominent over the skin level, the patient received liposuction of the pedicle flap. The patient further got physiotherapy and conservative scar treatment. Because of a relieving posture, the patient developed a shoulder contracture in 2018 and needed physiotherapy on a regular basis. (Figure 7).

*3.11. Free Tissue Transfer*

Due to technical advances in medicine and the improvement of microsurgical operating techniques, free tissue transfer has emerged as one of the most effective therapy methods for large wounds. Because of the better understanding of the free flap plasty, e.g., flap geometry, blood supply, and flap delay, new options were created to provide a wide range of tissue that could be transferred to the most distant locations of the human body. All types of tissues, including bone, tendon, muscle, fascia, fat, and skin can be used as free tissue transfer (Table 1). The pattern of the vascular supply determines the size, design, and thus the individual requirements for covering tissue defects. If there is no recipient vessel available e.g., in case of vascular diseases, severe scarring or irradiation, venous grafts or arteriovenous loops can be applied to provide recipient vessels for free flaps [36]. Due to the anatomical variations, the flap architecture and its vascular pattern are variable. Therefore, an initial magnetic resonance imaging (MRI) or computed tomography (CT)-angiography could help to develop an adequate strategy for applying free tissue transfer. Profound anatomical knowledge about the muscle origin, its insertion as well as vascular supply like perforator location or location of recipient's vessels is essential to provide the right indications for a free flap. We provide a systematic approach of free flaps regarding tissue requirements after scar excision (Table 1).

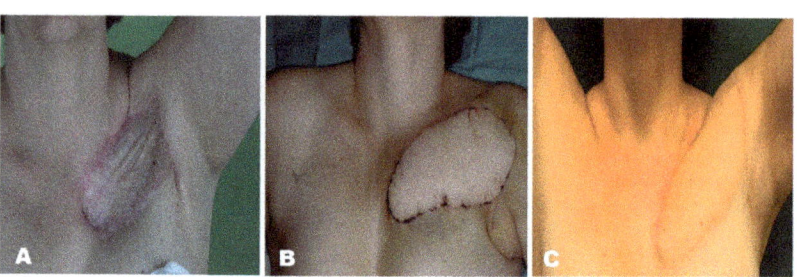

**Figure 7.** (**A**) Scar after skin graft transplantation, (**B**) 7 days postoperatively after pedicled latissimus dorsi muscle flap transfer, (**C**) Postoperative outcome after one year.

**Table 1.** Free flaps regarding tissue requirements after scar excision.

| Flap Type | Included Tissue | Examples | Blood Supply | Size |
|---|---|---|---|---|
| Arterial | Skin, subcutis and fascia | Radial arm flap | Radial artery | 8 × 16 cm |
| | | Dorsalis pedis flap | Dorsalis pedis artery | 3 × 7 cm |
| Muscle or myocutaneous | Skin, subcutis, muscle | Latissimus dorsi | Thoracodorsal artery | Muscle: 20 × 40; Skin: 12 × 20 |
| | | Rectus abdominis | Superior or inferior epigastric artery | Muscle: 25 × 6 cm Skin: large traverse or vertical paddle |
| Fascial, adipofascial and fasciocutaneous | Skin, subcutis, fascia | Serratus fascia | Serratus branch of thoracodorsal artery | 12 × 16 cm |
| | | Parascapular flap | Descending branch of the circumflex sapular artery | 15 × 25 cm |
| Perforator | Skin, subcutis and scubcutaneous fascia | Anterolateral thigh flap | Septocutaneous perforators from descending branch of the lateral femoral circumflex artery | 8 × 25 cm |
| | | Deep inferior epigastric perforator flap | Deep inferior epigastric artery | Variable skin paddle, similar size to TRAM |
| Specialized | Sensor tissue, differentiated structure and texture | Wrap around flap | First dorsal metatarsal artery | Big toe |
| | | Composite tissue allografts | No blood supply | e.g., finger tip |

3.11.1. Case Report 1

In 2003 the patient suffered from necrotizing fasciitis. Subsequently, the patient got a split-skin graft. However, the patient developed a fragile and painful scar on the left lower leg. In May 2013 the patient received a musculus latissimus dorsi free flap (MLD) after excision of the scar. Postoperatively, a small part of the free flap got necrotic. A debridement and removal of the necrotic tissue was necessary. However, a secondary wound closure was not possible, and a full-thickness skin graft and VAC-therapy were applied in June 2013. After VAC-therapy, another full-thickness skin graft was needed. In November 2014, lipofilling between the MLD and the split skin graft was performed. In September 2018, the patient suffered from a minor trauma at the lower leg and needed another split skin graft. Afterwards, the patient was satisfied and experienced no further complications (Figure 8).

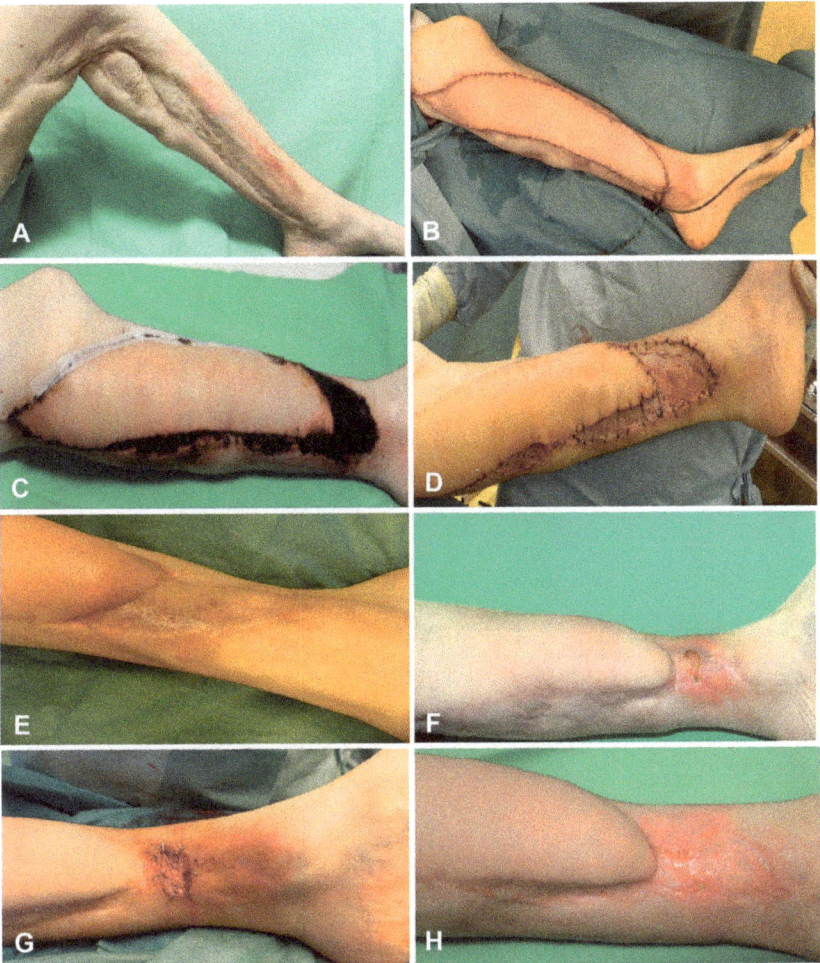

**Figure 8.** (**A**) Fragile and painful scar of the left leg, (**B**) Intraoperative picture after excision of the scar and reconstruction of the lower leg using latissimus dorsi muscle free flap, (**C**) Development of flap margin necrosis, (**D**) Excision of the flap margin necrosis and skin graft transplantation, (**E**) complete healing of the wound, (**F**) Development of a small wound, (**G**) Treatment of the wound using skin graft, (**H**) Final outcome.

### 3.11.2. Case Report 2

A 59-year-old patient suffered from multiple traumas including a femur fracture, ankle fracture type Weber B on the right side, commotio cerebri, and soft tissue defect anterior to the left thigh. The fractures were treated by trauma surgeons and the soft tissue defect was covered using a skin graft. Three years later the patient presented to our clinic with a scar in the area of the split-thickness skin graft. Since the skin graft was attached directly to the muscle, the scar was concerning functionally and aesthetically. To adequately reconstruct the soft tissue of the left thigh, the scar was excised and the wound was subsequently covered using a free DIEP flap. However, the flap developed marginal necrosis. After debridement of the necrosis, the remaining defect was covered using a split-skin graft. 1 year later the DIEP flap was thinned out, followed by a liposuction of the flap to improve contour. Finally, the flap and its adjacent area were aligned using liposuction (Figure 9).

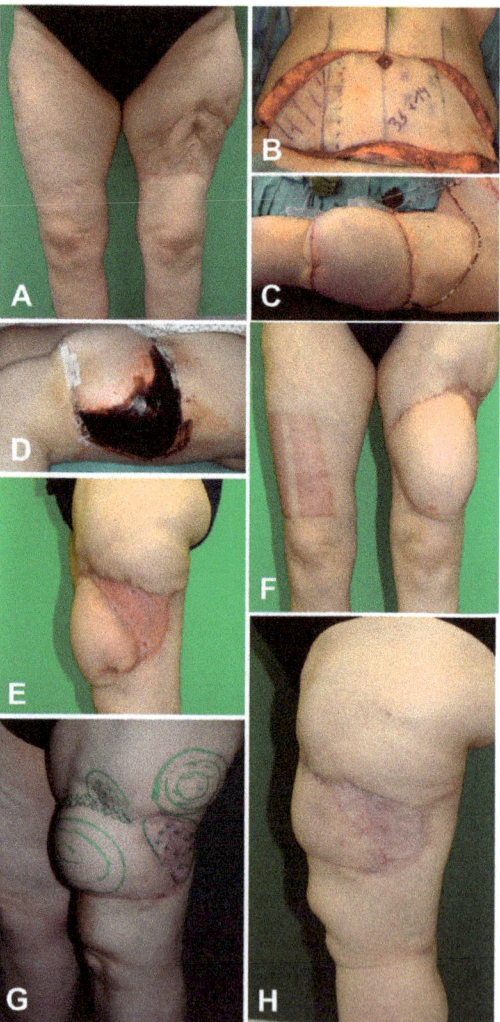

**Figure 9.** (**A**) Split-thickness skin graft scar, (**B**) Preparation of a DIEP flap, (**C**) Covering of the soft-tissue defect after scar excision, (**D**) Development of flap margin necrosis, (**E,F**) Postoperative image after excision of flap necrosis and skin graft transplantation, (**G**) Preoperative planning of liposuction of the flap, (**H**) Final outcome.

## 4. Discussion

The prevalence of scar tissue formation is on the rise. However, successful scar management has still remained elusive for many clinicians in light of a broad array of possible treatment modalities and the continuous evolution of new therapeutic options. Multiple well-established therapeutic modalities to treat scars have been described and treatment advances have allowed us to improve aesthetic and functional deficits due to scars. Efficient comprehensive scar treatment frequently incorporates conservative measures, physical therapy, injection of corticosteroids and antimetabolites, laser treatment, and surgical options. Based on our clinical experience with the presented scar treatment modalities, we have attempted to compose a treatment algorithm for the management of scars, in the hope that this paradigm will aid clinicians in their treatment evaluation. Based on the considerations depicted above, we present an extensively applicable algorithm for the treatment of a variety of scars (Figure 10).

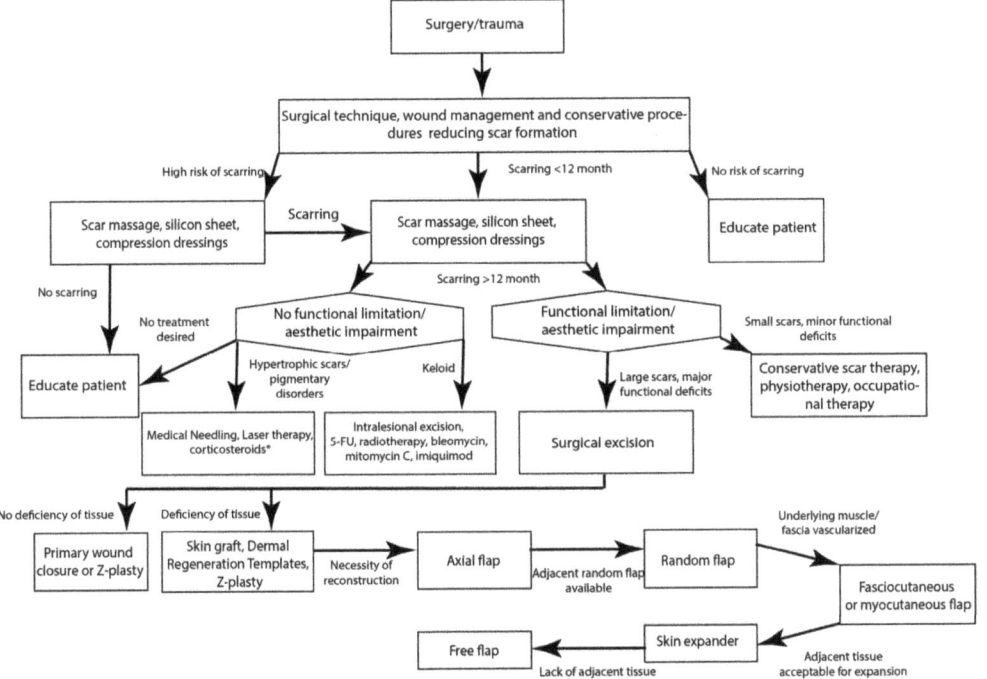

**Figure 10.** Algorithm for the treatment of scars.

During the initial consultation, we firstly aim to inform the patient of all the possible treatment options and their realistic outcomes. Early on, we highlight the frequent requirement of several treatment sessions and the possibility of remnants or recurrence of scar tissue. In general, patients presenting with scars prior to full scar maturation (12 months postoperatively/after trauma) are advised to take full advantage of available conservative treatment options comprising of scar massage, the application of silicone sheets and compression dressings. Particularly with an early application, this may aid in optimizing the aesthetic factor of scars and may render further treatment modalities unnecessary. Upon scar maturation and absence of scar regredience, scar re-evaluation takes place. In the case of remaining aesthetic impairments or hypertrophic scars, the application of laser therapy or corticosteroid injections may be a viable treatment option. For larger scar areas, such as post-burn scars or extensive self-injury scars, medical needling may be a promising treatment option, despite its invasiveness and the need for regional or general anaesthesia. Patients presenting with keloids usually undergo intralesional keloid excision and triamcinolone and antimetabolite injection. In our clinic, postoperative radiotherapy has been an integral step postoperatively to help minimize keloid recurrence.

In case of extensive functional deficits resulting from the scar tissue, we recommend scar excision and subsequent primary wound closure, when feasible. To reduce tension on the new scar, Z-plasties or skin grafts may need to be performed. Adhering to the principles of the reconstructive ladder, larger defects resulting from scar excisions will have to be addressed by local, regional or free flaps.

Naturally, patient education remains an integral part of the joint decision-making process throughout each step of the algorithm and all therapeutic measures should be based on a highly individualized approach to the patient's impairments and wishes. In clinical practice, the therapeutic endpoint is mostly based on patient satisfaction regarding scar improvement. Evidence-based therapeutic concepts should remain an integral part of the decision-making process as well as patient-dependent parameters.

**Author Contributions:** Conceptualization, K.D. and P.M.V.; Data curation, K.D., D.O., F.B., T.H. and K.I.K.; Formal analysis, K.D.; Investigation, K.D.; Methodology, K.D. and P.M.V.; Project administration, K.D. and P.M.V.; Resources, K.D.; Software, K.D.; Supervision, P.M.V.; Validation, K.D.; Visualization, K.D.; Writing—original draft, K.D. and D.O.; Writing—review & editing, K.D. and P.M.V. All authors have read and agreed to the published version of the manuscript.

**Funding:** This research received no external funding.

**Institutional Review Board Statement:** The study was conducted according to the guidelines of the Declaration of Helsinki. Not applicable due to the retrospective character of the study.

**Informed Consent Statement:** Informed consent was obtained from all subjects involved in the study. Written informed consent has been obtained from the patient(s) to publish this paper if applicable.

**Data Availability Statement:** The data presented in this study are available on request from the corresponding author.

**Conflicts of Interest:** The authors declare no conflict of interest.

## References

1. Sen, C.K. Human wound and its burden: Updated 2020 Compendium of Estimates. *Adv. Wound Care* **2021**, *10*, 281–292. [CrossRef] [PubMed]
2. De Lorenzi, F.; van der Hulst, R.; Boeckx, W. Free flaps in burn reconstruction. *Burns* **2001**, *27*, 603–612. [CrossRef]
3. Hogg, N.J.V. Primary and secondary management of pediatric soft tissue injuries. *Oral Maxillofac. Surg. Clin. N. Am.* **2012**, *24*, 365–375. [CrossRef] [PubMed]
4. Meaume, S.; Le Pillouer-Prost, A.; Richert, B.; Roseeuw, D.; Vadoud, J. Management of scars: Updated practical guidelines and use of silicones. *Eur. J. Dermatol.* **2014**, *24*, 435–443. [CrossRef] [PubMed]
5. Gold, M.H.; McGuire, M.; A Mustoe, T.; Pusic, A.; Sachdev, M.; Waibel, J.; Murcia, C. Updated international clinical recommendations on scar management: Part 2–algorithms for scar prevention and treatment. *Dermatol. Surg.* **2014**, *40*, 825–831. [PubMed]
6. Monstrey, S.; Middelkoop, E.; Vranckx, J.J.; Bassetto, F.; Ziegler, U.E.; Meaume, S.; Téot, L. Updated scar management practical guidelines: Non-invasive and invasive measures. *J. Plast. Reconstr. Aesthet. Surg.* **2014**, *67*, 1017–1025. [CrossRef] [PubMed]
7. Nast, A.; Eming, S.; Fluhr, J.; Fritz, K.; Gauglitz, G.; Hohenleutner, S.; Panizzon, R.G.; Sebastian, G.; Sporbeck, B.; Koller, J. German S2k guidelines for the therapy of pathological scars (hypertrophic scars and keloids). *J. Dtsch. Dermatol. Ges.* **2012**, *10*, 747–762. [CrossRef]
8. Tran, B.; Wu, J.J.; Ratner, D.; Han, G. Topical scar treatment products for wounds: A systematic review. *Dermatol. Surg.* **2020**, *46*, 1564–1571. [CrossRef] [PubMed]
9. Seago, M.; Shumaker, P.R.; Do, L.K.S.; Alam, M.; Al-Niaimi, F.; Anderson, R.R.; Artzi, O.; Bayat, A.; Cassuto, D.; Chan, H.H.L.; et al. Laser treatment of traumatic scars and contractures: 2020 international consensus recommendations. *Lasers Surg. Med.* **2020**, *52*, 96–116. [CrossRef] [PubMed]
10. Ward, R.E.; Sklar, L.R.; Eisen, D.B. Surgical and noninvasive modalities for scar revision. *Dermatol. Clin.* **2019**, *37*, 375–386. [CrossRef]

11. Cho, S.B.; Lee, S.J.; Oh, S.H.; Chung, W.S.; Kang, J.M.; Kim, Y.K.; Kim, D.H. Non-ablative 1550-nm erbium-glass and ablative 10 600-nm carbon dioxide fractional lasers for acne scars: A randomized split-face study with blinded response evaluation. *J. Eur. Acad. Dermatol. Venereol.* **2010**, *24*, 921–925. [CrossRef]
12. Blome-Eberwein, S.; Gogal, C.; Weiss, M.J.; Boorse, D.; Pagella, P. Prospective evaluation of fractional $CO_2$ laser treatment of mature burn scars. *J. Burn. Care Res.* **2016**, *37*, 379–387. [CrossRef]
13. Hochman, B.; Locali, R.F.; Matsuoka, P.K.; Ferreira, L.M. Intralesional Triamcinolone Acetonide for Keloid Treatment: A Systematic Review. *Aesthetic Plast. Surg.* **2008**, *32*, 705–709. [CrossRef]
14. Ud-Din, S.; Bowring, A.; Derbyshire, B.; Morris, J.; Bayat, A. Identification of steroid sensitive responders versus non-responders in the treatment of keloid disease. *Arch. Dermatol. Res.* **2013**, *305*, 423–432. [CrossRef]
15. Larrabee, W.F.; East, C.A.; Jaffe, H.S.; Stephenson, C.; Peterson, K.E. Intralesional interferon gamma treatment for keloids and hypertrophic scars. *Arch. Otolaryngol. Head Neck Surg.* **1990**, *116*, 1159–1162. [CrossRef]
16. Al-Attar, A.; Mess, S.; Thomassen, J.M.; Kauffman, C.L.; Davison, S.P. Keloid pathogenesis and treatment. *Plast. Reconstr. Surg.* **2006**, *117*, 286–300. [CrossRef]
17. Zhuang, Z.; Li, Y.; Wei, X. The safety and efficacy of intralesional triamcinolone acetonide for keloids and hypertrophic scars: A systematic review and meta-analysis. *Burns* **2021**, *47*, 987–998. [CrossRef]
18. Jiang, Z.-Y.; Liao, X.-C.; Liu, M.-Z.; Fu, Z.-H.; Min, D.-H.; Yu, X.-T.; Guo, G.-H. Efficacy and safety of intralesional triamcinolone versus combination of triamcinolone with 5-fluorouracil in the treatment of keloids and hypertrophic scars: A systematic review and meta-analysis. *Aesthetic Plast. Surg.* **2020**, *44*, 1859–1868. [CrossRef] [PubMed]
19. Demir, C.Y.; Ersoz, M.E.; Erten, R.; Kocak, O.F.; Sultanoglu, Y.; Basbugan, Y. Comparison of enalapril, candesartan and intralesional triamcinolone in reducing hypertrophic scar development: An experimental study. *Aesthetic Plast. Surg.* **2018**, *42*, 352–361. [CrossRef] [PubMed]
20. Riyat, H.; Touil, L.L.; Briggs, M.; Shokrollahi, K. Autologous fat grafting for scars, healing and pain: A review. *Scars Burn. Heal.* **2017**, *3*. [CrossRef] [PubMed]
21. Bassetto, F.; Scarpa, C.; Vindigni, V. Invasive techniques in scar management: Fat injections. In *Textbook on Scar Management*; Springer Nature: Berlin/Heidelberg, Germany, 2020; pp. 333–342.
22. Aust, M.C.; Fernandes, D.; Kolokythas, P.; Kaplan, H.M.; Vogt, P.M. Percutaneous collagen induction therapy: An alternative treatment for scars, wrinkles, and skin laxity. *Plast. Reconstr. Surg.* **2008**, *121*, 1421–1429. [CrossRef] [PubMed]
23. Busch, K.-H.; Aliu, A.; Walezko, N.; Aust, M. Medical needling: Effect on skin erythema of hypertrophic burn scars. *Cureus* **2018**, *10*, e3260. [CrossRef] [PubMed]
24. Aust, M.; Reimers, K.; Kaplan, H.; Stahl, F.; Repenning, C.; Scheper, T.; Jahn, S.; Schwaiger, N.; Ipaktchi, R.; Redeker, J.; et al. Percutaneous collagen induction–regeneration in place of cicatrisation? *J. Plast. Reconstr. Aesthetic Surg.* **2011**, *64*, 97–107. [CrossRef] [PubMed]
25. Hazani, R.; Whitney, R.; Wilhelmi, B.J. Article commentary: Optimizing aesthetic results in skin grafting. *Am. Surg.* **2012**, *78*, 151–154. [CrossRef]
26. Walden, J.L.; Garcia, H.; Hawkins, H.; Crouchet, J.R.; Traber, L.; Gore, D.C. Both dermal matrix and epidermis contribute to an inhibition of wound contraction. *Ann. Plast. Surg.* **2000**, *45*, 162–166. [CrossRef]
27. Tobin, G.R. The compromised bed technique. An improved method for skin grafting problem wounds. *Surg. Clin. N. Am.* **1984**, *64*, 653–658. [CrossRef]
28. Shahrokhi, S.; Arno, A.; Jeschke, M.G. The use of dermal substitutes in burn surgery: Acute phase. *Wound Repair Regen.* **2014**, *22*, 14–22. [CrossRef]
29. Pham, C.; Greenwood, J.; Cleland, H.; Woodruff, P.; Maddern, G. Bioengineered skin substitutes for the management of burns: A systematic review. *Burns* **2007**, *33*, 946–957. [CrossRef] [PubMed]
30. Cheshire, P.A.; Herson, M.R.; Cleland, H.; Akbarzadeh, S. Artificial dermal templates: A comparative study of NovoSorb™ Biodegradable Temporising Matrix (BTM) and Integra® Dermal Regeneration Template (DRT). *Burns* **2016**, *42*, 1088–1096. [CrossRef] [PubMed]
31. Li, A.; Dearman, B.L.; Crompton, K.E.; Moore, T.G.; Greenwood, J.E. Evaluation of a novel biodegradable polymer for the generation of a dermal matrix. *J. Burn Care Res.* **2009**, *30*, 717–728. [CrossRef]
32. Lo, C.H.; Brown, J.N.; Dantzer, E.J.; Maitz, P.K.; Vandervord, J.G.; Wagstaff, M.J.; Barker, T.M.; Cleland, H. Wound healing and dermal regeneration in severe burn patients treated with NovoSorb® Biodegradable Temporising Matrix: A prospective clinical study. *Burns* **2021**. [CrossRef] [PubMed]
33. Solanki, N.S.; York, B.; Gao, Y.; Baker, P.; Wong She, R.B. A consecutive case series of defects reconstructed using NovoSorb® Biodegradable Temporising Matrix: Initial experience and early results. *J. Plast. Reconstr. Aesthet. Surg.* **2020**, *73*, 1845–1853. [CrossRef] [PubMed]
34. Wagstaff, M.J.D.; Schmitt, B.J.; Coghlan, P.; Finkemeyer, J.P.; Caplash, Y.; Greenwood, J.E. A biodegradable polyurethane dermal matrix in reconstruction of free flap donor sites: A pilot study. *Eplasty* **2015**, *15*, e13.
35. Shockley, W.W. Scar revision techniques: Z-Plasty, W-Plasty, and geometric broken line closure. *Facial Plast. Surg. Clin. N. Am.* **2011**, *19*, 455–463. [CrossRef] [PubMed]
36. Vogt, P.M.; Alawi, S.A.; Ipaktchi, R. Free flaps in scar treatment. *Innov. Surg. Sci.* **2017**, *2*, 203–209. [CrossRef]

37. Staindl, O. Indications for free transplants for scar correction in the area of the head and neck. *Laryngol. Rhinol. Otol.* **1986**, *65*, 538–544. [CrossRef]
38. Robson, M.C.; Barnett, R.A.; Leitch, I.O.; Hayward, P.G. Prevention and treatment of postburn scars and contracture. *World J. Surg.* **1992**, *16*, 87–96. [CrossRef]
39. Grishkevich, V.M. Postburn shoulder medial-adduction contracture: Anatomy and treatment with trapeze-flap plasty. *Burns* **2013**, *39*, 341–348. [CrossRef]

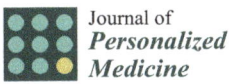 

*Review*

# Beyond the Knife—Reviewing the Interplay of Psychosocial Factors and Peripheral Nerve Lesions

Johannes C. Heinzel [1,\*], Lucy F. Dadun [1], Cosima Prahm [1], Natalie Winter [2], Michael Bressler [1], Henrik Lauer [1], Jana Ritter [1], Adrien Daigeler [1] and Jonas Kolbenschlag [1]

1 Department of Hand-, Plastic, Reconstructive and Burn Surgery, BG Klinik Tuebingen, University of Tuebingen, Schnarrenbergstraße 95, 72076 Tuebingen, Germany; lucy-felice.dadun@student.uni-tuebingen.de (L.F.D.); cprahm@bgu-tuebingen.de (C.P.); mbressler@bgu-tuebingen.de (M.B.); hlauer@bgu-tuebingen.de (H.L.); jana.ritter@comdesign24.de (J.R.); adaigeler@bgu-tuebingen.de (A.D.); jkolbenschlag@bgu-tuebingen.de (J.K.)
2 Department of Neurology, Hertie Institute for Clinical Brain Research (HIH), University of Tuebingen, Hoppe-Seyler-Str. 3, 72076 Tuebingen, Germany; natalie.winter@med.uni-tuebingen.de
\* Correspondence: jheinzel@bgu-tuebingen.de; Tel.: +49-7071-6061038

**Abstract:** Peripheral nerve injuries are a common clinical problem. They not only affect the physical capabilities of the injured person due to loss of motor or sensory function but also have a significant impact on psychosocial aspects of life. The aim of this work is to review the interplay of psychosocial factors and peripheral nerve lesions. By reviewing the published literature, we identified several factors to be heavily influenced by peripheral nerve lesions. In addition to psychological factors like pain, depression, catastrophizing and stress, social factors like employment status and worker's compensation status could be identified to be influenced by peripheral nerve lesions as well as serving as predictors of functional outcome themselves, respectively. This work sheds a light not only on the impact of peripheral nerve lesions on psychosocial aspects of life, but also on the prognostic values of these factors of functional outcome. Interdisciplinary, individualized treatment of patients is required to identify patient at risk for adverse outcomes and provide them with emotional support when adapting to their new life situation.

**Keywords:** peripheral nerve injury; psychosocial factor; nerve repair; neuroma; brachial plexus injury; compression neuropathy; pain; depression; disability; quality of life

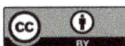

## 1. Introduction

Peripheral nerve injuries (PNIs) have annual incidence rates in the USA of 43.8/1,000,000 for PNIs of the upper extremities [1] and 13.3/1,000,000 of the lower extremities, respectively [2]. PNIs often have disastrous sequalae on the affected patients' qualities of life, especially in case of major nerve injuries and often required long and elaborate rehabilitation [3]. Therefore, surgical treatment options to restore sensibility and muscular function as well as to relieve pain are subject of a plethora of clinical and preclinical research efforts [4–8]. In addition to research efforts to deepen under understanding of the peripheral nervous systems anatomy, as well as the neurobiological and pathophysiological aspects of PNIs [9], novel treatment options and concepts are rapidly evolving in the wake of refined microsurgical techniques [10]. In addition to advances in neurobiological, anatomical and (micro)surgical aspects, the current body of knowledge regarding epidemiology of PNIs is also steadily evolving. About 25 years ago, Noble was one of the first to publish epidemiological data concerning PNI in patients with multiple injuries seen at a regional Level 1 trauma center [11] and in recent years, large multicenter studies have contributed to our knowledge and understanding of the epidemiology of lower and upper extremity PNIs [12,13]. Representative patients' characteristics and socioeconomic sequelae of PNIs have recently been described by Bergmeister and colleagues, approaching another important perspective of research regarding surgical treatment of peripheral nerve lesions. According to their observations in a study sample of 250 patients with 268 PNIs, acute in-patient treatment costs for upper extremity nerve damages ranged between 2650€ and 5000€ [14]. Although the overall incidence of PNI has decreased in recent year, treatment costs are steadily increasing [1,2].

The severity of PNIs and postoperative functional outcomes are usually assessed by quantitative biomedical measures and postoperative evaluations of strength, sensory function, and range of motion [15,16]. However, research shining a light on the psychosocial aspects of such injuries is yet sparse [17,18]. Psychosocial factors have been defined as "characteristics or facets that influence an individual psychologically and/or socially" by Thomas [19]. Their role has been extensively studied and reviewed in diseases and conditions such as extremity trauma [20,21] or isolated hand injuries [22–24]. It was also shown that negative emotions prior to surgery are associated with adverse pain outcomes and postoperative disability [25–29]. Besides psychological aspects, the social impact of upper extremity injuries, e.g., predictors of return to work in patients suffering from work-related injuries has been addressed before in regard to other trauma, e.g., hand lesions [30,31]. It has also been demonstrated that the ability to return to work after traumatic injury does not only depend on physical capability and health but also by other aspects including psychosocial factors like psychological distress, personal income, the educational level of the injured person or the presence of a strong social network [32–34]. There is yet no comprehensive review summarizing the interplay of psychosocial factors with peripheral nerve injury and functional outcome following surgical treatment of such lesions. Therefore, it is the aim of this work to compile the current body of knowledge to provide surgeons, hand therapists, occupational therapists and other disciplines involved in the treatment of peripheral nerve injuries with another perspective on psychosocial aspects of peripheral nerve injuries to enable an even more holistic treatment approach.

## 2. Methods

To gather eligible studies, a literature search on PubMed was performed using the search terms "peripheral nerve"; "peripheral nerve injuries"; "psychosocial "and "psychological". This yielded 95 results. After removal of duplicates, 90 papers remained for eligibility screening. Both original work and review papers were deemed fitting for discussion in this work. After removal of studies and reviews which addressed topics not related to our research questions and further reference screening of eligible work, 30 papers remained to be included in this review.

## 3. The Psychosocial Impact of Peripheral Nerve Lesions

Uvarov was among the first to publish his hypothesis that negative emotions are involved in the pathogenesis of peripheral nervous system disorders in Russian in the year 1971 [35]. However, the topic remained of little interest for the scientific community in the following years and decades. More than thirty years after Uvarov published his work, Jaquet et al. conducted a retrospective chart review of 107 patients with either median nerve injury, ulnar nerve injury, or combined injuries of both nerves. 94% of these patients experienced early psychological stress following nerve trauma. More than a third of the affected patients reported psychological symptoms of clinical depression. The authors found that combined nerve injuries had a significantly higher risk for early psychological stress following trauma when compared to isolated injuries of either the median or ulnar nerve. Severe psychological distress as assessed by means of the Impact of Event Scale (IES) was associated with more severe functional deficits, mean time off work and motor recovery. Additionally, patients with higher psychological stress had an Odds ratio of 3.32 for long-term incapacity for work. A higher education level was identified as a protective factor in regard to psychological distress following nerve injury [36]. Ultee's group reproduced these findings in a prospective study which evaluated early posttraumatic psychological stress in 61 patients with either isolated or combined injuries of the median and ulnar nerve.

The aforementioned authors found that >90% of patients experienced psychological stress one month postoperatively and about a fourth required psychological treatment based on their IES scores. Three months postoperatively, psychological stress was still reported by more than 83% of the patients, and around 13% qualified for psychological treatment. The authors identified a correlation of female gender, adult age, and combined nerve injuries with the occurrence of psychological stress symptoms 1 month postoperatively [37]. In regard to the impact of single or combined nerve injuries on the affected patients' work lives, Bruyns and colleagues analyzed potential predictors for return to work in 81 patients with median and/or ulnar nerve injuries in a retrospective study. Within a year after injury 59% of the patients returned to work after a mean time of work of 31 weeks. While 8 out of 10 patients with median nerve lesions were able to resume their work, this applied to less than 6 out of 10 and less than 3 out of 10 patients in the groups with ulnar nerve and combined nerve lesions, respectively. The ability to return to work (RTW) was significantly associated with the educational status of the participants and high rates of RTW were found in patients with white-collar employment, in comparison to those with blue-collar employment. Compliance to hand therapy was also found to result in odds ratio of 3.5 for RTW following nerve injury and repair [34]. Novak's group studied 158 patients who suffered from peripheral nerve injuries in the upper extremity and evaluated potential biomedical and psychosocial factors which correlated with disability. They found that patients who received worker's compensation, were involved in litigation or who were unemployed had significantly more severe disabilities of the affected extremity than their counterparts. These disabilities which were assessed by the Disabilities of Arm, Shoulder and Hand Questionnaire (DASH) score showed a significant correlation with the level of pain in these patients. In regard to potential predictors for post-injury disabilities, pain intensity, cold sensitivity, pain catastrophizing score, depression, employment status, worker's compensation and potential ongoing litigation were identified [18]. To summarize all aforementioned authors' findings, patients with combined median and ulnar nerve injuries are at higher risk for psychological stress and also not return to work as compared to patients with single site nerve lesions. Additionally, patients who report high levels of injury-related neuropathic pain, suffer from depression, are unemployed or have an ongoing lawsuit are also at higher risk for post-injury disability.

Besides the number of injured nerves, another point to consider in regard to the psychosocial impact is the severity of the respective lesion. In 2009, Bailey et al. aimed to evaluate the relationship between the degree of nerve damage in the upper extremity and psychosocial parameters such as activity participation, perceived quality of life (QoL), pain, and depression. Two individual groups were analyzed, one with compression neuropathies ($n = 25$), the other suffering from traumatic PNI of the upper extremity ($n = 24$). The authors observed that their study cohort of 49 individuals have given up about a fifth of their daily activities prior to their initial surgeon consultation and a significantly greater activity loss was observable in the group with traumatic PNI. Especially high-demand leisure activity such as physical exercise was reduced by almost 50% in the nerve injury group while social activities were reduced to 82%. In the group with compression neuropathies, leisure activities decreased by 30% and social activities were reduced to 87%, respectively. Pain intensity was reported as moderate among the studied patient sample with no significant differences between groups. The overall ratings for physical and psychological qualities of life were under average and almost 40% of the studied patients suffered from signs of depression secondary to the nerve damage. Interestingly, the cut-off for clinical depression was transgressed in the group with traumatic nerve injury only, but this difference was not statistically significant. Correlation analysis revealed a strong association between activity loss on the one hand and higher levels of depression as well lower perceived QoL on the other hand. Higher level of depression did also strongly correlate with lower perceived QoL. More severe pain was moderately associated with higher depression scores but only a weak correlation was found between the former and QoL. Interestingly, no correlation was observable between pain severity and physical QoL following peripheral nerve damage. In summary, more than 60% of the observed variance could be predicted by means of the two factors depression and activity participation, indicating that these two factors could be addressed as potential targets to improve the QoL in patients with upper extremity nerve damage, regardless of its genesis. However, it must be noted that the authors did not assess the manifestation of depression or other psychosocial factors prior to nerve damage, a potential confounder for the observed results [38]. Aiming to further differentiate the psychosocial impact of different types of nerve injuries, e.g., single site compression neuropathies from more complex pathologies like brachial plexus injuries and neuromas, Mackinnon's group performed a retrospective chart review of 490 patients presenting to their department between 2010 and 2012. The divided their patient sample into seven groups in accordance with their respective diagnosis: 1. Brachial plexus injuries; 2. Thoracic outlet syndrome (TOS); 3. single compression neuropathy; 4. dual compression neuropathy; 5. ulnar nerve lesions other than cubital tunnel syndrome; 6. compression mononeuropathy in the lower extremity and 7. neuroma. To distinguish between motor deficits due to compression of the common peroneal nerve and sensory disturbances caused by compressions of the cutaneus branches or the superficial or deep peroneal nerve, the sixth group was further subdivided. The authors reported a statistically significant difference regarding the pain-related decrease of QoL which was more severe in patients suffering from TOS, neuroma, or compression neuropathies of the superficial and deep branch of the peroneal nerve when compared to patients suffering from compression mononeuropathy in the upper extremity. Patients in the neuroma subgroup also reported significantly more stress at home as well as at work when compared to the patients with single compression mononeuropathies. Patients with dual compression neuropathies had reported higher stress levels and a decreased ability to cope with stress at work. Other factors which were identified as negative predictors for a significant decrease in QoL were female sex, smoking and anti-alcoholism. Female sex and anti-alcoholism were also associated with higher pain intensities. In regard to the reported stress-at-home, significantly higher levels were reported by female patients. Non-alcoholics had an increased risk for reduced coping abilities and higher stress-at-work levels [17]. Stonner, Mackinnon and Kaskutas conducted a retrospective cross-sectional study, including 627 patients with nerve disorders of the upper extremity. In the style of the aforementioned study conducted by Wojtkiewicz [17] patients were grouped based on the nerve disorder they were diagnosed with. The seven groups were categorized as follows: 1. lesions of the median nerve; 2. lesions of the ulnar nerve; 3. lesions of the radial nerve; 4. proximal lesions of either the axillary, long thoracic, suprascapular, or musculocutaneous nerve; 5. compression neuropathies of at least two different nerves; 6. TOS; 7. brachial plexus injuries. The authors found little difference in regard to post-injury work status when comparing the seven different groups with the exception of patients suffering from brachial plexus injuries. In this group only a fourth of the patients continued to work in their respective jobs on a daily basis and almost half of all patients did not work at all. More than ten percent of the entire study population of 627 received worker's compensation and more than half of these patients did not return to work. These participants reported significantly higher levels of depression and higher stress at home when compared to patients which did not receive worker's compensation and were not working. The latter group's proportion was also markedly smaller, comprising only 14% of the patients which did not receive worker's compensation. In regard to the overall disability following peripheral nerve lesions as assessed by the DASH score, the studied patients reported a significantly higher degree of disability in comparison to the general population. A quarter of all patients were unable to work as they wanted to. Both general disability as well as work-related disability were more severe in patient who were unemployed, received worker's compensation or reported depression ratings which were significantly higher than the general population's mean. While patients with brachial plexus lesions scored highest in the DASH, median nerve lesions were associated with lowest disability ratings. Both the mean mental and physical QoL were significantly lower in the participants when compared to the general population and lowest scores were observed in the patients with brachial plexus injuries. Poorer QoL ratings were associated with female sex, unemployment, worker's compensation status and above-mean depression ratings. Final stepwise linear regression analysis yielded ten variables which accounted for more than 60% of the observed variability in reported disability ratings. Among them were 7 psychosocial factors: 1. depression; 2. the level of pain; 3. momentary unemployment; 4. difficulties in sleeping; 5. affection of intimate relationships; 6. modified job demands and 7. stress at work. 46% of variance regarding work disability could be predicted by five variables: 1. affection of intimate relationships; 2. performance of household chores by others; 3. performance of a reduced amount of household chores; 4. difficulties with sleeping and 5. performance of the same level of household chores but with pain. Around 50% of physical QoL scores were predictable by: 1. DASH score; 2. the level of pain; 3. number of medications and 4. Work DASH scores. Slightly less than 50% of variability in mental QoL scores could be explained by: 1. the ability to cope with stress at home; 2. DASH score; 3. stress at home and 4. sleeping difficulties [39]. In accordance with the aforementioned authors' findings, Yannascoli et al. found significantly increased rates of coded depression and coded anxiety in their study sample of >1800 patients suffering from brachial plexus injury as compared to >18,000 healthy subjects. While 46% of the control patients had coded depression and/or anxiety, this rate was 54% in the group of patients suffering from brachial plexus injuries. Additionally, there were significantly increased incidences of new-onset postoperative depression (20%) and anxiety (12%) in the latter group when compared to the healthy controls [40]. Landers et al. reported that about one fifth of their study population of 21 patients with brachial plexus injuries met criteria for posttraumatic stress disorder (PTSD) and exhibited clinical depression, respectively. Most concerningly, about a third of the studied patients reported suicidal ideation [41]. In regard to the impact of injury severity in case of isolated hand injuries, Tezel's group found no correlation between psychological morbidities and injury severity and hand function, respectively in patients suffering from traumatic hand injury with major nerve involvement. The hand injury severity as assessed by the modified Hand Injury Severity Score (MHISS) correlated significantly with the patients' ability to return to work following hand trauma [42]. In conclusion, the reviewed studies indicate, that traumatic nerve injuries are more likely to have a strong psychosocial impact as compared to compression mononeuropathies. Notably, severe nerve lesions, especially brachial plexus injuries, have devastating consequences for the affected patients both in regard to employment status and work life as well as mental health [43].

In addition to upper extremity nerve lesions, the impact of PNI has also been studied in patients with lower extremity nerve damage, e.g., peroneal mononeuropathy. Aprile assessed QoL by means of the SF-36 in 69 patients with peroneal mononeuropathy and found significantly lower scores for the aspects of vitality, social function and is emotional role in their study sample as compared to healthy subjects. However, when stratification was performed to exclude patients with peroneal mononeuropathy which reported predisposing factors which were likely to affects QoL, no significant differences between the healthy sample and the sample with peroneal mononeuropathy were found [44].

### 4. Psychosocial Factors as Predictors of Functional Outcome Following Treatment of Peripheral Nerve Lesions

*4.1. Surgical Repair of Traumatic Nerve Injuries*

Hundepool et al. conducted a prospective multicenter study in 61 patients, aiming to identify prognostic factors for functional recovery in the first postoperative year following injuries of the median nerve ($n = 28$), ulnar nerve ($n = 27$) or combined lesions ($n = 6$) at forearm level. The majority of patients (85%) were blue-collar workers and the median educational score equaled a high-school degree. One year after injury, 84.6% of patients had returned to work. Besides the identification of the DASH score, power grip and sensibility of the hand as best prognostic factors, the aforementioned authors found gender, level of education as well as posttraumatic levels of stress at one- and three months post-injury as highly predictive in regard to functional recovery [45]. Building on the aforementioned authors' work, Goswami and colleagues evaluated ten patients with isolated or combined transection lesions of the median and ulnar nerve three weeks and approximately one year following surgical treatment of their injuries, aiming to identify potential predictors for the observed functional outcome. The patients completed the Brief Pain Inventory (BPI) Short Form, NEO Five Factor Inventory (NEO-FFI), and Pain Catastrophizing Scale (PCS) and the McGill Pain Questionnaire (MPQ) at both postoperative time points. Ten healthy individuals served as control group and were evaluated by means of the NEO and PCS. The authors found that pain-catastrophizing was correlated both with the reported pain intensity as well as the occurrence of neuropathic pain. The level of pain-catastrophizing at the first postoperative time-point served as predictor for cold pain thresholds twelve months postoperatively. The level of chronic pain reported at the second assessment time point was also related to the level of pain-catastrophizing as assessed by the PCS which in turn showed correlation with cold pain threshold at this time point [46]. Logically related to Goswami's research question, Mackinnon's group investigated the relationship between psychosocial factors and pain relief following peripheral nerve surgery. 331 patients who underwent surgery for peripheral nerve injuries or compression neuropathies and returned for at least two postoperative follow-ups were included. On the one hand, an increased impact of pain on QoL or reported anger, respectively were significant predictors of next-visit pain. On the other hand, self-reported hopefulness, sadness, and depression were not found to be predictive of next-visit pain. Patients who suffered from upper extremity PNI and refused to comment on a possible history of childhood trauma had a significant association with both same-visit pain and next-visit pain. The level of pain served a significant predictor of the reported impact of pain on QoL, sadness, depression, anger, and hopefulness during the next visit. Lower extremity nerve injury was predictive of anger during the next visit, whereas upper extremity nerve injury had no predictive value. Female sex served as a significant predictor for next-visit sadness and anger. Next-visit sadness and depression could be predicted in case the patient reported a positive history of childhood trauma, which was the case in 7.9% of study sample. While 89.3% of the patients denied childhood trauma, 2.8% refused to comment on this question [47]. In conclusion, the listed studies' results suggest that surgeons should be aware of the fact that functional recovery following repair of peripheral nerve lesions can be significantly influenced by the prevalence of postoperative stress and pain-catastrophizing. In regard to the psychosocial Sadness and depression, although not predictive of functional outcome in the limited number of studies investigating this relationship, are more likely in patients suffering from PNI and have a positive or suspected positive history of childhood trauma.

### 4.2. Surgical Treatment of Compression Neuropathies

Besides cases of traumatic nerve injuries, patients suffering from compression neuropathies also frequently require surgical treatment. In consequence, predictors of functional outcomes following peripheral nerve decompression have been studies by several groups. A retrospective study aiming to identify outcomes of care and predictors of disability and health status in adults with peripheral nerve injuries included >360 patients with PNI which underwent surgical treatment. Included patients presented with 1. median nerve compression; 2. ulnar neuropathy; 3. mixed median and ulnar nerve compression; 4. radial nerve palsy; 5. thoracic outlet syndrome or 6. brachial plexus injury. About 80% of the patients were treated operatively and 70% of these underwent nerve release while the remaining 20% received conservative treatment. The authors found that while health status changed minimally, significant improvements in disability, work disability, pain, depression, and stress were observable following any treatment. At discharge, 57% of employed patients had resumed their work. No significant differences were observable between patients who were treated surgically or those who underwent conservative therapy. Disability was most significantly increased in patients with brachial plexus injuries. More favorable outcomes were observable in patients who pursued gainful employment and had reported symptoms less than six months prior to treatment. Post-treatment functional outcomes could be predicted by psychosocial factors like work status, household management, pain, depression, stress, and difficulty sleeping [48]. In addition to Stonner's comprehensive analysis of patients with different compression neuropathies, other authors have evaluated cohorts of patients suffering from one distinctive nerve compression syndrome alone with the results summarized in the following paragraphs.

4.2.1. Peroneal Nerve Decompression

In 2019, Wilson et al. published the results of a retrospective study aiming to identify potential predictors of functional outcome following peroneal nerve decompression at the level of the fibular head. The working status of the included patients was also evaluated in regard to a possible correlation with functional outcome. However, no statistically significant correlation could be identified [49].

4.2.2. Ulnar Nerve Decompression

Gaspar's group aimed to evaluate predictors for revision surgery both following in situ ulnar nerve decompression [50] as well as medial epicondylectomy [51] in patients with cubital tunnel syndrome. While revision surgery following in situ decompression of the ulnar nerve was required in 3.2% of the analyzed 216 cases, patient age < 50 years was the only significant predictor of revision surgery. Neither gender nor workers 'compensation status had any predictive significance. In regard to patients who underwent medial epicondylectomy, 13.3% of the 82 cases required revision surgery. In accordance with the aforementioned study, younger age was identified as predictive factor. Workers' compensation claims, lesser disease severity, and preoperative opioid use were identified as additional significant predictors.

4.2.3. Treatment of Carpal Tunnel Syndrome

In 2017, Jerosch-Herold and colleagues published the results of large multicenter study aiming to identify prognostics factors for functional outcome and resulting costs for carpal tunnel syndrome either treated by surgical decompression or corticosteroid injection. They found a highly significant correlation between the patient-reported carpal tunnel symptom severity, depression, anxiety and the health-related QoL as assessed by the EQ-5D-3L (3-level version of EuroQol-5 dimension). The level of anxiety was also correlated with the objective carpal tunnel syndrome severity as assessed by electrophysiological evaluations, but there was no correlation of electrophysiological findings and depression [52]. Straub's group evaluated 100 hands of 67 patients, respectively, who underwent endoscopic carpal tunnel release, aiming to identify patient- and psychosocial factors associated with unsatisfactory outcomes. Out of the 8% percent of hands which were classified as unsatisfactory 75% were covered by the worker's compensatory system and in 21% of cases which were involved in litigation an unsatisfactory result was reported. Interestingly, the author concluded that various comorbid factors which were assessed, e.g., obesity, smoking or working in a job at risk did neither in isolation nor in combination result in an increased likelihood for unsatisfactory results. However, psychological factors, e.g., use of psychotropic medications or active psychiatric treatment, which were found positive in 20% of the study population, were associated with lower patient satisfaction both in isolation and combination [53]. In 2008, Lozano Calderón and colleagues conducted a retrospective survey to evaluate patient satisfaction following open carpal tunnel release and included 82 participants. They found that greater levels of depression were associated with more severe dissatisfaction following surgery and perceived disability could be predicted by depression and pain catastrophizing. The authors concluded that depression and perceived disability after carpal tunnel release can be predicted primarily by psychosocial factors like depression and insufficient coping skills [54]. Das De et al. found a significant correlation between DASH scores of patients suffering from carpal tunnel syndrome and psychosocial factors such as depression, catastrophic thinking, kinesiophobia and a punishing response by the respective patient's partner. Conversely, pain anxiety as well as solicitous or distracting responses by the respective patient's partner did not correlate with disabilities of the upper extremity in patients with carpal tunnel syndrome [55]. To summarize, these studies indicate that disease severity in patients with carpal tunnel syndrome is often directly linked to psychosocial aspects of life on the one hand whereas patients suffering from depression or anxiety are likely to experience adverse functional outcomes following carpal tunnel release.

### 4.3. Recovery of Donor Site Morbidity following Nerve Harvest

Ehretsman and colleagues evaluated subjective healing of nerve donor site morbidity following nerve graft harvest by means of a telephone survey. The authors evaluated possible correlations between satisfaction with donor site morbidity, both in regard to functional and cosmetic factors, and patient factors such as age, gender, involvement of worker's compensation and/or ongoing litigation. However, no statistically significant correlation with patient factors was observable [56]. Another study conducted by Miloro's group assessed patient satisfaction following sural nerve harvesting in 47 patients. In accordance with Ehretsman's results these authors did not observe any correlation between patient factor like age, gender and legal involvement and satisfaction level in regard to the donor site [57].

### 4.4. Treatment of Painful Neuroma

Stokvis et al. conducted a literature review aiming to identify possible prognostics factors for insufficient pain relief following neuroma treatment in 2009 [58]. They extracted ongoing worker's compensation, employment status and active litigation as predictive factors for unsuccessful treatment attempts. However, the authors stated that these factors are very difficult to consider separately, given the fact that employment status is likely more important regarding the outcome of patients undergoing surgery for painful neuroma [59,60]. Stovkis' group also emphasized Dellon's and Mackinnon's observation, that the duration of preoperative pain was significantly longer in patients who reported poor pain relief following surgery when compared to patients with satisfactory postoperative amelioration of pain [58,60]. In 2019, Lans and colleagues retrospectively analyzed 33 painful neuromas in 29 patients who underwent surgical therapy. Comparing the three treatment concepts of 1. neuroma excision with consecutive nerve repair or reconstruction; 2. neuroma excision with implantation of the proximal stump and 3. neuroma excision alone. In their study population the mean PROMIS Upper Extremity score was $45.2 \pm 11.2$, the mean PROMIS Pain Interference score was $54.3 \pm 10.7$, and the median numeric rating scale pain score was 3 (interquartile range, 1 to 5). Higher PROMIS depression scores and the surgical concept of neuroma excision alone were both independently significantly correlated with lower PROMIS Upper Extremity scores. Postoperative PROMIS Upper Extremity scores were lower in patients who underwent neuroma excision with nerve stump implantation, but this was not statistically significant. Neuroma excision alone and neuroma excision with nerve stump implantation as well as higher PROMIS Depression scores were all independently associated with higher, e.g., more severe PROMIS Pain Interference scores. Higher numeric rating scale pain scores showed a significant correlation with neuroma excision alone and neuroma excision and implantation whereas neuroma excision with consecutive nerve repair or reconstruction was associated with lower numeric rating scale pain scores [61].

## 5. A Perspective on Experimental Insights

In addition to clinical studies, psychosocial aspects of peripheral nerve injuries have also been studied in preclinical models, e.g., rodents. Using a spared nerve injury (SNI) model Norman et al. tested the hypotheses that peripheral nerve injury is causative for depression by induction of inflammatory processes in the brain and these neuroinflammatory changes are further exacerbated in case of stress exposure prior to nerve injury. The authors found their presumptions to be confirmed as they observed that injury of the common peroneal and tibial nerve caused mechanical allodynia and depressive behavior in mice, as well as an increased expression of interleukin-1b (IL-1b) and glial fibrillary acidic protein (GFAP). The mechanical allodynia was more severe in mice which were exposed to increased stress by chronic physical constraint two weeks prior to the experimental surgery. Treatment of these animals with a corticosteroid synthesis inhibitor prior to physical constraint eliminated the aforementioned effects, proving that psychosocial factors, e.g., the experience of increased stress directly influences the severity of symptoms following peripheral nerve injury [62].

Besides individual psychological factors like depression, social factors have also been identified to play an important role in symptom severity in rats with peripheral nerve injury. Raber and Devor used a neuroma model of neuropathic pain caused by sciatic nerve injury to investigate pain phenotype in two distinct rat strains. When rats with high (HA) and low (LA) pain phenotype and autotomy-behavior, e.g., gnawing of the toes or entire paws in consequence to nerve injury, were housed together, LA rats showed high levels of autotomy even when they were familiar with the HA preoperatively. The observed autotomy in LA rats was also independent of the performance of autotomy by the HA rats. Interestingly, even the contact with cage bedding soiled by HA rats was sufficient to induce moderate levels of autotomy in LA rats even in the absence of HA rats [63]. Another study investigated the effects of ongoing social stress (OSS) on mechanical sensitivity and cold allodynia in a rat model of chronic constriction injury (CCI) of the sciatic nerve. Rats which experienced ongoing social stress by twice-weekly exchange of their cage mates did not display significant changes in mechanical sensitivity. In regard to cold allodynia, rats with CCI and OSS were less susceptible during the early phase of the observation period when compared to rats which underwent CCI surgery only. At later time points however, rats with CCI + OSS were more susceptible to cold stimuli compared to the CCI rats. In addition, in the former group enhanced glial cell activation, pro-inflammatory cytokine expression and higher neurotrophic factor mRNA levels were observable [64].

## 6. Discussion

In this work we reviewed the current body of knowledge in regard to the interplay of psychosocial factors and peripheral nerve lesions as well as these factors' predictive value of functional outcome following peripheral nerve injury. Our work emphasizes that psychological factors like depression, pain-catastrophizing and anxiety are both influenced by peripheral nerve lesions and also significant predictors of functional recovery and QoL after peripheral nerve surgery in patients suffering from PNI. The same applies to social factors, e.g., employment status or worker's compensation. These findings underpin the need for personalized treatment concepts involving not only surgeons but also psychologists, occupational therapists, and others. As was pointed out by Kaltenbrunner and other authors [65,66] there are large differences between countries in regard to the regulatory framework of disability cases and rehabilitation measures to facilitate the affected individuals return to work. Notably, this not only applies to the transatlantic comparison, but also within the smaller perimeter of the European Union, indicating the need to consider the country-dependent differences when developing treatment and rehabilitation concepts for patients with PNIs.

Patients with depression, pain catastrophizing and anxiety are usually at risk to experience poor outcomes following PNI, reporting higher levels of pain and disability as well as lower satisfaction [54]. Vice versa, the rate of symptoms of clinical depression among patients suffering from PNI is alarmingly high, reaching almost 40%, which is more than twice the numbers reported in the general population, ranging between 10% and 20%, depending on the studied population [38,67,68]. In case of brachial plexus injuries, even more than 50% of patients could be suffering from depression, underpinning the need for adequate treatment strategies beyond surgical intervention in this group of patients [69,70]. In conclusion, screening for depression and referral of patients for psychological and/or psychiatric counseling or treatment is advised for surgeons and any other profession involved in the treatment of patients with PNIs, especially in case of a planned operative intervention [38]. However, it might be demanding to identify such patients since they might show a tendency to conceal their depression, afraid of the social stigma which might come with diagnosed mental illness [17,71]. Circling back to the aforementioned cross-country differences regarding post-injury rehabilitation and return to work, the same applies to mental health care systems. Again, significant differences are not only observable when comparing mental health care systems worldwide [72] but also within the European Union [73]. These observations emphasize that the interplay of psychosocial factors and peripheral nerve lesions extends beyond the affected patients' ways of living but are also heavily influenced by significant differences between countries regarding their health care system.

In our opinion, the findings reported by Ehretsman [56] and Miloro [57] deserve special emphasis, as both authors reported that donor site morbidity following nerve harvest was not correlated with any of the psychosocial factors they assessed. Although nerve graft harvesting can be considered as nerve lesion, it is interesting to note that sequalae of these "non-accidental" nerve injuries seem not to be correlated with psychosocial factors as it is the case with traumatic nerve lesions or compression neuropathies. As possible explanation for this observation we would like to suggest that patients who undergo nerve graft harvest choose this procedure voluntarily and without the experience of a "loss of control" associated with traumatic nerve injuries. It was shown that the feelings of uncontrollability or helplessness are associated with an increase in psychological vulnerabilities [74–76] and pain levels [77,78]. The patient's impression of being in control of the situation leading to a nerve lesion, e.g., sural nerve harvest, might be protective of adverse functional outcome following these procedures.

Another interesting finding was the correlation between picking "no comment" when asked about a possible childhood trauma and pain reported at the current and next visit. The same applies to the predictive value of a positive history childhood trauma for next-visit sadness and depression. It has been suggested that this correlation is caused by trauma-induced changes to the brain of abused or traumatized children [47,79,80]. In this context, one should consider the fact that about 10% of American youth have experienced at least one episode of sexual assault and 9–19% were subject to physical abuse or a physical assault by the respective caregiver [81]. Although a history of childhood trauma does not necessarily cause pain, sadness and depression, the likelihood of seeing an abused person with PNI at the inpatient or outpatient clinic is relatively high.

As several studies reviewed in this work have pointed out there are distinct variations regarding the impact of PNIs on psychosocial factors depending on their severity. Patients with distal, single-site compression neuropathies will likely experience fewer negative psychosocial effects that patients with distal traumatic injuries of both the median and ulnar nerve, dual compression neuropathies or TOS. As was emphasized by Wojtkiewicz these findings bear several implications for clinical practice, as patients suffering from the aforementioned conditions should be counseled regarding the impact of such PNIs on their psychosocial and occupational status prior to surgical treatment [17]. The ability to return to work (RTW) is another exemplary psychosocial factor, as it is primarily affected by PNI but also has an impact on functional recovery in patients with PNI. Knowledge of this interplay is of high value when an individual treatment and rehabilitation plan is conceptualized for the patient as patients with more complex injuries, e.g., combined nerve injuries of the upper extremity are at high risk not to return to work. In consequence functional recovery in these patients might also be poor, given their inability to pursue their profession as desired [34]. Considering the exorbitant indirect costs of low productivity which exceed direct health costs by more than 100% in case of upper extremity PNIs [14,82–84] an adequate prognostic assessment and a personalized interdisciplinary treatment are of outmost relevance. A battery of structured preoperative assessment tools such as the PROMIS-29 and EQ-5D [85] are suited to determine the impact of peripheral nerve injuries on patient-reported QoL. The healthcare team involved in treatment of patients with

PNI should consist of expert not only in surgical treatment of nerve injuries, but also specialist for physical as well as emotional adaptation and resilience, e.g., hand therapists, occupational therapists, psychologist, and social workers [86].

Wojtkiewicz summarized the evidence gathered in the literature regarding the influence of pain caused by PNIs on patient-reported disability [17,18,38,87–90]. Pain levels can be assessed by the BPI Short Form, NEO-FFI, PCS and the MPQ. A more personalized pain-assessment is possible via pain drawings [91]. It was shown that these drawings are affected by pain and depression in patients with cervical degenerative disc disease [92] or cervical spine nerve involvement in chronic whiplash-associated disorders [93]. They are also a feasible and reliable tool to assess neuropathic pain following spinal cord injury [94]. Pain drawings are also predictive of functional outcome in patients undergoing surgical treatment for degenerative disc disease in the cervical spine [95]. Use of a related assessment-tool named CALA to visualize pain in upper limbs amputees has been published by Prahm et al. [96], but there is yet no published large patient sample study evaluating the value of pain drawings in patient with peripheral nerve lesions in general. Given the high prevalence of neuropathic pain of up to 10% in society and its deleterious impact on physical and psychical function [47], a more personalized assessment tool might be a valuable addition to the armamentarium of diagnostic and prognostic instruments.

To summarize our findings, coaching, and providing emotional support to patients suffering from PNI can be effective to help them adapting a positive mindset, overcome severe psychological distress, and eventually adapting to their new situation, even if the functional outcome following surgical treatment is not more than mediocre. It must be emphasized that objective impairment, e.g., severe paresis, or diminished sensibility does not inevitably result in the same level of subjective disability. This observation has been beautifully condensed by Ring who had reconstructed the median nerve in a female nurse following complete iatrogenic laceration: "Credit goes to her (the patient's) spirit, adaptation and resiliency; not my knife or suture" [86].

## 7. Conclusions

Psychosocial factors play an important role in case of PNI. They are not only directly affected by PNI but also have significant predictive value of functional outcome following surgical treatment. Careful psychological assessment can help to identify patients at risk for unsatisfactory functional recovery and persistent disability following surgical treatment. The interplay of psychosocial factors and PNIs should be kept in mind in regard to personalized treatment concepts for these patients.

**Author Contributions:** Conceptualization, J.C.H., C.P., J.K. and A.D.; methodology and literature research, J.C.H., L.F.D. and J.R.; writing—original draft preparation, J.C.H., L.F.D., N.W., M.B. and J.R.; writing—review and editing, H.L., C.P., J.K. and A.D.; supervision, J.K. and A.D. All authors have read and agreed to the published version of the manuscript.

**Funding:** This research received no external funding.

**Acknowledgments:** We acknowledge support by Open Access Publishing Fund of University of Tübingen.

**Conflicts of Interest:** The authors declare no conflict of interest.

## References

1. Karsy, M.; Watkins, R.; Jensen, M.R.; Guan, J.; Brock, A.A.; Mahan, M.A. Trends and Cost Analysis of Upper Extremity Nerve Injury Using the National (Nationwide) Inpatient Sample. *World Neurosurg.* **2019**, *123*, e488–e500. [CrossRef] [PubMed]
2. Foster, C.H.; Karsy, M.; Jensen, M.R.; Guan, J.; Eli, I.; Mahan, M.A. Trends and Cost-Analysis of Lower Extremity Nerve Injury Using the National Inpatient Sample. *Neurosurgery* **2019**, *85*, 250–256. [CrossRef] [PubMed]
3. Robinson, M.D.; Shannon, S. Rehabilitation of peripheral nerve injuries. *Phys. Med. Rehabil. Clin.* **2002**, *13*, 109–135. [CrossRef]
4. Carvalho, C.R.; Oliveira, J.M.; Reis, R.L. Modern Trends for Peripheral Nerve Repair and Regeneration: Beyond the Hollow Nerve Guidance Conduit. *Front. Bioeng. Biotechnol.* **2019**, *7*, 337. [CrossRef] [PubMed]

5. Raza, C.; Riaz, H.A.; Anjum, R.; Shakeel, N.U.A. Repair strategies for injured peripheral nerve: Review. *Life Sci.* **2020**, *243*, 117308. [CrossRef]
6. Vela, F.J.; Martinez-Chacon, G.; Ballestin, A.; Campos, J.L.; Sanchez-Margallo, F.M.; Abellan, E. Animal models used to study direct peripheral nerve repair: A systematic review. *Neural Regen. Res.* **2020**, *15*, 491–502. [CrossRef] [PubMed]
7. Haastert-Talini, K. Appropriate Animal Models for Translational Nerve Research. In *Peripheral Nerve Tissue Engineering and Regeneration*; Phillips, J., Hercher, D., Hausner, T., Eds.; Springer International Publishing: Cham, Switzerland, 2020; pp. 1–17. [CrossRef]
8. Mohanty, C.B.; Bhat, D.I.; Devi, B.I. Use of animal models in peripheral nerve surgery and research. *Neurol India* **2019**, *67*, S100–S105. [CrossRef] [PubMed]
9. Saffari, S.; Saffari, T.M.; Moore, A.M.; Shin, A.Y. Peripheral Nerve Basic Science Research-What Is Important for Hand Surgeons to Know? *J. Hand Surg.* **2021**, *46*, 608–618. [CrossRef]
10. Pan, D.; Mackinnon, S.E.; Wood, M.D. Advances in the repair of segmental nerve injuries and trends in reconstruction. *Muscle Nerve* **2020**, *61*, 726–739. [CrossRef] [PubMed]
11. Noble, J.; Munro, C.A.; Prasad, V.S.; Midha, R. Analysis of upper and lower extremity peripheral nerve injuries in a population of patients with multiple injuries. *J. Trauma Acute Care Surg.* **1998**, *45*, 116–122. [CrossRef]
12. Huckhagel, T.; Nuchtern, J.; Regelsberger, J.; Lefering, R.; TraumaRegister, D.G.U. Nerve injury in severe trauma with upper extremity involvement: Evaluation of 49,382 patients from the TraumaRegister DGU(R) between 2002 and 2015. *Scand. J. Trauma Resusc. Emerg. Med.* **2018**, *26*, 76. [CrossRef]
13. Huckhagel, T.; Nüchtern, J.; Regelsberger, J.; Gelderblom, M.; Lefering, R.; TraumaRegister, D. Nerve trauma of the lower extremity: Evaluation of 60,422 leg injured patients from the TraumaRegister DGU® between 2002 and 2015. *Scand. J. Trauma Resusc. Emerg. Med.* **2018**, *26*, 40. [CrossRef] [PubMed]
14. Bergmeister, K.D.; Große-Hartlage, L.; Daeschler, S.C.; Rhodius, P.; Böcker, A.; Beyersdorff, M.; Kern, A.O.; Kneser, U.; Harhaus, L. Acute and long-term costs of 268 peripheral nerve injuries in the upper extremity. *PLoS ONE* **2020**, *15*, e0229530. [CrossRef] [PubMed]
15. Rayner, M.L.D.; Brown, H.L.; Wilcox, M.; Phillips, J.B.; Quick, T.J. Quantifying regeneration in patients following peripheral nerve injury. *J. Plast. Reconstr. Aesthetic Surg.* **2020**, *73*, 201–208. [CrossRef] [PubMed]
16. Wilcox, M.; Brown, H.; Quick, T. Clinical Outcome Measures Following Peripheral Nerve Repair. In *Peripheral Nerve Tissue Engineering and Regeneration*; Phillips, J., Hercher, D., Hausner, T., Eds.; Springer International Publishing: Cham, Switzerland, 2020; pp. 1–46. [CrossRef]
17. Wojtkiewicz, D.M.; Saunders, J.; Domeshek, L.; Novak, C.B.; Kaskutas, V.; Mackinnon, S.E. Social impact of peripheral nerve injuries. *Hand* **2015**, *10*, 161–167. [CrossRef]
18. Novak, C.B.; Anastakis, D.J.; Beaton, D.E.; Mackinnon, S.E.; Katz, J. Biomedical and psychosocial factors associated with disability after peripheral nerve injury. *J. Bone Joint Surg.* **2011**, *93*, 929–936. [CrossRef] [PubMed]
19. Thomas, K.; Nilsson, E.; Festin, K.; Henriksson, P.; Lowen, M.; Lof, M.; Kristenson, M. Associations of Psychosocial Factors with Multiple Health Behaviors: A Population-Based Study of Middle-Aged Men and Women. *Int. J. Environ. Res. Public Health* **2020**, *17*, 1239. [CrossRef] [PubMed]
20. Archer, K.R.; Abraham, C.M.; Obremskey, W.T. Psychosocial Factors Predict Pain and Physical Health After Lower Extremity Trauma. *Clin. Orthop. Relat. Res.* **2015**, *473*, 3519–3526. [CrossRef] [PubMed]
21. Jayakumar, P.; Overbeek, C.L.; Lamb, S.; Williams, M.; Funes, C.J.; Gwilym, S.; Ring, D.; Vranceanu, A.M. What Factors Are Associated with Disability after Upper Extremity Injuries? A Systematic Review. *Clin. Orthop. Relat. Res.* **2018**, *476*, 2190–2215. [CrossRef]
22. Bongers, P.M.; Kremer, A.M.; ter Laak, J. Are psychosocial factors, risk factors for symptoms and signs of the shoulder, elbow, or hand/wrist?: A review of the epidemiological literature. *Am. J. Ind. Med.* **2002**, *41*, 315–342. [CrossRef] [PubMed]
23. Gustafsson, M.; Ahlström, G. Emotional distress and coping in the early stage of recovery following acute traumatic hand injury: A questionnaire survey. *Int. J. Nurs. Stud.* **2006**, *43*, 557–565. [CrossRef]
24. Gustafsson, M.; Persson, L.O.; Amilon, A. A qualitative study of stress factors in the early stage of acute traumatic hand injury. *J. Adv. Nurs.* **2000**, *32*, 1333–1340. [CrossRef] [PubMed]
25. Busse, J.W.; Heels-Ansdell, D.; Makosso-Kallyth, S.; Petrisor, B.; Jeray, K.; Tufescu, T.; Laflamme, Y.; McKay, P.; McCabe, R.E.; Le Manach, Y.; et al. Patient coping and expectations predict recovery after major orthopaedic trauma. *Br. J. Anaesth.* **2019**, *122*, 51–59. [CrossRef]
26. Marek, R.J.; Lieberman, I.; Derman, P.; Nghiem, D.M.; Block, A.R. Validity of a pre-surgical algorithm to predict pain, functional disability, and emotional functioning 1 year after spine surgery. *Psychol. Assess.* **2021**, *33*, 541–551. [CrossRef] [PubMed]
27. Qi, A.; Lin, C.; Zhou, A.; Du, J.; Jia, X.; Sun, L.; Zhang, G.; Zhang, L.; Liu, M. Negative emotions affect postoperative scores for evaluating functional knee recovery and quality of life after total knee replacement. *Braz. J. Med. Biol. Res.* **2016**, *49*, e4616. [CrossRef] [PubMed]
28. Davis, G.; Curtin, C.M. Management of Pain in Complex Nerve Injuries. *Hand Clin.* **2016**, *32*, 257–262. [CrossRef] [PubMed]
29. Schaefer, C.; Sadosky, A.; Mann, R.; Daniel, S.; Parsons, B.; Tuchman, M.; Anschel, A.; Stacey, B.R.; Nalamachu, S.; Nieshoff, E. Pain severity and the economic burden of neuropathic pain in the United States: BEAT Neuropathic Pain Observational Study. *Clin. Outcomes Res.* **2014**, *6*, 483–496.

30. Akbarzadeh Khorshidi, H.; Marembo, M.; Aickelin, U. Predictors of Return to Work for Occupational Rehabilitation Users in Work-Related Injury Insurance Claims: Insights from Mental Health. *J. Occup. Rehabil.* **2019**, *29*, 740–753. [CrossRef] [PubMed]
31. Ash, P.; Goldstein, S.I. Predictors of returning to work. *J. Am. Acad. Psychiatry Law* **1995**, *23*, 205–210.
32. MacKenzie, E.J.; Shapiro, S.; Smith, R.T.; Siegel, J.H.; Moody, M.; Pitt, A. Factors influencing return to work following hospitalization for traumatic injury. *Am. J. Public Health* **1987**, *77*, 329–334. [CrossRef]
33. Crook, J.; Moldofsky, H.; Shannon, H. Determinants of disability after a work related musculetal injury. *J. Rheumatol.* **1998**, *25*, 1570–1577. [PubMed]
34. Bruyns, C.N.; Jaquet, J.B.; Schreuders, T.A.; Kalmijn, S.; Kuypers, P.D.; Hovius, S.E. Predictors for return to work in patients with median and ulnar nerve injuries. *J. Hand Surg.* **2003**, *28*, 28–34. [CrossRef] [PubMed]
35. Uvarov, M.G. Negative emotions in the pathogenesis of peripheral nerve system disorders. *Voenno-meditsinskii zhurnal* **1971**, *8*, 78–79. [PubMed]
36. Jaquet, J.B.; Kalmijn, S.; Kuypers, P.D.; Hofman, A.; Passchier, J.; Hovius, S.E. Early psychological stress after forearm nerve injuries: A predictor for long-term functional outcome and return to productivity. *Ann. Plast. Surg.* **2002**, *49*, 82–90. [CrossRef]
37. Ultee, J.; Hundepool, C.A.; Nijhuis, T.H.; van Baar, A.L.; Hovius, S.E. Early posttraumatic psychological stress following peripheral nerve injury: A prospective study. *J. Plast. Reconstr. Aesthetic Surg.* **2013**, *66*, 1316–1321. [CrossRef] [PubMed]
38. Bailey, R.; Kaskutas, V.; Fox, I.; Baum, C.M.; Mackinnon, S.E. Effect of upper extremity nerve damage on activity participation, pain, depression, and quality of life. *J. Hand Surg.* **2009**, *34*, 1682–1688. [CrossRef] [PubMed]
39. Stonner, M.M.; Mackinnon, S.E.; Kaskutas, V. Predictors of Disability and Quality of Life With an Upper-Extremity Peripheral Nerve Disorder. *Am. J. Occup. Ther.* **2017**, *71*, 7101190050p1–7101190050p8. [CrossRef]
40. Yannascoli, S.M.; Stwalley, D.; Saeed, M.J.; Olsen, M.A.; Dy, C.J. A Population-Based Assessment of Depression and Anxiety in Patients With Brachial Plexus Injuries. *J. Hand Surg.* **2018**, *43*, 1136.e1–1136.e9. [CrossRef]
41. Landers, Z.A.; Jethanandani, R.; Lee, S.K.; Mancuso, C.A.; Seehaus, M.; Wolfe, S.W. The Psychological Impact of Adult Traumatic Brachial Plexus Injury. *J. Hand Surg.* **2018**, *43*, 950.e1–950.e6. [CrossRef] [PubMed]
42. Tezel, N.; Can, A. The association between injury severity and psychological morbidity, hand function, and return to work in traumatic hand injury with major nerve involvement: A one-year follow-up study. *Turk. J. Trauma Emerg. Surg.* **2020**, *26*, 905–910. [CrossRef] [PubMed]
43. Hill, J.R.; Lanier, S.T.; Brogan, D.M.; Dy, C.J. Management of Adult Brachial Plexus Injuries. *J Hand Surg Am* **2021**, *46*, 778–788. [CrossRef]
44. Aprile, I.; Caliandro, P.; La Torre, G.; Tonali, P.; Foschini, M.; Mondelli, M.; Bertolini, C.; Piazzini, D.B.; Padua, L. Multicenter study of peroneal mononeuropathy: Clinical, neurophysiologic, and quality of life assessment. *J. Peripher. Nerv. Syst.* **2005**, *10*, 259–268. [CrossRef] [PubMed]
45. Hundepool, C.A.; Ultee, J.; Nijhuis, T.H.; Houpt, P.; Hovius, S.E. Prognostic factors for outcome after median, ulnar, and combined median-ulnar nerve injuries: A prospective study. *J. Plast. Reconstr. Aesthetic Surg.* **2015**, *68*, 1–8. [CrossRef]
46. Goswami, R.; Anastakis, D.J.; Katz, J.; Davis, K.D. A longitudinal study of pain, personality, and brain plasticity following peripheral nerve injury. *Pain* **2016**, *157*, 729–739. [CrossRef] [PubMed]
47. Heary, K.O.; Wong, A.W.K.; Lau, S.C.L.; Dengler, J.; Thompson, M.R.; Crock, L.W.; Novak, C.B.; Philip, B.A.; Mackinnon, S.E. Quality of Life and Psychosocial Factors as Predictors of Pain Relief Following Nerve Surgery. *Hand* **2020**. [CrossRef] [PubMed]
48. Stonner, M.M.; Mackinnon, S.E.; Kaskutas, V. Predictors of functional outcome after peripheral nerve injury and compression. *J. Hand Ther.* **2020**, *34*, 369–375. [CrossRef] [PubMed]
49. Wilson, C.; Yaacoub, A.P.; Bakare, A.; Bo, N.; Aasar, A.; Barbaro, N.M. Peroneal nerve decompression: Institutional review and meta-analysis to identify prognostic associations with favorable and unfavorable surgical outcomes. *J. Neurosurg. Spine* **2019**, *30*, 714–721. [CrossRef] [PubMed]
50. Gaspar, M.P.; Kane, P.M.; Putthiwara, D.; Jacoby, S.M.; Osterman, A.L. Predicting Revision Following In Situ Ulnar Nerve Decompression for Patients With Idiopathic Cubital Tunnel Syndrome. *J. Hand Surg.* **2016**, *41*, 427–435. [CrossRef] [PubMed]
51. Gaspar, M.P.; Jacoby, S.M.; Osterman, A.L.; Kane, P.M. Risk factors predicting revision surgery after medial epicondylectomy for primary cubital tunnel syndrome. *J. Shoulder Elb. Surg.* **2016**, *25*, 681–687. [CrossRef]
52. Jerosch-Herold, C.; Houghton, J.; Blake, J.; Shaikh, A.; Wilson, E.C.; Shepstone, L. Association of psychological distress, quality of life and costs with carpal tunnel syndrome severity: A cross-sectional analysis of the PALMS cohort. *BMJ Open* **2017**, *7*, e017732. [CrossRef] [PubMed]
53. Straub, T.A. Endoscopic carpal tunnel release: A prospective analysis of factors associated with unsatisfactory results. *Arthroscopy* **1999**, *15*, 269–274. [CrossRef]
54. Lozano Calderón, S.A.; Paiva, A.; Ring, D. Patient satisfaction after open carpal tunnel release correlates with depression. *J. Hand Surg.* **2008**, *33*, 303–307. [CrossRef]
55. Das De, S.; Vranceanu, A.M.; Ring, D.C. Contribution of kinesophobia and catastrophic thinking to upper-extremity-specific disability. *J. Bone Joint Surg.* **2013**, *95*, 76–81. [CrossRef] [PubMed]
56. Ehretsman, R.L.; Novak, C.B.; Mackinnon, S.E. Subjective recovery of nerve graft donor site. *Ann. Plast. Surg.* **1999**, *43*, 606–612. [CrossRef] [PubMed]
57. Miloro, M.; Stoner, J.A. Subjective outcomes following sural nerve harvest. *J. Oral Maxillofac. Surg.* **2005**, *63*, 1150–1154. [CrossRef] [PubMed]

58. Stokvis, A.; Coert, J.H.; van Neck, J.W. Insufficient pain relief after surgical neuroma treatment: Prognostic factors and central sensitisation. *J. Plast. Reconstr. Aesthetic Surg.* **2010**, *63*, 1538–1543. [CrossRef]
59. Dworkin, R.H.; Handlin, D.S.; Richlin, D.M.; Brand, L.; Vannucci, C. Unraveling the effects of compensation, litigation, and employment on treatment response in chronic pain. *Pain* **1985**, *23*, 49–59. [CrossRef]
60. Mackinnon, S.E.; Dellon, A.L. Results of treatment of recurrent dorsoradial wrist neuromas. *Ann. Plast. Surg.* **1987**, *19*, 54–61. [CrossRef]
61. Lans, J.; Hoftiezer, Y.; Lozano-Calderón, S.A.; Heng, M.; Valerio, I.L.; Eberlin, K.R. Risk Factors for Neuropathic Pain Following Major Upper Extremity Amputation. *J. Reconstr. Microsurg.* **2021**, *37*, 413–420. [CrossRef] [PubMed]
62. Norman, G.J.; Karelina, K.; Zhang, N.; Walton, J.C.; Morris, J.S.; Devries, A.C. Stress and IL-1beta contribute to the development of depressive-like behavior following peripheral nerve injury. *Mol. Psychiatry* **2010**, *15*, 404–414. [CrossRef] [PubMed]
63. Raber, P.; Devor, M. Social variables affect phenotype in the neuroma model of neuropathic pain. *Pain* **2002**, *97*, 139–150. [CrossRef]
64. Le Coz, G.M.; Genty, J.; Anton, F.; Hanesch, U. Chronic Social Stress Time-Dependently Affects Neuropathic Pain-Related Cold Allodynia and Leads to Altered Expression of Spinal Biochemical Mediators. *Front Behav Neurosci* **2017**, *11*, 70. [CrossRef] [PubMed]
65. Kaltenbrunner Bernitz, B.; Grees, N.; Jakobsson Randers, M.; Gerner, U.; Bergendorff, S. Young adults on disability benefits in 7 countries. *Scand. J. Public Health* **2013**, *41*, 3–26. [CrossRef]
66. Muijzer, A.; Groothoff, J.W.; de Boer, W.E.; Geertzen, J.H.; Brouwer, S. The assessment of efforts to return to work in the European Union. *Eur. J. Public Health* **2010**, *20*, 689–694. [CrossRef] [PubMed]
67. Radloff, L.S. The CES-D Scale:A Self-Report Depression Scale for Research in the General Population. *Appl. Psychol. Meas.* **1977**, *1*, 385–401. [CrossRef]
68. Busch, M.A.; Maske, U.E.; Ryl, L.; Schlack, R.; Hapke, U. Prevalence of depressive symptoms and diagnosed depression among adults in Germany: Results of the German Health Interview and Examination Survey for Adults (DEGS1). *Bundesgesundheitsblatt Gesundh. Gesundh.* **2013**, *56*, 733–739. [CrossRef] [PubMed]
69. Pejkova, S.; Filipce, V.; Peev, I.; Nikolovska, B.; Jovanoski, T.; Georgieva, G.; Srbov, B. Brachial Plexus Injuries—Review of the Anatomy and the Treatment Options. *Pril. Makedon. Akad. Nauk. Umet. Oddel. Med. Nauk.* **2021**, *42*, 91–103. [CrossRef] [PubMed]
70. Bhandari, P.S.; Maurya, S. Recent advances in the management of brachial plexus injuries. *Indian J. Plast. Surg.* **2014**, *47*, 191–198. [CrossRef]
71. Yokoya, S.; Maeno, T.; Sakamoto, N.; Goto, R.; Maeno, T. A Brief Survey of Public Knowledge and Stigma Towards Depression. *J. Clin. Med. Res.* **2018**, *10*, 202–209. [CrossRef]
72. Volpe, U.; Mihai, A.; Jordanova, V.; Sartorius, N. The pathways to mental healthcare worldwide: A systematic review. *Curr. Opin. Psychiatry* **2015**, *28*, 299–306. [CrossRef] [PubMed]
73. Gutiérrez-Colosía, M.R.; Salvador-Carulla, L.; Salinas-Pérez, J.A.; García-Alonso, C.R.; Cid, J.; Salazzari, D.; Montagni, I.; Tedeschi, F.; Cetrano, G.; Chevreul, K.; et al. Standard comparison of local mental health care systems in eight European countries. *Epidemiol. Psychiatr. Sci.* **2019**, *28*, 210–223. [CrossRef]
74. Hancock, L.; Bryant, R.A. Posttraumatic stress, stressor controllability, and avoidance. *Behav. Res. Ther.* **2020**, *128*, 103591. [CrossRef] [PubMed]
75. Hancock, L.; Bryant, R.A. Perceived control and avoidance in posttraumatic stress. *Eur. J. Psychotraumatol.* **2018**, *9*, 1468708. [CrossRef]
76. Hancock, L.; Bryant, R.A. Posttraumatic stress, uncontrollability, and emotional distress tolerance. *Depress. Anxiety* **2018**, *35*, 1040–1047. [CrossRef] [PubMed]
77. Müller, M.J. Helplessness and perceived pain intensity: Relations to cortisol concentrations after electrocutaneous stimulation in healthy young men. *BioPsychoSoc. Med.* **2011**, *5*, 8. [CrossRef]
78. Samwel, H.J.; Evers, A.W.; Crul, B.J.; Kraaimaat, F.W. The role of helplessness, fear of pain, and passive pain-coping in chronic pain patients. *Clin. J. Pain* **2006**, *22*, 245–251. [CrossRef] [PubMed]
79. Tesarz, J.; Eich, W.; Treede, R.D.; Gerhardt, A. Altered pressure pain thresholds and increased wind-up in adult patients with chronic back pain with a history of childhood maltreatment: A quantitative sensory testing study. *Pain* **2016**, *157*, 1799–1809. [CrossRef]
80. Sachs-Ericsson, N.; Kendall-Tackett, K.; Hernandez, A. Childhood abuse, chronic pain, and depression in the National Comorbidity Survey. *Child Abus. Negl.* **2007**, *31*, 531–547. [CrossRef] [PubMed]
81. Saunders, B.E.; Adams, Z.W. Epidemiology of traumatic experiences in childhood. *Child. Adolesc. Psychiatr. Clin.* **2014**, *23*, 167–184. [CrossRef]
82. Tate, D.G. Workers' disability and return to work. *Am. J. Phys. Med. Rehabil.* **1992**, *71*, 92–96. [CrossRef]
83. MacKenzie, E.J.; Morris, J.A., Jr.; Jurkovich, G.J.; Yasui, Y.; Cushing, B.M.; Burgess, A.R.; DeLateur, B.J.; McAndrew, M.P.; Swiontkowski, M.F. Return to work following injury: The role of economic, social, and job-related factors. *Am. J. Public Health* **1998**, *88*, 1630–1637. [CrossRef] [PubMed]
84. Hong, T.S.; Tian, A.; Sachar, R.; Ray, W.Z.; Brogan, D.M.; Dy, C.J. Indirect Cost of Traumatic Brachial Plexus Injuries in the United States. *J. Bone Joint Surg.* **2019**, *101*, e80. [CrossRef]

85. Pan, T.; Mulhern, B.; Viney, R.; Norman, R.; Tran-Duy, A.; Hanmer, J.; Devlin, N. Evidence on the relationship between PROMIS-29 and EQ-5D: A literature review. *Qual. Life Res.* **2021**. [CrossRef]
86. Ring, D. Symptoms and disability after major peripheral nerve injury. *Hand Clin.* **2013**, *29*, 421–425. [CrossRef] [PubMed]
87. Boogaard, S.; De Vet, H.C.; Faber, C.G.; Zuurmond, W.W.; Perez, R.S. An overview of predictors for persistent neuropathic pain. *Expert Rev. Neurother.* **2013**, *13*, 505–513. [CrossRef]
88. Cocito, D.; Paolasso, I.; Pazzaglia, C.; Tavella, A.; Poglio, F.; Ciaramitaro, P.; Scarmozzino, A.; Cossa, F.M.; Bergamasco, B.; Padua, L. Pain affects the quality of life of neuropathic patients. *Neurol Sci.* **2006**, *27*, 155–160. [CrossRef]
89. Novak, C.B.; Anastakis, D.J.; Beaton, D.E.; Katz, J. Patient-reported outcome after peripheral nerve injury. *J. Hand Surg.* **2009**, *34*, 281–287. [CrossRef] [PubMed]
90. Burke, S.; Shorten, G.D. When pain after surgery doesn't go away. *Biochem. Soc. Trans.* **2009**, *37*, 318–322. [CrossRef]
91. Rankine, J.J.; Fortune, D.G.; Hutchinson, C.E.; Hughes, D.G.; Main, C.J. Pain drawings in the assessment of nerve root compression: A comparative study with lumbar spine magnetic resonance imaging. *Spine* **1998**, *23*, 1668–1676. [CrossRef]
92. MacDowall, A.; Robinson, Y.; Skeppholm, M.; Olerud, C. Anxiety and depression affect pain drawings in cervical degenerative disc disease. *Upsala J. Med Sci.* **2017**, *122*, 99–107. [CrossRef] [PubMed]
93. Bernhoff, G.; Landén Ludvigsson, M.; Peterson, G.; Bertilson, B.C.; Elf, M.; Peolsson, A. The pain drawing as an instrument for identifying cervical spine nerve involvement in chronic whiplash-associated disorders. *J. Pain Res.* **2016**, *9*, 397–404. [CrossRef]
94. Rosner, J.; Lütolf, R.; Hostettler, P.; Villiger, M.; Clijsen, R.; Hohenauer, E.; Barbero, M.; Curt, A.; Hubli, M. Assessment of neuropathic pain after spinal cord injury using quantitative pain drawings. *Spinal Cord* **2021**, *59*, 529–537. [CrossRef] [PubMed]
95. MacDowall, A.; Robinson, Y.; Skeppholm, M.; Olerud, C. Pain drawings predict outcome of surgical treatment for degenerative disc disease in the cervical spine. *Upsala J. Med Sci.* **2017**, *122*, 194–200. [CrossRef]
96. Prahm, C.; Bauer, K.; Sturma, A.; Hruby, L.; Pittermann, A.; Aszmann, O. 3D Body Image Perception and Pain Visualization Tool for Upper Limb Amputees. In Proceedings of the 2019 IEEE 7th International Conference on Serious Games and Applications for Health (SeGAH), Kyoto, Japan, 5–7 August 2019; pp. 1–5.

Article

# Indocyanine Green for Leakage Control in Isolated Limb Perfusion

Isabel Zucal [1,2], Sebastian Geis [1], Lukas Prantl [1], Silke Haerteis [2,†] and Thiha Aung [1,2,3,*,†]

1. Centre of Plastic, Aesthetic, Hand and Reconstructive Surgery, University Clinic of Regensburg, 93053 Regensburg, Germany; isabel.zucal@ksa.ch (I.Z.); sebastian.geis@ukr.de (S.G.); lukas.prantl@ukr.de (L.P.)
2. Institute for Molecular and Cellular Anatomy, University of Regensburg, 93053 Regensburg, Germany; silke.haerteis@ur.de
3. Faculty of Applied Healthcare Science, Deggendorf Institute of Technology, 94469 Deggendorf, Germany
* Correspondence: thiha.aung@ur.de
† Shared last-authorship.

**Abstract:** Sarcomas are characterized by a high metastatic potential and aggressive growth. Despite surgery, chemotherapy plays an important role in the treatment of these tumors. Optimal anti-cancer therapy with maximized local efficacy and minimized systemic side effects has been the object of many studies for a long time. To improve the local efficacy of anti-tumor therapy, isolated limb perfusion with high-dose cytostatic agents has been introduced in surgical oncology. In order to control the local distribution of substances, radiolabeled cytostatic drugs or perfusion solutions have been applied but often require the presence of specialized personnel and result in a certain exposure to radiation. In this study, we present a novel strategy using indocyanine green to track tumor perfusion with high-dose cytostatic therapy. In a rat cadaver model, the femoral vessels were cannulated and connected to a peristaltic pump to provide circulation within the selected limb. The perfusion solution contained indocyanine green and high-dose doxorubicin. An infrared camera enabled the visualization of indocyanine green during limb perfusion, and subsequent leakage control was successfully performed. Histologic analysis of sections derived proximally from the injection site excluded systemic drug dispersion. In this study, the application of indocyanine green was proven to be a safe and cost- and time-efficient method for precise leakage control in isolated limb perfusion with a high-dose cytostatic agent.

**Keywords:** cytostatic agents; doxorubicin; indocyanine green; oncology; perfusion; surgical oncology

## 1. Introduction

Sarcomas are tumors that are characterized by an aggressive growth pattern, early metastasis, and poor prognosis [1–3]. Oncologic surgery comprises many medical disciplines and therapeutic approaches. Surgical resection is an important aspect in cancer treatment and often involves additional lymphadenectomy of sentinel lymph nodes and downstream lymph node stations [4]. In some cases, radiotherapy is performed for local disease control and to increase functional outcomes [5]. However, despite lymph node resection, radiation increases the risk of lymphatic vessel damage and lymphatic complications [6,7]. Moreover, an exclusively surgical approach often results in the loss of the entire limb. In the last few decades, neoadjuvant chemotherapy and adjuvant chemotherapy have been added to the treatment protocols of sarcomas. A combination of doxorubicin, cisplatin, and methotrexate with leucovorin and ifosfamide represents the most commonly used combination of chemotherapeutic agents for the treatment of sarcomas [8]. However, systemic drug application is accompanied by systemic toxicity.

In the past few years, there has been a great effort within oncologic research to develop improved drug delivery systems and application modes that enable a high local efficacy while keeping systemic toxic effects at the lowest level possible. In this regard, isolated limb perfusion (ILP) has been described as a technique that permits the local application of high-dose cytostatic drugs into tumors or metastases located within extremities [9–11]. The technique is mostly used for the treatment of locally advanced melanoma and unresectable primary or recurrent sarcomas of the limb [12–14]. Depending on the affected limb, the perforating vessels are cannulated and connected to an extracorporeal device, which provides circulation to the affected limb with high doses of cytostatic agents. The vessels can be cannulated at different levels: iliac, iliofemoral, femoropopliteal, and popliteal [15]. Additionally, local hyperthermia is achieved by placing a thermal blanket around the affected extremity to increase the cytotoxic effects [12,15].

Radionuclide-labeled cytostatic drugs or perfusion solutions have been used for adequate leakage control at the cannulation site and for the control of the correct application of such procedures [16,17]. After the correct cannulation is confirmed, high-dose cytostatic drugs, such as TNFα + melphalan [9,18] are added to the solution, which is subsequently injected into the chosen region. However, this results in a certain amount of exposure to radiation [19,20], high costs, and the requirement of specialized personnel to carry out this procedure.

Doxorubicin, an anthracycline antibiotic, represents a substantial pillar in treatment protocols for solid tumors such as sarcomas [21]. However, cardiotoxicity and nephrotoxicity are some of the most common systemic side effects [21]. As these solid tumors usually affect the extremities, a limb salvage procedure is highly desirable. ILP presents one possibility to increase operability and to preserve functionality. Isolated limb infusion with doxorubicin has been described for the treatment of soft tissue sarcomas with promising results in this regard [22]. Due to the fluorescent property of doxorubicin, it can be visualized and traced by fluorescence microscopy, making it very suitable for preclinical and clinical studies. Here, we propose a simple, safe, and cost- and time-efficient technique for leakage control in ILP with high-dose doxorubicin.

## 2. Materials and Methods

Rat cadaver models were placed on a corkboard in a supine position underneath a microscope; the skin was incised longitudinally on the medial part of the thigh. The femoral vessels were carefully prepared, dissected, and cannulated. Cannulas were kept in place with clamps and were attached to a 12,000 Varioperpex peristaltic pump (LKB Bromma, Sweden) that provided circulation within the cannulated extremity. The maximum perfusion speed was 5 mL/min. A plastic loop was placed around the groin and served as a tourniquet. The femoral artery was utilized for inflow and the femoral vein for outflow of the perfusion fluid. The dissection and cannulation of the vessels were performed under a Leica M205A stereomicroscope, which conveys a maximal resolution of 1050 lp/mm and a zoom range of 7.8×–160×. Two different beam path lengths provide a high level of depth of focus, whereby orientation within a multidimensional space is enabled. For the microsurgical dissection and cannulation of the femoral vessels, customized instruments from Redam instruments GmbH were utilized. The rat cadavers we used were Munich–Wistar–Froemter rats, aged between 7 and 10 weeks, previously used for other experiments. The procedures were carried out within 1–4 h after the death of the rats. If the experiment could not be carried out immediately after death, the rats were placed in the freezer at −20 °C and thawed in a water bath for 1 h at 37 °C.

The peristaltic pump perfused the circulatory system of the cannulated limb with approximately 50 mL of perfusion solution containing 47 mL of 1× PBS (Sigma Aldrich, St. Louis, MO, USA), 1000 IU of heparin with a concentration of 5000 IU/mL (B. Braun Melsungen AG, Melsungen, Germany), 2 mL of indocyanine green (ICG) with a concentration of 2.5 mg/mL (Diagnostic Green GmbH, Aschheim, Germany), and high-dose doxorubicin (2 mg/mL). The Elevision IR (VSIII) fluorescence system (Medtronic, Minneapolis, MN, USA) was used for the fluorescence imaging in perfusion recognition modes to visualize and trace the injected ICG. The same camera conditions were used for all acquisitions:

exposure time was 40 Hz (=2.5 ms), and gain was 1. Fluorescence level was dependent on penetration depth and camera focus. ICG served as an indicator of leakage and confirmed the correct drug application. To provide a comparison between ILP and whole-body perfusion, the femoral vessels were also cannulated in the inverted direction, and after perfusion with the same solution, fluorescent imaging was performed. Perfusion time was between 15 and 20 min. The experiment was repeated five times.

*Fluorescence Microscopy*

For further proof of correct drug application, tissue samples (thigh muscle) were taken from anatomical regions proximal to the cannulation site and from the contralateral limb to exclude leakage and systemic dispersion. As a positive control, three samples were obtained from the perfused limb. These samples were immerged in 4% PFA in PBS (pH 7.4) for 16 days, then washed in PBS three times for 30 min, and immersed in EDTA decalcification solution for 90 min. Then, samples were embedded in Neg-50™ frozen section medium (Thermo Fisher Scientific, Waltham, MA, USA). Finally, samples were cryosectioned and analyzed by fluorescence microscopy with Axiovert 200 M (Zeiss, Oberkochen, Germany). Microscopic analysis enabled the visualization of doxorubicin via fluorescence after excitation at 560 nm (100 ms, mCherry mode) with DAPI counterstain (20 ms, DAPI mode) at 40× magnification. Magnification was further increased to 200× utilizing ImageJ (LOCI, University of Wisconsin, Madison, WI, USA).

## 3. Results

The femoral vessels were successfully dissected and cannulated in all rats. Each limb was perfused after connecting the cannulas to the peristaltic pump. ICG-fluorescence imaging showed locally restricted distribution of the perfusion fluid containing the cytostatic drug by causing the cannulated limb to emit a glowing signal (Figure 1A,B). No leakage was observed. In contrast to ILP, ICG-fluorescence imaging of whole-body perfusion after inverting the cannulation direction of the femoral vessels showed a glowing signal over the entire body (Figure 1C,D). In areas with less or no fur or skin, such as the paws, the belly, the tail, or the cannulation site, a higher fluorescence level was recorded. Fur contamination with perfusion fluid around the cannulation site also resulted in an increased fluorescence level.

Fluorescence microscopy of samples derived proximally from the injection site of the contralateral limb showed no intracellular doxorubicin accumulation (Figure 2, first two rows), giving proof of no systemic drug dispersion. On the other hand, microscopic analysis of the samples obtained from the perfused limb showed intracellular doxorubicin accumulation (Figure 2, last two rows).

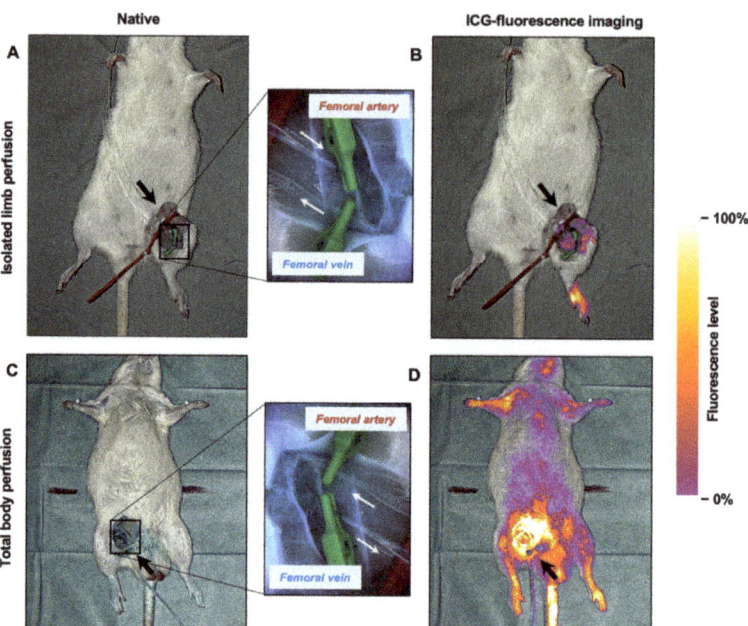

**Figure 1.** ICG-fluorescence imaging as indicator of ILP. (**A**) The native image shows the cannulation site: the femoral artery and vein are cannulated for perfusion inflow and outflow. The arrow indicates the direction of the flow. Clamps are used to keep the cannulas in place, and a magnification (4×) of the cannulation site is provided for a better overview. (**B**) ILP is demonstrated with ICG fluorescence imaging. (**C**) For comparison, a native picture of a rat cadaver with whole-body perfusion is shown. In this case, the direction of flow is inverted (arrow). A magnification of the cannulation site is provided (4×). (**D**) ICG fluorescence imaging of whole-body perfusion evokes a glowing signal of the entire body, while the cannulated extremity is spared. Fluorescence level is indicated by brightness and color: areas with the smallest penetration depth result in the highest fluorescence signal, e.g., areas uncovered by fur or skin, such as the cannulation site.

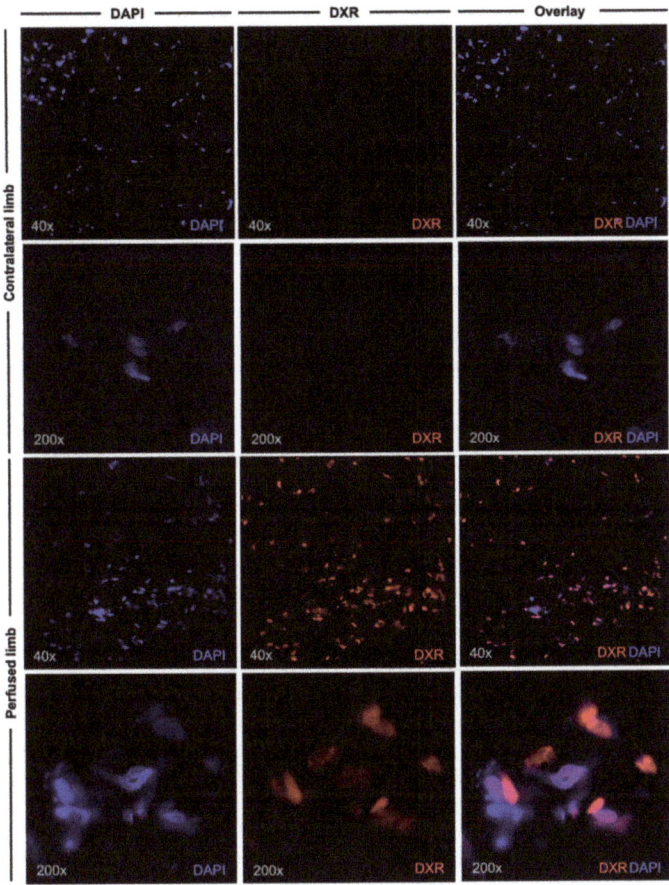

**Figure 2.** Fluorescence microscopy. In the first and second row, images of the sample derived from the contralateral limb are shown at 40× and 200× magnification, respectively. No intracellular doxorubicin (DXR) accumulation was observed, and nuclei were counterstained with DAPI. In the third and fourth row, fluorescence images of a sample from the perfused limb are displayed. Microscopic analysis displays intracellular doxorubicin accumulation.

## 4. Discussion

Sarcomas are aggressive tumors that often affect the extremities with high risk of metastatic spread. Among the different types of sarcomas, one differentiates between soft tissue sarcoma; bone tumors, such as osteosarcoma, chondrosarcoma, or Ewing-sarcoma; and gastrointestinal stromal tumors. Sarcomas are characterized by high inter- and intra-tumoral diversity at a genetic level, rendering treatment very difficult. Because of their aggressiveness and the potential for early metastasis, a safe tumor resection and lymphadenectomy of affected lymph nodes in combination with neoadjuvant and adjuvant chemotherapy are crucial. However, this radical surgical removal results in a high rate of lymphatic complications despite the risk of limb loss. With regard to complications related to the lymphatic system, an incidence of lymphedema of about 29% has been found following limb salvage of soft tissue sarcoma located within extremities [23]. The number of resected lymph nodes [24–26], tumor localization within the thigh, tumor depth, and size > 5 cm were identified as risk factors for the development of lymphedema [23,27]. Moreover, for local disease control, patients frequently undergo radiotherapy [28], and, as mentioned before, this also contributes to the development of lymphatic complications. To treat lymphatic complications, surgery such as lymphovenous anastomosis is often required [29]. Furthermore, limb preservation remains highly desirable, and complex microsurgical functional reconstructions have been developed for this purpose, such as the Borggreve rotationplasty, which provides a reconstruction of the knee joint after resection of osteosarcoma of the distal femur [30,31], or the Winkelmann procedure, which consists of a clavicula-based reconstruction of the humerus [32].

In Third World countries, such complex treatments and associated costs are neither available nor sustainable. For instance, amputation is still the most common therapy of osteosarcoma in Third World countries, whereas limb salvage procedures in combination with adjuvant and neoadjuvant chemotherapy became the momentary standard therapy in surgical oncology [33]. Poor countries in particular may profit from cost-, time-, and personnel-efficient techniques of cytostatic drug application, such as ILP.

Cancer therapy often requires the application of high-dose cytostatic drugs in order to cause antitumoral effects, but, on the other hand, this also carries the risk of serious side effects. Thus, in the past few decades, there has been an increased effort to develop therapies that avoid these side effects, such as the administration of corticosteroids and colony stimulating factors [34,35]. ILP has been developed to minimize systemic effects of cytostatic agents and maximize the local drug concentration [9–11]. Additional hyperthermia is thought to enhance the uptake of cytostatic agents, thereby increasing the effects on the tumor [12]. However, for safe application of these highly concentrated cytostatic agents, leakage control is of utmost importance. In this regard, the addition of radionuclides to the perfusion solution has already been described as a method for sufficient leakage control [16,17], but this causes a certain amount of radiation and requires specialized personnel [19,20]. Although doxorubicin has been used for decades, it was recently replaced by TNF$\alpha$ + melphalan, which is now the standard therapy in ILP for sarcomas. In fact, higher toxicities and less activity are attributed to the application of doxorubicin compared to TNF$\alpha$ + melphalan [36]. In our experiments, we used doxorubicin because of its fluorescent property to track drug dispersion after ILP. Cytostatic drug toxicity in ILP is related to the amount of leakage into systemic circulation, and, in addition to local leakage control, high intravenous hydration promotes the washout effect of these drugs, reducing systemic toxicity. Local complications affecting the perfused limb include deep venous thrombosis [37], limb edema, and erythema, deep tissue damage with functional impairment and compartment syndrome [38]. In our experiments, we observed limb edema in all rats. No blisters or epidermolysis were present. However, as we performed the experiment on rat cadavers, complications such as functional impairment or compartment syndrome could not be assessed.

The innovative aspect of this experiment is the utilization of ICG for leakage control in isolated limb perfusion. In a rat cadaver model, the femoral vessels were cannulated and attached to a peristaltic pump for the establishment of circulation within the cannulated extremity. The perfusion fluid contained PBS, 1000 IE of heparin, 2 mL of ICG, and high doses of doxorubicin. An infrared camera was used to visualize ICG, which served as an indicator of leakage and depicted the localized drug application in ILP. Histologic analysis of anatomical regions proximal to the cannulated limb provided proof of the correct application of the drug by indicating that there was no systemic dispersion. Another innovative aspect of this experiment is the usage of rat cadaver models. Fluid-resuscitated rat cadavers represent an animal-friendly research model with regard to the 3R principles of replacement, refinement, and reduction of animal models in research and medical training. Therefore, this model could be used for further infusion/perfusion studies in the future.

ICG has a broad application spectrum in surgery. It is an amphiphilic fluorescence dye, which is used for the purpose of intravenous injection into patients. Once in the circulatory system, 98% of the injected ICG binds to plasma protein, and 2% remains free in the blood serum until it is metabolized by the liver and subsequently excreted into bile [39]. The dye has a half-life of generally 3–4 min that depends on the vascularity of the investigated organ [39]. Because of the rapid clearance rate, the dye can be used for several injections during one procedure [39]. In addition, ICG is a well-established substance in clinics and surgery and is also characterized by a low side effect profile, ensuring the safety of its application [40,41]. Moreover, it is easily available and applicable to the perfusion solution used for ILP. For instance, it is well established in supermicrosurgery, as it permits the visualization of lymphatics, and in reconstructive surgery where it is used to assess the perforators, tissue perfusion, and the viability of microvascular anastomoses [41–43]. In oncologic surgery, it is used for sentinel lymph node mapping and intraoperative identification of tumors [44]. Due to intratumoral injection, exact tumor margins can be visualized, ensuring safe resection without damage of surrounding tissue [45,46]. Moreover, it can be injected into the epineurium of nerves to improve the intraoperative visualization and to avoid accidental damage [47]. An important limitation of the use of ICG, however, is the depth of detection. In fact, structures deeper than 5–8 mm cannot be visualized [48]. Nevertheless, the detection depth is sufficient for leakage control of the cannulation site.

This study has some limitations. Although no systemic cytostatic drug dispersion was found in our experiments after approximately 15 min of infusion, systemic dispersion will likely occur due to the vascular collaterals if no tourniquet is placed at the level of the groin or the axillary fossa. Another limitation of this model is post-mortem clot formation and incomplete limb and/or whole-body perfusion. Although our perfusion fluid contained heparin, complete thrombus dissolution was not always possible, especially in thawed rat cadavers. We observed that the longer we waited after the rats had deceased, the higher the probability of clot formation. Freezing rat cadavers allowed for preservation for weeks or months, but the probability of vascular obstruction was higher compared to unfrozen and rapidly perfused rats. According to Okazaki et al., heparinization was described post-mortem in transplanted canine lungs for the prevention of microthrombi [49]. In this study, the optimal post-mortem heparinization time was 30 min after cardiac arrest [49]. Moreover, Marchioro et al. described the use of heparin in extracorporeal perfusion for the obtainment of post-mortem homografts in animal models [50].

As an alternative to the more invasive ILP, requiring open dissection of the vessels and the use of large-caliber catheters, isolated limb infusion has been suggested as a valid, minimally invasive, and safe alternative. In addition, when performing isolated limb infusion, small-caliber catheters are placed percutaneously [12,13]. Moreover, perfusion fluid is not oxygenated in isolated limb infusion, providing a hypoxic milieu, which enhances cytotoxic drug effects [12]. In our experiment, a percutaneous procedure could not be performed due to the small diameter of the femoral vessels of rats (approximately 0.54–0.56 mm [51]).

## 5. Conclusions

The use of ICG for leakage control in ILP for cancer treatment enables a safe application of high-dose cytostatic drugs by avoiding the application of radionuclides for this purpose. This makes it a more cost-, time-, and personnel-efficient technique, and no cooperation with nuclear medicine specialists is required.

**Author Contributions:** Conceptualization, T.A. and S.H.; methodology, T.A.; formal analysis, T.A., S.H. and I.Z.; investigation, I.Z.; resources, S.H. and L.P.; data curation, I.Z.; writing—original draft preparation, I.Z.; writing—review and editing, T.A., S.H., L.P. and S.G.; visualization, I.Z.; supervision, S.H. and L.P.; funding acquisition, S.H. and L.P. All authors have read and agreed to the published version of the manuscript.

**Funding:** This research received no external funding.

**Institutional Review Board Statement:** Not applicable.

**Informed Consent Statement:** Not applicable.

**Data Availability Statement:** The data presented in this study are available on request from the corresponding author.

**Acknowledgments:** We thank Cand. med. Eric Pion, Lucia Denk, and Dipl. Biol. Manfred Depner for their support.

**Conflicts of Interest:** The authors declare no conflict of interest.

## References

1. Vodanovich, D.A.; Choong, P.F.M. Soft-tissue Sarcomas. *Indian J. Orthop.* **2018**, *52*, 35–44. [CrossRef]
2. Skubitz, K.M.; D'Adamo, D.R. Sarcoma. *Mayo Clin. Proc.* **2007**, *82*, 1409–1432. [CrossRef]
3. Hoang, N.T.; Acevedo, L.A.; Mann, M.J.; Tolani, B. A review of soft-tissue sarcomas: Translation of biological advances into treatment measures. *Cancer Manag. Res.* **2018**, *10*, 1089–1114. [CrossRef]
4. Faries, M.B.; Morton, D.L. Surgery and sentinel lymph node biopsy. *Semin. Oncol.* **2007**, *34*, 498–508. [CrossRef] [PubMed]
5. Kaushal, A.; Citrin, D. The role of radiation therapy in the management of sarcomas. *Surg. Clin. N. Am.* **2008**, *88*, 629–646. [CrossRef] [PubMed]
6. Allam, O.; Park, K.E.; Chandler, L.; Mozaffari, M.A.; Ahmad, M.; Lu, X.; Alperovich, M. The impact of radiation on lymphedema: A review of the literature. *Gland Surg.* **2020**, *9*, 596–602. [CrossRef]
7. Togami, S.; Kawamura, T.; Fukuda, M.; Yanazume, S.; Kamio, M.; Kobayashi, H. Risk factors for lymphatic complications following lymphadenectomy in patients with cervical cancer. *Jpn. J. Clin. Oncol.* **2018**, *48*, 1036–1040. [CrossRef] [PubMed]
8. He, H.; Ni, J.; Huang, J. Molecular mechanisms of chemoresistance in osteosarcoma (Review). *Oncol. Lett.* **2014**, *7*, 1352–1362. [CrossRef]
9. Eggermont, A.M.; Koops, H.S.; Klausner, J.M.; Kroon, B.B.; Schlag, P.M.; Liénard, D.; van Geel, A.N.; Hoekstra, H.J.; Meller, I.; Nieweg, O.E.; et al. Isolated limb perfusion with tumor necrosis factor and melphalan for limb salvage in 186 patients with locally advanced soft tissue extremity sarcomas. The cumulative multicenter European experience. *Ann. Surg.* **1996**, *224*, 756–764. [CrossRef]
10. Moreno-Ramirez, D.; de la Cruz-Merino, L.; Ferrandiz, L.; Villegas-Portero, R.; Nieto-Garcia, A. Isolated limb perfusion for malignant melanoma: Systematic review on effectiveness and safety. *Oncologist* **2010**, *15*, 416–427. [CrossRef]
11. Duprat Neto, J.P.; Oliveira, F.; Bertolli, E.; Molina, A.S.; Nishinari, K.; Facure, L.; Fregnani, J.H. Isolated limb perfusion with hyperthermia and chemotherapy: Predictive factors for regional toxicity. *Clinics* **2012**, *67*, 237–241. [CrossRef]
12. Teras, J.; Carr, M.J.; Zager, J.S.; Kroon, H.M. Molecular Aspects of the Isolated Limb Infusion Procedure. *Biomedicines* **2021**, *9*, 163. [CrossRef]
13. Kroon, H.M.; Thompson, J.F. Isolated limb infusion: A review. *J. Surg. Oncol.* **2009**, *100*, 169–177. [CrossRef]
14. Brady, M.S.; Brown, K.; Patel, A.; Fisher, C.; Marx, W. A phase II trial of isolated limb infusion with melphalan and dactinomycin for regional melanoma and soft tissue sarcoma of the extremity. *Ann. Surg. Oncol.* **2006**, *13*, 1123–1129. [CrossRef] [PubMed]
15. Martin-Tellez, K.S.; van Houdt, W.J.; van Coevorden, F.; Colombo, C.; Fiore, M. Isolated limb perfusion for soft tissue sarcoma: Current practices and future directions. A survey of experts and a review of literature. *Cancer Treat. Rev.* **2020**, *88*, 102058. [CrossRef]
16. Sprenger, H.J.; Markwardt, J.; Schlag, P.M. Quantitative radionuclide leakage control during isolated limb perfusion. *Nuklearmedizin* **1994**, *33*, 248–253. [PubMed]
17. Paulsen, I.F.; Chakera, A.H.; Schmidt, G.; Drejøe, J.; Klyver, H.; Oturai, P.S.; Hesse, B.; Drzewiecki, K.; Mortensen, J. Radionuclide leakage monitoring during hyperthermic isolated limb perfusion for treatment of local melanoma metastasis in an extremity. *Clin. Physiol. Funct. Imaging* **2015**, *35*, 301–305. [CrossRef] [PubMed]
18. Rastrelli, M.; Campana, L.G.; Valpione, S.; Tropea, S.; Zanon, A.; Rossi, C.R. Hyperthermic isolated limb perfusion in locally advanced limb soft tissue sarcoma: A 24-year single-centre experience. *Int. J. Hyperth.* **2016**, *32*, 165–172. [CrossRef]
19. Barnaby, F.; Boeker, E. Is technetium-99 (Tc-99) radiologically significant? *Med. Confl. Surviv.* **1999**, *15*, 57–70. [CrossRef]
20. Santos-Oliveira, R.; Machado, M. Pitfalls with radiopharmaceuticals. *Am. J. Med. Sci.* **2011**, *342*, 50–53. [CrossRef] [PubMed]
21. Johnson-Arbor, K.; Dubey, R. Doxorubicin. In *StatPearls*; StatPearls Publishing: Treasure Island, FL, USA, 2020.
22. Hegazy, M.A.; Kotb, S.Z.; Sakr, H.; El Dosoky, E.; Amer, T.; Hegazi, R.A.; Farouk, O. Preoperative isolated limb infusion of Doxorubicin and external irradiation for limb-threatening soft tissue sarcomas. *Ann. Surg. Oncol.* **2007**, *14*, 568–576. [CrossRef]
23. Friedmann, D.; Wunder, J.S.; Ferguson, P.; O'Sullivan, B.; Roberge, D.; Catton, C.; Freeman, C.; Saran, N.; Turcotte, R.E. Incidence and Severity of Lymphoedema following Limb Salvage of Extremity Soft Tissue Sarcoma. *Sarcoma* **2011**, *2011*, 289673. [CrossRef]
24. Boughey, J.C.; Hoskin, T.L.; Cheville, A.L.; Miller, J.; Loprinzi, M.D.; Thomsen, K.M.; Maloney, S.; Baddour, L.M.; Degnim, A.C. Risk factors associated with breast lymphedema. *Ann. Surg. Oncol.* **2014**, *21*, 1202–1208. [CrossRef] [PubMed]
25. DiSipio, T.; Rye, S.; Newman, B.; Hayes, S. Incidence of unilateral arm lymphoedema after breast cancer: A systematic review and meta-analysis. *Lancet Oncol.* **2013**, *14*, 500–515. [CrossRef]
26. McLaughlin, S.A.; Bagaria, S.; Gibson, T.; Arnold, M.; Diehl, N.; Crook, J.; Parker, A.; Nguyen, J. Trends in risk reduction practices for the prevention of lymphedema in the first 12 months after breast cancer surgery. *J. Am. Coll. Surg.* **2013**, *216*, 380–389. [CrossRef] [PubMed]
27. Wu, P.; Elswick, S.M.; Arkhavan, A.; Molinar, V.E.; Mohan, A.T.; Curiel, D.; Sim, F.H.; Martinez-Jorge, J.; Saint-Cyr, M. Risk Factors for Lymphedema after Thigh Sarcoma Resection and Reconstruction. *Plast. Reconstr. Surg. Glob. Open* **2020**, *8*, e2912. [CrossRef]
28. Tiong, S.S.; Dickie, C.; Haas, R.L.; O'Sullivan, B. The role of radiotherapy in the management of localized soft tissue sarcomas. *Cancer Biol. Med.* **2016**, *13*, 373–383. [CrossRef]

29. Scaglioni, M.F.; Fontein, D.B.Y.; Arvanitakis, M.; Giovanoli, P. Systematic review of lymphovenous anastomosis (LVA) for the treatment of lymphedema. *Microsurgery* **2017**, *37*, 947–953. [CrossRef]
30. Heise, U.; Minet-Sommer, S. The Borggreve rotation-plasty. A surgical method in therapy of malignant bone tumors and functional results. *Z. Orthop. Ihre Grenzgeb.* **1993**, *131*, 452–460. [CrossRef]
31. Borggreve, J. Kniegelenkersatz durch das in der Beinlängsachse um 180 Grad gedrehte Fußgelenk. *Arch. Für Orthopädische Und Unf.-Chir.* **1930**, *28*, 175–178. [CrossRef]
32. Winkelmann, W.W. Clavicula pro humero—a new surgical method for malignant tumors of the proximal humerus. *Z. Orthop. Ihre Grenzgeb.* **1992**, *130*, 197–201. [CrossRef] [PubMed]
33. Askari, R.; Umer, M. Our experience with Van Nes Rotationplasty for locally advanced lower extremity tumours. *JPMA J. Pak. Med. Assoc.* **2014**, *64*, S139–S143. [PubMed]
34. Lossignol, D. A little help from steroids in oncology. *J. Transl. Int. Med.* **2016**, *4*, 52–54. [CrossRef] [PubMed]
35. Metcalf, D. The colony-stimulating factors and cancer. *Nat. Rev. Cancer* **2010**, *10*, 425–434. [CrossRef]
36. Wray, C.J.; Benjamin, R.S.; Hunt, K.K.; Cormier, J.N.; Ross, M.I.; Feig, B.W. Isolated limb perfusion for unresectable extremity sarcoma: Results of 2 single-institution phase 2 trials. *Cancer* **2011**, *117*, 3235–3241. [CrossRef]
37. Eroğlu, A.; Ozcan, H.; Eryavuz, Y.; Kocağlu, H.; Demirci, S.; Aytac, S.K. Deep venous thrombosis of the extremity diagnosed by color Doppler ultrasonography after isolated limb perfusion. *Tumori* **2001**, *87*, 187–190. [CrossRef]
38. Wieberdink, J.; Benckhuysen, C.; Braat, R.P.; van Slooten, E.A.; Olthuis, G.A. Dosimetry in isolation perfusion of the limbs by assessment of perfused tissue volume and grading of toxic tissue reactions. *Eur. J. Cancer Clin. Oncol.* **1982**, *18*, 905–910. [CrossRef]
39. Reinhart, M.B.; Huntington, C.R.; Blair, L.J.; Heniford, B.T.; Augenstein, V.A. Indocyanine Green: Historical Context, Current Applications, and Future Considerations. *Surg. Innov.* **2016**, *23*, 166–175. [CrossRef] [PubMed]
40. Alander, J.T.; Kaartinen, I.; Laakso, A.; Pätilä, T.; Spillmann, T.; Tuchin, V.V.; Venermo, M.; Välisuo, P. A review of indocyanine green fluorescent imaging in surgery. *Int. J. Biomed. Imaging* **2012**, *2012*, 940585. [CrossRef]
41. Burnier, P.; Niddam, J.; Bosc, R.; Hersant, B.; Meningaud, J.P. Indocyanine green applications in plastic surgery: A review of the literature. *J. Plast. Reconstr. Aesthet. Surg.* **2017**, *70*, 814–827. [CrossRef]
42. Liu, D.Z.; Mathes, D.W.; Zenn, M.R.; Neligan, P.C. The application of indocyanine green fluorescence angiography in plastic surgery. *J. Reconstr. Microsurg.* **2011**, *27*, 355–364. [CrossRef] [PubMed]
43. Ludolph, I.; Horch, R.E.; Arkudas, A.; Schmitz, M. Enhancing Safety in Reconstructive Microsurgery Using Intraoperative Indocyanine Green Angiography. *Front. Surg.* **2019**, *6*, 39. [CrossRef]
44. Schaafsma, B.E.; Mieog, J.S.; Hutteman, M.; van der Vorst, J.R.; Kuppen, P.J.; Löwik, C.W.; Frangioni, J.V.; van de Velde, C.J.; Vahrmeijer, A.L. The clinical use of indocyanine green as a near-infrared fluorescent contrast agent for image-guided oncologic surgery. *J. Surg. Oncol.* **2011**, *104*, 323–332. [CrossRef] [PubMed]
45. Predina, J.D.; Keating, J.; Newton, A.; Corbett, C.; Xia, L.; Shin, M.; Frenzel Sulyok, L.; Deshpande, C.; Litzky, L.; Nie, S.; et al. A clinical trial of intraoperative near-infrared imaging to assess tumor extent and identify residual disease during anterior mediastinal tumor resection. *Cancer* **2019**, *125*, 807–817. [CrossRef] [PubMed]
46. Mahjoub, A.; Morales-Restrepo, A.; Fourman, M.S.; Mandell, J.B.; Feiqi, L.; Hankins, M.L.; Watters, R.J.; Weiss, K.R. Tumor Resection Guided by Intraoperative Indocyanine Green Dye Fluorescence Angiography Results in Negative Surgical Margins and Decreased Local Recurrence in an Orthotopic Mouse Model of Osteosarcoma. *Ann. Surg. Oncol.* **2019**, *26*, 894–898. [CrossRef]
47. Kwon, J.G.; Choi, Y.J.; Kim, S.C.; Hong, J.P.; Jeong, W.S.; Oh, T.S. A technique for safe deep facial tissue dissection: Indocyanine green-assisted intraoperative real-time visualization of the vasa nervorum of facial nerve with a near-infrared camera. *J. Craniomaxillofac. Surg.* **2019**, *47*, 1819–1826. [CrossRef]
48. Vahrmeijer, A.L.; Hutteman, M.; van der Vorst, J.R.; van de Velde, C.J.; Frangioni, J.V. Image-guided cancer surgery using near-infrared fluorescence. *Nat. Rev. Clin. Oncol.* **2013**, *10*, 507–518. [CrossRef]
49. Okazaki, M.; Date, H.; Inokawa, H.; Okutani, D.; Aokage, K.; Nagahiro, I.; Aoe, M.; Sano, Y.; Shimizu, N. Optimal time for post-mortem heparinization in canine lung transplantation with non-heart-beating donors. *J. Heart Lung Transpl.* **2006**, *25*, 454–460. [CrossRef]
50. Marchioro, T.L.; Huntley, R.T.; Waddell, W.R.; Starzl, T.E. Extracorporeal perfusion for obtaining postmortem homografts. *Surgery* **1963**, *54*, 900–911.
51. Liu, H.L. Microvascular anastomosis of submillimeter vessels-a training model in rats. *J. Hand Microsurg.* **2013**, *5*, 14–17. [CrossRef]

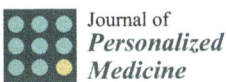 

Article

# New Approach to the Old Challenge of Free Flap Monitoring—Hyperspectral Imaging Outperforms Clinical Assessment by Earlier Detection of Perfusion Failure

Daniel G. E. Thiem *, Paul Römer, Sebastian Blatt, Bilal Al-Nawas and Peer W. Kämmerer

Department of Oral and Maxillofacial Surgery, University Medical Centre Mainz, 55131 Mainz, Germany; paul.roemer@unimedizin-mainz.de (P.R.); sebastian.blatt@unimedizin-mainz.de (S.B.); bilal.al-nawas@unimedizin-mainz.de (B.A.-N.); peer.kaemmerer@unimedizin-mainz.de (P.W.K.)
* Correspondence: daniel.thiem@uni-mainz.de; Tel.: +49-(0)-613-117-5459

**Abstract:** In reconstructive surgery, free flap failure, especially in complex osteocutaneous reconstructions, represents a significant clinical burden. Therefore, the aim of the presented study was to assess hyperspectral imaging (HSI) for monitoring of free flaps compared to clinical monitoring. In a prospective, non-randomized clinical study, patients with free flap reconstruction of the oro-maxillofacial-complex were included. Monitoring was assessed clinically and by using hyperspectral imaging (TIVITA™ Tissue-System, DiaspectiveVision GmbH, Pepelow, Germany) to determine tissue-oxygen-saturation [$StO_2$], near-infrared-perfusion-index [NPI], distribution of haemoglobin [THI] and water [TWI], and variance to an adjacent reference area (Δreference). A total of 54 primary and 11 secondary reconstructions were performed including fasciocutaneous and osteocutaneous flaps. Re-exploration was performed in 19 cases. A total of seven complete flap failures occurred, resulting in a 63% salvage rate. Mean time from flap inset to decision making for re-exploration based on clinical assessment was 23.1 ± 21.9 vs. 18.2 ± 19.4 h by the appearance of hyperspectral criteria indicating impaired perfusion ($StO_2$ ≤ 32% OR $StO_2$Δreference > −38% OR NPI ≤ 32.9 OR NPIΔreference ≥ −13.4%) resulting in a difference of 4.8 ± 5 h ($p < 0.001$). HSI seems able to detect perfusion compromise significantly earlier than clinical monitoring. These findings provide an interpretation aid for clinicians to simplify postoperative flap monitoring.

**Keywords:** HSI; objective; hyperspectral signature; timely recognition; reconstruction; head and neck; non-invasive; non-contact

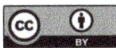

## 1. Introduction

In reconstructive oral and maxillofacial surgery, free flap transfer represents one of the most important and frequently performed methods for defect reconstruction of the head and neck region. Flap survival as the primary criterion for success after free flap transfer is generally considered to be very good at approximately 96% [1]. However, this is largely based on studies using less complex flap types such as fasciocutaneous radial or ulnar forearm flaps (R/UFFF) and does not generally apply to more compound flaps such as the osteocutaneous fibular flap (8% failure), scapular flap (6% failure), anterolateral thigh (ALT) or gracilis flap (5% failure) [2–4]. This is in contrast to the results of a recent study which showed flap survival of 98% in 157 fibular flaps used for mandibular reconstruction [5]. In addition to the flap type and its complexity, there are numerous other relevant factors (e.g., duration of surgery >8 h, need for intraoperative re-anastomosis, anatomically complex flap sites, challenging microanastomoses, arterial > venous thrombosis) that may contribute to the need for flap revision or even complete early flap failure [6]. Partial and complete flap loss, mainly due to impaired perfusion (venous > arterial), means a significant increase in morbidity and mortality for the affected patients due to prolonged wound healing, necessary second interventions, delay of adjuvant therapy (radio- and/or chemotherapy) and prolonged hospital stay [7,8]. In addition, the above-mentioned complications lead to a relevant additional financial burden on health care systems [9]. In this context, close perioperative flap monitoring has been established as the only effective tool allowing early detection of malperfusion and thus providing the possibility of timely re-exploration. Although several valid monitoring methods have been developed in recent years, clinical assessment, though subjective and poorly reproducible, is still considered the gold standard for flap monitoring [10]. The medical application of hyperspectral imaging (HSI) is an overall new and still quite unexplored field. Previous studies by our group have demonstrated the successful usage of medical hyperspectral imaging in the fields of wound diagnostics [11], perfusion monitoring after microsurgical anastomotic suturing in the rat hind limb and visualisation and quantification of the vasoactive effect of vasoconstrictor-containing local anaesthetics [12,13]. Following preliminary animal experiments [12], we were able to demonstrate the successful use of HSI to monitor free flaps in humans as part of a feasibility study [1]. The main limitation of this feasibility study was the limited number of compromised flaps, being the relevant variable to evaluate monitoring techniques. Therefore, the aim of this clinical study was to compare HSI and clinical monitoring in terms of their ability for early detection of impaired free flap perfusion.

## 2. Materials and Methods

### 2.1. Patients

In this prospective, non-randomized, clinical study, patients with free flaps for reconstruction of the oro-maxillofacial complex were included. The patient population consists of 40 males and 23 females. The average patient age was $62.2 \pm 12.6$ years. Due to its design, the sensor unit of the hyperspectral camera system was not able to image the posterior portion of the oropharynx. Therefore, free flaps of the anterior-lateral region of the maxilla and mandible, as well as exposed flaps of the facial region, were included in the present study. All flaps that did not have regular monitoring (t0–t10 for HSI and t4–t10 for clinical monitoring) were not included.

### 2.2. Monitoring

#### 2.2.1. Clinical Monitoring

Clinical monitoring started with the first postoperative control (t4) and was always performed prior to hyperspectral imaging to avoid examination bias. The measurement time points are shown in Figure 1. In each case, clinical parameters of flap perfusion (color, temperature, re-capillarization time and tissue turgor) were assessed and documented by an experienced physician. Point values were assigned to each clinical category (color, temperature, re-capillarization time, turgor). Criteria for surgical re-exploration were met if total was $\geq 9$ OR two variables scored 6 points OR flap color remained pale white or blue >60 min AND re-capillarization time was not detectable or <1 s (Table 1). Because clinical monitoring is still considered the gold standard, the final decision for re-exploration was always based on clinical assessment.

**Table 1.** Clinical flap evaluation system with point values.

| Flap Color | Flap Temperature | Re-Capillarization Time | Flap Turgor | Total |
|---|---|---|---|---|
| Pale white (3) | Cold (2) | Approx. 1 s (2) | Soft (2) | |
| Pink (1) | Body temperature (1) | >2 s (1) | Elastic (1) | |
| Red (2) | Superheated (2) | <1 s (3) | Plump (2) | |
| Blue (3) | | No capillary refill (3) | | |

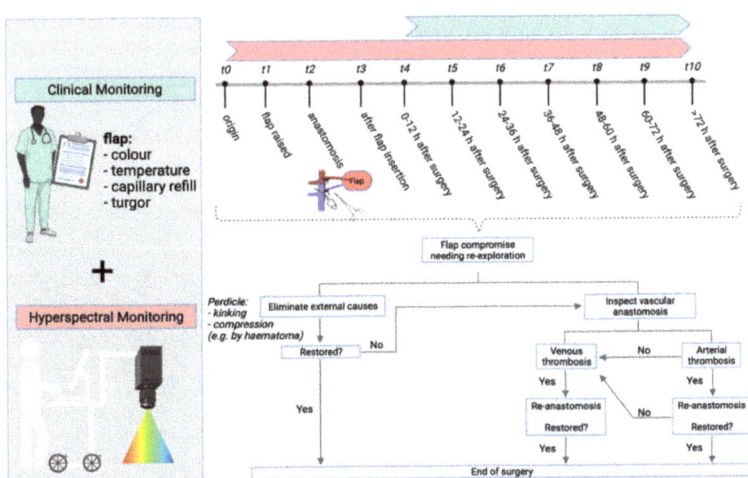

**Figure 1.** Graphical study protocol shows the measurement time points (t0–t3) and time intervals (t4–t10), as well as the process of decision making for re-exploration surgery. Created with BioRender.com (accessed on 13 October 2021).

2.2.2. Hyperspectral Monitoring

In this study, a hyperspectral sensor system (TIVITA™ Tissue System, Diaspective Vision GmbH, Pepelow, Germany) was used. The HSI sensors generate a three-dimensional (3D) data cube (hyperspectral cube), with the spatial information contained in the first two dimensions (resolution: 0.1 mm/pixel at 50 cm distance) and the spectral information in the third dimension (resolution: 5 nm). The method includes conventional as well as spectroscopic approaches to capture both spatial and spectral information of an image scene. While conventional RGB methods (red, green and blue) cover a limited wavelength spectrum, HSI is able to process electromagnetic wavelength spectra > 740 nm [14]. Briefly, HSI is based on the assessment of contiguous spectra (i.e., light of different wavelengths) individually re-emitted by molecules. These physicochemical raw data are then processed by computerized algorithms, specific for the respective molecule of interest (hyperspectral signatures), particularly haemoglobin, oxygenated haemoglobin and water [15,16]. Following HS-image recording over 10 s (s), additional 8 s are needed to compute a RGD (red, green and blue) truecolor image and additional four pseudo-color images, representing the parameters: tissue oxygen saturation [$StO_2$ (0–100%)], near infrared perfusion index [NPI as arbitrary units (0–100)] as well as distribution of haemoglobin [THI as arbitrary units (0–100)] and water [TWI as arbitrary units (0–100)] (Figure 2) [1,17]. Haemoglobin and its differentiation between its oxygenated and deoxygenated form plays a central role in HSI perfusion monitoring [15]. Since the absorbance of haemoglobin in the range from 570 to 590 nm is high, electromagnetic radiation of a shorter wavelength shows a lower penetration depth into tissue, thus microcirculation is detected at a depth up to 1 mm. $StO_2$ describes the relative oxygen saturation of blood in the microcirculatory system within superficial tissue layers, captures arterial and venous blood, and shows changes in oxygen supply and consumption directly in the tissue area measured. Thus, $StO_2$ represents the tissue oxygen saturation, which is mainly based on the blood volume in the venous part (75%) of the microcirculation and its oxygen saturation after delivery of oxygen to the tissue. Reference values are between 50–70% [18]. However, there are no thresholds, although corresponding studies are currently being conducted. Near-Perfusion-Index (NPI) describes the quality of blood flow which is determined by the relative oxygen saturation of the haemoglobin and the relative haemoglobin content in deep tissue layers (4 to 6 mm) [1]. In the software from the manufacturer, parameters are displayed in false colors from red = high, through yellow and green, to blue = low. The Tissue-Haemoglobin-Index (THI) describes the relative amount of haemoglobin in the microcirculatory system. This parameter gives information on inflow and/or outflow disorders. Tissue Water Index (TWI) describes the relative water content in the assessed region of interest. We have described the importance of the parameters and their combination for perfusion assessment in detail in a previous publication [1].

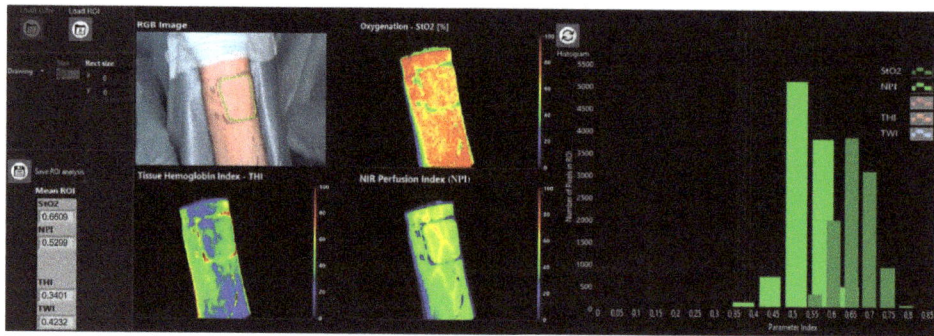

**Figure 2.** HSI shows the blood flow measured in the left ulnar flap raise site (t0) with the region of interest (ROI) marked manually (green line, RGB image). The quality of blood flow is indicated by false colors ranging from blue (low) to red (high). On the left, quantification of ROI is listed and shows mean values of the respective parameters (StO$_2$, NPI, THI, TWI). The number of assessed pixels and the corresponding amount of StO$_2$ and NPI within ROI (Y-axis) is represented as a bar chart.

*2.3. Statistics*

Raw data sets were saved in Excel® sheets (Microsoft Corporation, Redmond, WA, USA) and subsequently transferred into SPSS Statistics® (version 23.0.0.2, MacOS X; SPSS Inc., IBM Corporation, Armonk, NY, USA). Data were expressed as mean (m), standard deviation (SD±), minimum (min), maximum (max) and standard error of the mean (SEM). Normal distribution was checked using non-parametric Shapiro–Wilk-test(+) and Kolmogorov–Smirnov Test. In addition to the descriptive analysis, the dependency analysis included tests to detect/exclude differences and correlations. Results were analysed for statistical significance by the use of analysis of variance (ANOVA(#)), unpaired non-parametric Mann–Whitney U-tests($), Wilcoxon Signed Ranks test(§) and Students' *t*-test(*). To investigate whether the means of several dependent samples differ, Wilcoxon matched-pairs signed rank tests(**) were performed. Correlations between two categorical variables were tested using the Pearson Chi-Square Test(+) or, in the case of expected cell frequencies < 5, using Fisher's Exact Test(++). The eta-squared coefficient as a measure of correlation measures the extent to which the total variance of a dependent metric variable is explained by an independent nominal variable. The partial Eta square (Eta) shows how much % of the variation of "Duration of surgery" can be explained by the revision status (Group-1 vs. Group-2). The *p*-values of ≤0.05 were termed significant. Line charts with plotted means ±SD, pie charts, aligned dot plots and boxplots were used for illustration purposes. Due to the small number of similar studies, as well as the lack of cut-off values, case number planning could not be performed [19,20].

## 3. Results

A total of 54 primary and 11 secondary reconstructions were performed. Flaps included Radial-(RFF, 24) and Ulnar-(UFF, 16) Forearm flaps, Osteocutaneous Fibula flaps (OMFF, 16), Latissimus Dorsi flaps (LDF, 4), Osteocutaneous Scapula flaps (OMSF, 3) and 2 Upper Arm flaps (UAF). Affected regions included the tongue (4), cheek (18), floor of the mouth (10), alveolar ridge (2), soft (3) and hard palate (4), mandible (18), midface (4) and neurocranium (2). Recipient vessels were as follows: superior thyroid (43) (end-to-end), lingual (11) (end-to-end), external carotid (7) (end-to-side) and the facial artery (4) (end-to-end). Out of 65 flaps (two patients received 2 microvascular flaps each), re-exploration was performed in 19 cases (Group-2$^{(R+)}$) due to a clinically apparent perfusion disturbance, of which in one case no cause could be found intraoperatively. In the latter, because there was improved flap perfusion after reopening of the neck in both, clinical assessment and HSI, this case was considered kinking of the pedicle. A total of seven complete flap failures occurred, resulting in a salvage rate of 63% regardless of cause (haematoma, kinking, arterial or venous thrombosis). There was no correlation between the reconstruction regime (primary or secondary)$^{(++)}$, the irradiation status$^{(++)}$, the arterial recipient vessel type$^{(+)}$ or the duration of surgery (Eta = 0.06) and the occurrence of poor perfusion (need for revision) (Table 2).

Table 2. Baseline data showing patient and flap characteristics.

| | Group-1$^{(R+)}$ No Revision | Group-2$^{(R+)}$ Revision | Total (N) | p-Value |
|---|---|---|---|---|
| N | 46 | 19 | 65 | |
| Age | 64.2 ± 11.7 | 53.6 ± 18 | | 0.48$^{(+)}$ |
| Gender | | | | 0.10$^{(++)}$ |
| male | 26 (63%) | 15 (37%) | 41 | |
| female | 20 (83%) | 4 (17%) | 24 | |
| Indication | | | | |
| Malignant | 43 (73%) | 16 (27%) | 59 | |
| Benign | 1 (50%) | 1 (50%) | 2 | |
| Chronic wound | 2 (50%) | 2 (50%) | 4 | |
| Flap types | | | | 0.27$^{(+)}$ |
| RFF | 16 (66.6%) | 8 (33.3%) | 24 | |
| UFF | 13 (81%) | 3 (19%) | 16 | |
| OMFF | 13 (81.3%) | 3 (18.7%) | 16 | |
| LDF | 1 (25%) | 3 (75%) | 4 | |
| OMSF | 2 (66.6%) | 1 (33.3%) | 3 | |
| UAF | 1 (50%) | 1 (50%) | 2 | |
| Reconstruction regime | | | | 0.72$^{(++)}$ |
| Primary reconstruction | 39 (72%) | 15 (28%) | 54 | |
| Secondary reconstruction | 7 (63.6%) | 4 (36.4%) | 11 | |
| After radiotherapy | 6 (66.7%) | 3 (33.3%) | 9 | 0.71$^{(++)}$ |
| Recipient vessel (artery) | | | | 0.99$^{(+)}$ |
| Superior thyroid | 30 (70%) | 13 (30%) | 43 | |
| Lingual | 8 (72.7%) | 3 (27.3%) | 11 | |
| External carotid | 5 (71%) | 2 (29%) | 7 | |
| Facial | 3 (75%) | 1 (25%) | 4 | |
| Duration of surgery (minutes) | 543.7 ± 126.5 | 527.3 ± 128.1 | | 0.06$^{(Eta)}$ |
| Cause for malperfusion | | | | |
| Venous thrombosis | | 8 (42.1%) | 8 | |
| Arterial thrombosis | | 8 (36.8%) | 8 | |
| Haematoma | | 3 (4.6%) | 3 | |
| Kinking | | 1 (5.3%) | 1 | |

$^{+}$ = Chi-Square test; $^{++}$ = Fisher's Exact Test; $^{Eta}$ = Partial Eta square (explained in Section 2.3. *Statistics*).

## 3.1. Monitoring

### 3.1.1. Clinical Monitoring Characteristics

The true-positive rate of clinical assessment for detection of perfusion defect was 100% with 19/19 flaps. The distribution of scores obtained using the clinical scoring system is shown in Figure 3.

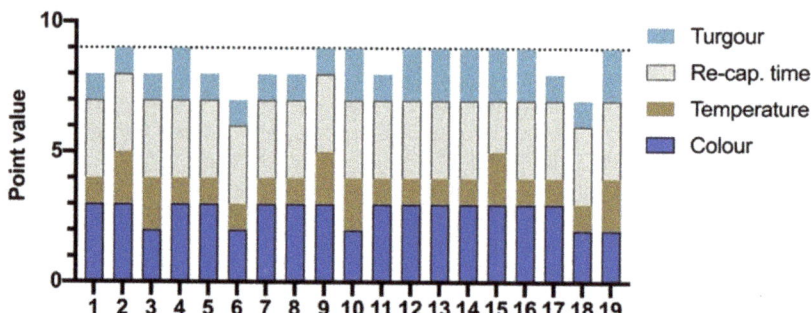

**Figure 3.** Bar chart shows the point total of clinical assessment from each impaired flap (Group-2(R+)) that led to re-exploration.

### 3.1.2. General HSI Characteristics for Non-Revised and Revised Flaps
Oxygen Saturation of Haemoglobin ($StO_2$)

Except t0 (origin), t1 (flap raise), t2 (anastomosis) and t3 (flap inset), $StO_2$ was significantly lower in Group-2(R+) at any time after flap inset including t4 (0–12 h; $p < 0.001$), t5 (12–24 h; $p = 0.034$), t6 (24–36 h; $p < 0.001$), t7 (36–48 h; $p = 0.008$), t8 (48–60 h, $p < 0.001$), and t10 (>72 h, $p = 0.004$) (Figure 4A). Compared with the reference site ($StO_2\Delta$reference), $StO_2$ decreased (%) significantly in Group-2(R+) during t4 ($p = 0.004$), t5 ($p < 0.001$), t6 ($p < 0.001$), t7 ($p = 0.002$), t8 ($p = 0.002$), and t10 ($p = 0.006^{(*)}$) compared to Group-1(R−) (Figure 4B). Compared with flap inset (t3), $StO_2$ significantly ($p = 0.011^{(*)}$) decreased at t4 in Group-2(R+) when compared to Group-1(R−) (Figure 4C). Regarding the difference to the pre-value ($StO_2\Delta$pre-value), $StO_2$ decreased significantly in Group-2(R+) during t4 ($p < 0.001^{(*)}$), t5 ($p = 0.021^{(*)}$), and t6 ($p < 0.001^{(*)}$) when compared to Group-1(R−), respectively (Figure 4D).

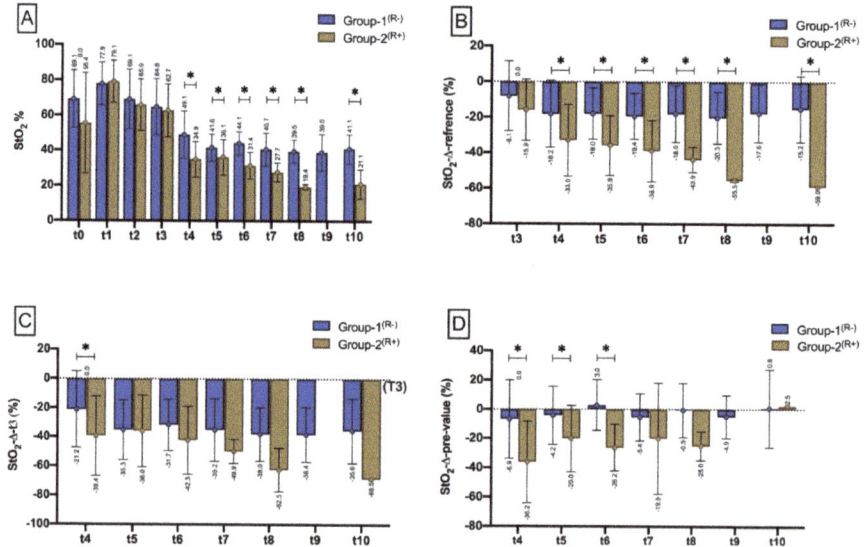

**Figure 4.** Bar chart with means (±SD) show $StO_2$ at different measurement timepoints (T0–T3)/time intervals (t4–t10) as (**A**) ($StO_2$ mean), (**B**) $StO_2$ drop to reference (%) $StO_2$ drop to the respective reference site ($StO_2\Delta$reference), (**C**) $StO_2$ drop to t3 ($StO_2\Delta$t3), and (**D**) in relation to the pre-measurement ($StO_2\Delta$pre-value). Means are shown scalar. Asterisk (*) marks existing significance.

NIR-Perfusion Index (NPI)

There was no difference in Near-Infrared Perfusion Index (NIR-P) between Group-1$^{(R-)}$ and Group-2$^{(R+)}$ before flap harvesting (T0), after flap raise (t1), after microvascular anastomosis (t2), and after flap insertion (t3). Within the first 12 h after flap inset, the Near-Infrared Perfusion-Index (NPI) was significantly lower in Group-2$^{(R+)}$ compared to Group-1$^{(R-)}$ ($p = 0.024^{(*)}$). The same was seen within t6 ($p = 0.008^{(*)}$) and t8 ($p = 0.045^{(*)}$), with the latter period containing only two compromised flaps that were subsequently re-explored (Figure 5A). Compared with the reference measurement site, Group-2$^{(R+)}$ revealed a significantly greater decrease in NPI (%) (NPIΔreference) at t4 ($p = 0.023^{(*)}$) compared to Group-1$^{(R-)}$ (Figure 5B). Compared with t3 (NPIΔt3), NPI decreased significantly more in Group-2$^{(R+)}$ at t4 ($p = 0.016^{(*)}$) and t6 ($p = 0.011^{(*)}$) than in Group-1$^{(R-)}$ (Figure 5C). Compared with the pre-measurement (NPIΔpre-value), the NPI drop was significantly higher in Group-2$^{(R+)}$ within the measurement intervals t4 ($p < 0.001^{(*)}$), t6 ($p = 0.044^{(\$)}$) and t8 ($p = 0.002^{(*)}$) than in Group-1$^{(R-)}$ (Figure 5D).

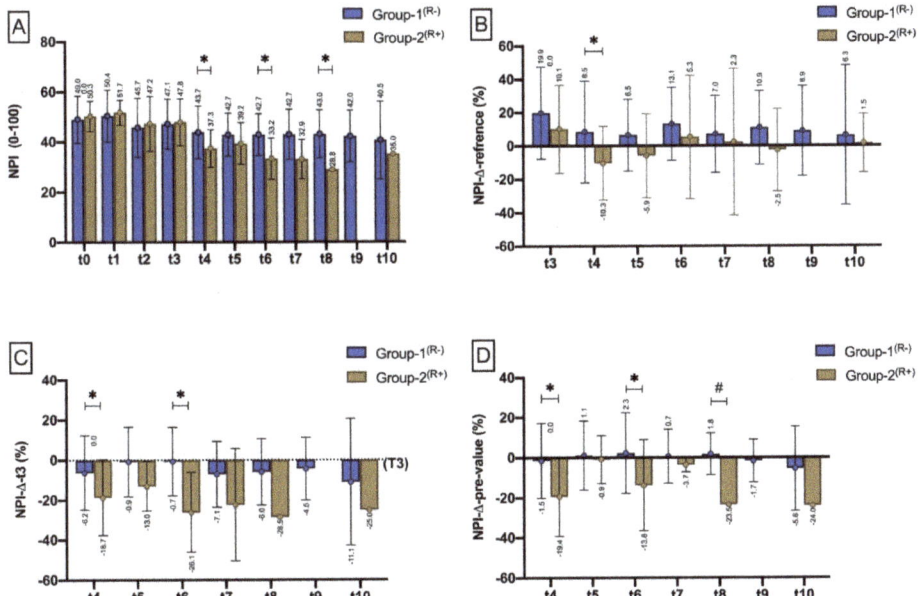

**Figure 5.** Bar chart with means (±SD) show NPI at different measurement timepoints (t0–t3)/time intervals (t4–t10) as (**A**) (NPI mean), (**B**) NPI drop to reference (%) NPI drop to the respective reference site (NPIΔreference), (**C**) NPI drop to t3 (NPIΔt3), and (**D**) in relation to the pre-measurement (NPIΔpre-value). Means are shown scalar. Asterisk (*) marks existing significance. ANOVA (#).

Tissue-Haemoglobin-Index (THI)

At the measurement time points (T0-t3)/within the measurement intervals (t4 and t5), the Tissue-Haemoglobin Index (THI) was not different between Group-2$^{(R+)}$ and Group-1$^{(R-)}$. At t6 ($p = 0.010^{(*)}$), t7 ($p = 0.006^{(*)}$) and t8 ($p = 0.033^{(*)}$), THI was significantly increased in Group-2$^{(R+)}$ (Figure 6A). In proportion to the reference site (THIΔreference), THI was significantly increased in Group-2$^{(R+)}$ compared with Group-1$^{(R)}$ during t6 ($p = 0.048^{(\$)}$) and t7 ($p = 0.048^{(\$)}$) (Figure 6B). Compared with flap inset (THIΔt3), THI was significantly higher in Group-2$^{(R+)}$ than in Group-1$^{(R-)}$ during t4 ($p = 0.011^{(\$)}$) and t7 ($p = 0.012^{(\$)}$) (Figure 6C). Compared with the pre-measurement (THIΔpre-value), the percentage increase in THI was significantly higher in Group-2$^{(R+)}$ within the measurement interval t4 ($p < 0.001^{(\$)}$) than in Group-1$^{(R-)}$ (Figure 6D).

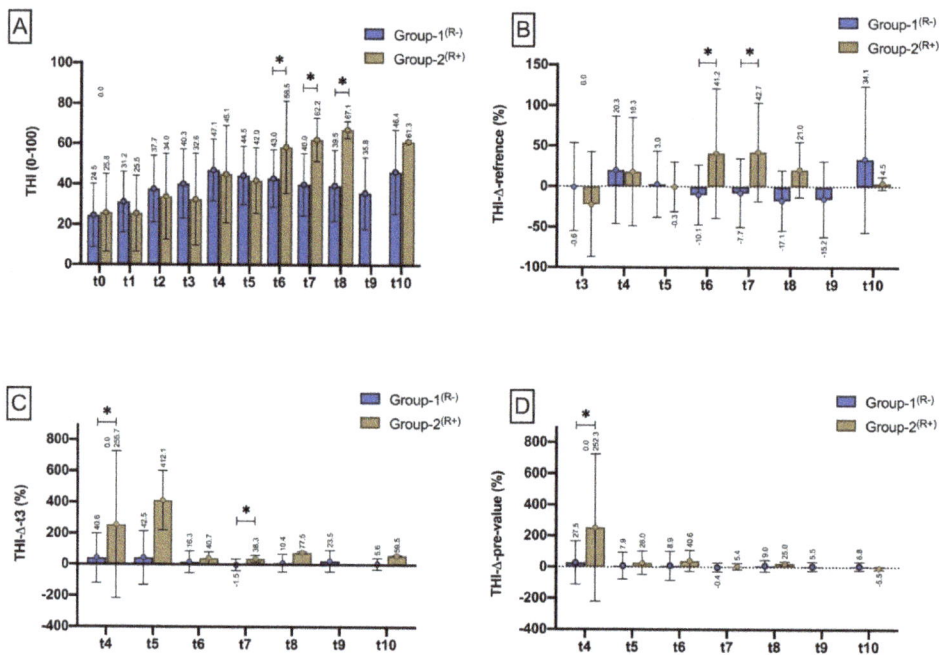

**Figure 6.** Bar chart with means (±SD) show THI at different measurement timepoints (t0–t3)/time intervals (t4–t10) as (**A**) (THI mean), (**B**) THI drop to reference (%) THI drop to the respective reference site (THIΔreference), (**C**) THI drop to t3 (THIΔt3), and (**D**) in relation to the pre-measurement (THIΔpre-value). Means are shown scalar. Asterisk (*) marks existing significance.

Tissue-Water-Index (TWI)

From t0 to t6, there was no difference in the water content (TWI) comparing Group-1[R−] and Group-2[R+]. At t7 and t8, TWI was found to be significantly lower ($p = 0.045$[*]; $p = 0.007$[*]) in the group of poorly perfused flaps (Figure 7A). Compared with the reference site (TWIΔreference), TWI was significantly lower at t8 ($p = 0.035$[$]) in Group-2[R+] than in Group-1[R−] (Figure 7B). Compared to flap inset (THIΔt3), TWI was significantly lower in Group-2[R+] at t6 ($p = 0.015$[$]), t7 ($p = 0.008$[$]) and t8 ($p = 0.002$[$]) (Figure 7C). Compared with the pre-measurement (TWIΔpre-value), TWI decreased significantly more in Group-2[R+] at t8 ($p = 0.002$[$]) (Figure 7D).

Duration until Signs of Malperfusion

Independent of the time point/interval, mean values of $StO_2$ and NPI as well as their drop rate (Δreference) differed significantly between Group-1[R−] and Group-2[R+] (Figure 8). $StO_2$, as well as $StO_2$Δreference were significantly lower in Group-2[R+] (32.6% ± 9.8; −38.1% ± 18.2) than in Group-1[R−] (43.2% ± 10.3; −18.3% ± 15.9) ($p < 0.001$). The same was seen with NPI (Group-1[R−]: 42.8 ± 9.8; Group-2[R+]: 32.9 ± 12.8) and NPIΔreference (Group-1[R−]: 8.8 ± 25.7; Group-2[R+]: −13.4% ± 36.9) ($p < 0.001$[*]).

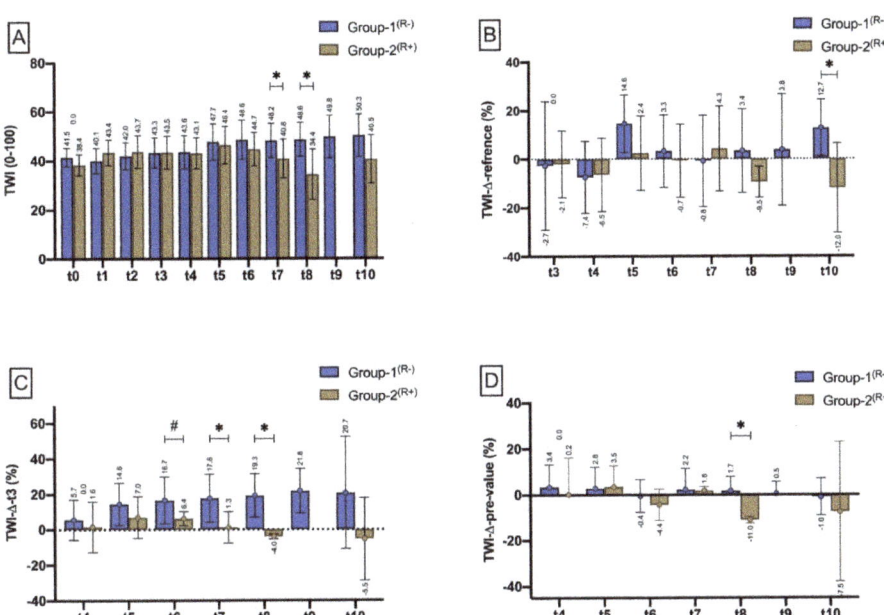

**Figure 7.** Bar chart with means (±SD) show TWI at different measurement timepoints (t0–t3)/time intervals (t4–t10) as (**A**) (TWI mean), (**B**) TWI drop to reference (%) TWI drop to the respective reference site (TWIΔreference), (**C**) TWI drop to t3 (TWIΔt3), and (**D**) in relation to the pre-measurement (TWIΔpre-value). Means are shown scalar. Asterisk (*) marks existing significance. ANOVA (#).

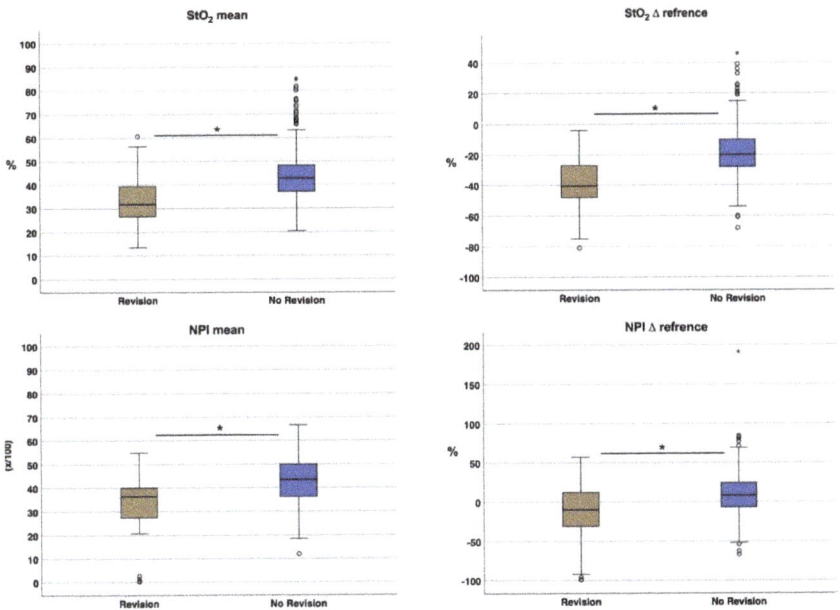

**Figure 8.** Boxplot showing the distribution of StO2, StO2Δreference, NPI and NPIΔreference comparing flaps with and without revision following poor perfusion. Asterisk (*) marks existing significance.

Of a total of 19 compromised flaps, 12 (36.8%) occurred within the first 24 h postoperatively. The exact distribution is shown in Figure 9A. To calculate the duration from flap inset (t3) to the detection of malperfusion in HSI, the mean values of $StO_2$ (32.6%), $StO_2\Delta$reference (−38.1%), NPI (32.9) and NPI$\Delta$reference (−13.4%) were used for dichotomization. If there was a negative deviation (<$StO_2$; <NPI; >$StO_2\Delta$reference; >NPI$\Delta$reference) from one of the parameters, the respective measurement time was counted as the detection time. Overall, the mean time from flap inset to decision making for re-exploration based on clinical assessment was 23.1 ± 21.9 h. In contrast, the average time from flap insertion to the appearance of hyperspectral criteria of inferior perfusion ($StO_2 \leq 32\%$ OR $StO_2$ diff > −38% OR NPI ≤ 32.9 OR NPI diff. ≥ −13.4%) was 18.2 ± 19.4 h, resulting in a difference of 4.8 ± 5 h ($p < 0.001^{(**)}$) (Figure 9B).

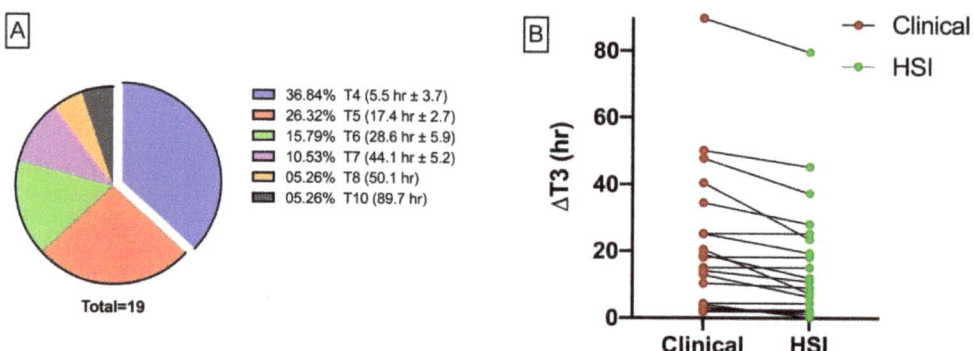

**Figure 9.** (**A**) Pie chart showing actual duration to clinical manifestation of flap malperfusion and subsequent re-exploration with associated time interval. (**B**) Aligned dot plot shows duration (h) from flap insertion to clinical (left) and hyperspectral detection of flap malperfusion.

## 4. Discussion

In this study, monitoring of free flap perfusion in the head and neck region was compared between clinical assessment and hyperspectral imaging. As the major finding, malperfusion could be detected at a mean of 4.8 h earlier with the help of Hyperspectral Imaging (HSI) when compared to clinical examination. In addition, general information on the perfusion characteristics of the included flap types were presented.

Postoperative flap monitoring is a key component for successful free tissue transfer whereby early detection of malperfusion is the pivotal criterion for treatment success as only early detection can ensure timely re-exploration to avoid flap failure [21]. One measure of this is the overall salvage rate which is reported to be from 60% up to 80% on average (63% in the present study) [22,23]. However, this neglects the subdivision according to the underlying cause (venous or arterial), with the salvage rate being significantly lower for arterial thrombosis [24]. To overcome the issue of delayed re-exploration due to late detection of malperfusion, several monitoring methods have been developed during the last decades, including the implantable Doppler, color duplex sonography, near-infrared spectroscopy, laser Doppler flowmetry, fluorescence angiography and microdialysis [10,25–28]. The ideal flap monitoring technique should be continuous, accurate, cost-efficient, non-invasive, safe, objective, recordable, reliable, reproducible, sensitive, highly spatially resolved, easy to use/interpret and applicable to all flap types [29]. As currently no single traditional monitoring technique meets all these requirements, clinical examination, as the least reproducible and little to no objective technique, still remains the most frequently used [10]. However, clinical assessment depends on evaluator experience and it is only reliable when the flap color changes significantly into pale or blueish [30]. In addition, technical monitoring support is only used by 30% of the surgeons whereas the Doppler (handheld or implanted) is the most commonly used method for free flap monitoring [31]. In addition to increased costs due to consumables and acquisition, the experience-dependent classification of measurement results is also cited as a limitation of technology-based monitoring techniques [30]. When color duplex ultrasound is used, microanastomotic vessels can also be visualized in embedded flaps. It is a non-invasive and quantitative flap monitoring technique, whereby its use requires special training. The implantable doppler is placed distal to an anastomosis in contact to the vessel, to allow continuous measurement of blood flow [32]. However, it is an invasive technique that does not allow quantitative measurement. Laser Doppler flowmetry (LDF) is also frequently used for monitoring of free flaps whereby probes are implanted or applied to the flap surface. In this context, Yoshino et al. could not distinguish between arterial and venous malperfusion when monitoring 37 intraoral free flaps with LDF [33]. In contrast, Muecke et al. demonstrated in an animal study that the combination of at least two different technical monitoring methods (ICG and flowmeter) improved the monitoring of critical and/or buried flaps, whereas the use of the multispectral technique (O2C) diminished the predictive value [34]. In contrast, Hölzle et al. described the successful use of O2C (Oxygen-to-see, LEA-Medizintechnik GmbH, Giessen, Germany), a device combination of laser doppler flowmeter and tissue spectrophotometry, to monitor free flaps and to detect flap malperfusion at an early stage [35]. Compared to multispectral methods, the use of the complete and high-resolution spectrum (hyperspectral) results in significantly increased reliability and reproducibility of parameter determination [36]. Providing non-contact, non-invasive measurements, HSI allows perfusion monitoring status in different tissue layers/depths through pictorial representation of parameters calculated from the spectra (tissue oxygenation saturation ($StO_2$), Near-Infrared Perfusion Index (NPI), Tissue Haemoglobin Index (THI), and Tissue Water Index (TWI)). Using the THI, additional conclusions can be drawn about the underlying cause of perfusion failure (venous versus arterial perfusion compromise) [1]. However, in the present study there was no significant correlation between $StO_2$ or NPI and THI. There were no signs of impaired flap perfusion at flap origin (t0), at flap/pedicle preparation (t1), directly after anastomosis (t2) or after flap inset (t3), as $StO_2$, NPI, THI and TWI did not differ significantly between Group $1^{(R-)}$ and $2^{(R+)}$. The characteristics of the blood flow dynamic of free flaps prior to the actual tissue transfer as well as its possible reasons have already been presented in a previous publication [1]. During t4, $StO_2$ was significantly lower on average in Group $2^{(R+)}$ (34.9 ± 10%) than in Group $1^{(R-)}$ (49.1 ± 13.5% $p < 0.001$). This, in turn, is in line with the earlier findings of our group, as well as with those of Kohler et al., defining 40% as the lower limit of $StO_2$ in normal perfused flaps [1,37]. In both of these pilot studies, the low number of malperfused flaps (<10) must be taken into account with regard to their significance. Deep tissue perfusion (represented by NPI) was also significantly lower (37.3 ± 7.5 $p < 0.001$) in Group $2^{(R+)}$ within the first 12 h (t4) in contrast to Group $1^{(R-)}$ (43.75 ± 10.52). No significant differences were found for THI and TWI.

Since $StO_2$ and NPI are not independent of systemic total haemoglobin (regarding the relationship between Hb and $StO_2$), we consider the drop rate (Δreference), as a measure of the systemic blood flow situation (adjacent reference site), providing high predictive value. This is in accordance with Keller et al. who stated the drop rate as a meaningful instrument [38]. In comparison between group $1^{(R-)}$ and $2^{(R+)}$, both $StO_2^{\Delta reference}$ and $NPI^{\Delta reference}$ were overall (t4–t10) significantly lower in group $2^{(R+)}$ (Figure 8). Previous studies on medical HSI were able to investigate its application in the field of visceral surgery, as well as plastic reconstructive surgery. In this context Barberio et al. implemented HSI as an intraoperative surgical guidance tool, using its capability of accurate detection and visualization of perfusion changes in the region of ischemic bowel segments [39]. The same group was able to demonstrate the successful usage of HSI and confocal laser endomicroscopy (CLE) for perfusion monitoring in esophageal surgery [40]. In a preclinical animal study, Chin et al. demonstrated the successful use of hyperspectral imaging for early detection of malperfusion in random axial flaps [41], as well as Grambow et al.

revealed real-time perfusion monitoring of the rats' hind limb after vessel transection and re-anastomosis [12]. Recent approaches have been able to successfully perform automated tissue classification and differentiation ex- and in-vivo based on hyperspectral cubes using deep learning algorithms (neural networks and computer vision) [14,42,43].

Disadvantages of HSI are a relevant dependence on ambient illumination, as well as the lack of applicability in heavily pigmented individuals due to extended light absorption. The issue of illumination particularly affects intraoral skin islands, but these can probably be better examined in the near future with a newly developed endoscope variant of the system used. Furthermore, the number of microvascular flaps included must be mentioned as a study-specific limitation, although the crucial number of poorly perfused flaps (19), presents a valuable and representative collective of the main subject. While the sensitivity to detect malperfusion is the same for clinical monitoring and HSI (100%), we demonstrated that HSI indicates poor perfusion significantly earlier (4.8 h).

## 5. Conclusions

On average, evidence of critical flap perfusion occurred 4.8 h earlier in hyperspectral imaging when compared to clinical assessment. Therefore, our findings provide an interpretation aid for clinicians to simplify postoperative flap monitoring.

**Author Contributions:** Conceptualization, D.G.E.T. and P.W.K.; methodology, D.G.E.T., P.R. and S.B.; validation, D.G.E.T., P.R., S.B. and P.W.K.; formal analysis, D.G.E.T., P.W.K., P.R. and S.B., investigation, D.G.E.T., S.B. and P.R.; resources, D.G.E.T. and P.W.K.; data curation, D.G.E.T.; writing—original draft preparation, D.G.E.T., P.W.K. and B.A.-N.; writing—review and editing, D.G.E.T., S.B., P.W.K., B.A.-N. and P.R.; visualization, D.G.E.T.; supervision, D.G.E.T. and P.W.K.; project administration, D.G.E.T., P.W.K. and B.A.-N. All authors have read and agreed to the published version of the manuscript.

**Funding:** This research received no external funding.

**Institutional Review Board Statement:** The study was approved by the local ethic committee of Rhineland-Palate (registration-number: 2019-14312) and was conducted in accordance with the protocol and in compliance with the moral, ethical, and scientific principles governing clinical research as set out in the Declaration of Helsinki of 1975 as revised in 1983.

**Informed Consent Statement:** Informed consent was obtained from all subjects involved in the study.

**Data Availability Statement:** All raw data on which this study is based will be made available by the corresponding author upon request.

**Conflicts of Interest:** The authors declare no conflict of interest.

## References

1. Thiem, D.G.E.; Frick, R.W.; Goetze, E.; Gielisch, M.; Al-Nawas, B.; Kammerer, P.W. Hyperspectral analysis for perioperative perfusion monitoring-a clinical feasibility study on free and pedicled flaps. *Clin. Oral Investig.* 2021, 25, 933–945. [CrossRef] [PubMed]
2. Rendenbach, C.; Holterhoff, N.; Hischke, S.; Kreutzer, K.; Smeets, R.; Assaf, A.T.; Heiland, M.; Wikner, J. Free flap surgery in Europe: An interdisciplinary survey. *Int. J. Oral Maxillofac. Surg.* 2018, 47, 676–682. [CrossRef] [PubMed]
3. Frederick, J.W.; Sweeny, L.; Carroll, W.R.; Peters, G.E.; Rosenthal, E.L. Outcomes in head and neck reconstruction by surgical site and donor site. *Laryngoscope* 2013, 123, 1612–1617. [CrossRef]
4. Kansy, K.; Mueller, A.A.; Mucke, T.; Koersgen, F.; Wolff, K.D.; Zeilhofer, H.F.; Holzle, F.; Pradel, W.; Schneider, M.; Kolk, A.; et al. Microsurgical reconstruction of the head and neck region: Current concepts of maxillofacial surgery units worldwide. *J. Craniomaxillofac. Surg.* 2015, 43, 1364–1368. [CrossRef]
5. Aksoyler, D.; Losco, L.; Bolletta, A.; Ercan, A.; Chen, S.H.; Velazquez-Mujica, J.; Tang, Y.B.; Chen, H.C. Three salvage strategies in microvascular fibula osteocutaneous flap for mandible reconstruction with vascular compromise and establishment of an algorithm. *Microsurgery* 2021, 41, 223–232. [CrossRef] [PubMed]
6. Sweeny, L.; Curry, J.; Crawley, M.; Cave, T.; Stewart, M.; Luginbuhl, A.; Heffelfinger, R.; Krein, H.; Petrisor, D.; Bender-Heine, A.; et al. Factors impacting successful salvage of the failing free flap. *Head Neck* 2020, 42, 3568–3579. [CrossRef]
7. Zeng, Y.C.; Bongrani, S.; Bronzetti, E.; Cadel, S.; Ricci, A.; Valsecchi, B.; Amenta, F. Influence of long-term treatment with L-deprenyl on the age-dependent changes in rat brain microanatomy. *Mech. Ageing Dev.* 1994, 73, 113–126. [CrossRef]

8. Chang, C.S.; Chu, M.W.; Nelson, J.A.; Basta, M.; Gerety, P.; Kanchwala, S.K.; Wu, L.C. Complications and Cost Analysis of Intraoperative Arterial Complications in Head and Neck Free Flap Reconstruction. *J. Reconstr. Microsurg.* **2017**, *33*, 318–327. [CrossRef]
9. Sweeny, L.; Rosenthal, E.L.; Light, T.; Grayson, J.; Petrisor, D.; Troob, S.H.; Greene, B.J.; Carroll, W.R.; Wax, M.K. Outcomes and cost implications of microvascular reconstructions of the head and neck. *Head Neck* **2019**, *41*, 930–939. [CrossRef]
10. Kohlert, S.; Quimby, A.E.; Saman, M.; Ducic, Y. Postoperative Free-Flap Monitoring Techniques. *Semin. Plast. Surg.* **2019**, *33*, 13–16. [CrossRef]
11. Holmer, A.; Marotz, J.; Wahl, P.; Dau, M.; Kammerer, P.W. Hyperspectral imaging in perfusion and wound diagnostics—Methods and algorithms for the determination of tissue parameters. *Biomed. Tech. Eng.* **2018**, *63*, 547–556. [CrossRef]
12. Grambow, E.; Dau, M.; Holmer, A.; Lipp, V.; Frerich, B.; Klar, E.; Vollmar, B.; Kammerer, P.W. Hyperspectral imaging for monitoring of perfusion failure upon microvascular anastomosis in the rat hind limb. *Microvasc. Res.* **2018**, *116*, 64–70. [CrossRef] [PubMed]
13. Thiem, D.G.E.; Hans, L.; Blatt, S.; Römer, P.; Heimes, D.; Al-Nawas, B.; Kämmerer, P.W. Hyperspectral Imaging to Study Dynamic Skin Perfusion after Injection of Articaine-4% with and without Epinephrine—Clinical Implications on Local Vasoconstriction. *J. Clin. Med.* **2021**, *10*, 3411. [CrossRef] [PubMed]
14. Halicek, M.; Fabelo, H.; Ortega, S.; Callico, G.M.; Fei, B. In-Vivo and Ex-Vivo Tissue Analysis through Hyperspectral Imaging Techniques: Revealing the Invisible Features of Cancer. *Cancers* **2019**, *11*, 756. [CrossRef]
15. Chen, P.C.; Lin, W.C. Spectral-profile-based algorithm for hemoglobin oxygen saturation determination from diffuse reflectance spectra. *Biomed. Opt. Express* **2011**, *2*, 1082–1096. [CrossRef] [PubMed]
16. Steinke, J.M.; Shepherd, A.P. Effects of temperature on optical absorbance spectra of oxy-, carboxy-, and deoxyhemoglobin. *Clin. Chem.* **1992**, *38*, 1360–1364. [CrossRef]
17. Bashkatov, A.N.; Genina, E.A.; Kochubey, V.I.; Tuchin, V.V. Optical properties of human skin, subcutaneous and mucous tissues in the wavelength range from 400 to 2000 nm. *J. Phys. D Appl. Phys.* **2005**, *38*, 2543–2555. [CrossRef]
18. Bickler, P.E.; Feiner, J.R.; Rollins, M.D. Factors affecting the performance of 5 cerebral oximeters during hypoxia in healthy volunteers. *Anesth. Analg.* **2013**, *117*, 813–823. [CrossRef]
19. McAdams, D.R.; Stapels, C.J.; Kolodziejski, N.J.; Chung, Y.G.; Vishwanath, K.; Helton, M.C.; Pakela, J.M.; Lee, S.Y. Compact dual-mode diffuse optical system for blood perfusion monitoring in a porcine model of microvascular tissue flaps. *J. Biomed. Opt.* **2017**, *22*, 1–14. [CrossRef]
20. Khan, M.; Pretty, C.G.; Amies, A.C.; Balmer, J.; Banna, H.E.; Shaw, G.M.; Geoffrey Chase, J. Proof of concept non-invasive estimation of peripheral venous oxygen saturation. *Biomed. Eng. Online* **2017**, *16*, 60. [CrossRef]
21. Mucke, T.; Rau, A.; Merezas, A.; Loeffelbein, D.J.; Wagenpfeil, S.; Mitchell, D.A.; Wolff, K.D.; Steiner, T. Identification of perioperative risk factor by laser-doppler spectroscopy after free flap perfusion in the head and neck: A prospective clinical study. *Microsurgery* **2014**, *34*, 345–351. [CrossRef]
22. Chae, M.P.; Rozen, W.M.; Whitaker, I.S.; Chubb, D.; Grinsell, D.; Ashton, M.W.; Hunter-Smith, D.J.; Lineaweaver, W.C. Current evidence for postoperative monitoring of microvascular free flaps: A systematic review. *Ann. Plast. Surg.* **2015**, *74*, 621–632. [CrossRef] [PubMed]
23. Kudpaje, A.; Thankappan, K.; Rajan, R.P.; Vidhyadharan, S.; Balasubramanian, D.; Wakure, A.; Mathew, J.; Sharma, M.; Iyer, S. Outcomes of Re-exploration Procedures After Head and Neck Free Flap Reconstruction. *Indian J. Surg. Oncol.* **2021**, *12*, 530–537. [CrossRef]
24. Bui, D.T.; Cordeiro, P.G.; Hu, Q.-Y.; Disa, J.J.; Pusic, A.; Mehrara, B.J. Free Flap Reexploration: Indications, Treatment, and Outcomes in 1193 Free Flaps. *Plast. Reconstr. Surg.* **2007**, *119*, 2092–2100. [CrossRef]
25. Holzle, F.; Rau, A.; Loeffelbein, D.J.; Mucke, T.; Kesting, M.R.; Wolff, K.D. Results of monitoring fasciocutaneous, myocutaneous, osteocutaneous and perforator flaps: 4-year experience with 166 cases. *Int. J. Oral Maxillofac. Surg.* **2010**, *39*, 21–28. [CrossRef]
26. Abdel-Galil, K.; Mitchell, D. Postoperative monitoring of microsurgical free-tissue transfers for head and neck reconstruction: A systematic review of current techniques–part II. Invasive techniques. *Br. J. Oral Maxillofac. Surg.* **2009**, *47*, 438–442. [CrossRef] [PubMed]
27. Dakpe, S.; Colin, E.; Bettoni, J.; Davrou, J.; Diouf, M.; Devauchelle, B.; Testelin, S. Intraosseous microdialysis for bone free flap monitoring in head and neck reconstructive surgery: A prospective pilot study. *Microsurgery* **2020**, *40*, 315–323. [CrossRef]
28. Hitier, M.; Cracowski, J.L.; Hamou, C.; Righini, C.; Bettega, G. Indocyanine green fluorescence angiography for free flap monitoring: A pilot study. *J. Craniomaxillofac. Surg.* **2016**, *44*, 1833–1841. [CrossRef] [PubMed]
29. Chao, A.H.; Lamp, S. Current approaches to free flap monitoring. *Plast. Surg. Nurs.* **2014**, *34*, 52–56. [CrossRef] [PubMed]
30. Kwasnicki, R.M.; Noakes, A.J.; Banhidy, N.; Hettiaratchy, S. Quantifying the Limitations of Clinical and Technology-based Flap Monitoring Strategies using a Systematic Thematic Analysis. *Plast. Reconstr. Surg. Glob. Open* **2021**, *9*, e3663. [CrossRef]
31. Patel, U.A.; Hernandez, D.; Shnayder, Y.; Wax, M.K.; Hanasono, M.M.; Hornig, J.; Ghanem, T.A.; Old, M.; Jackson, R.S.; Ledgerwood, L.G.; et al. Free Flap Reconstruction Monitoring Techniques and Frequency in the Era of Restricted Resident Work Hours. *JAMA Otolaryngol. Head Neck Surg.* **2017**, *143*, 803–809. [CrossRef]
32. Leibig, N.; Ha-Phuoc, A.; Stark, G.B.; Schmelzeisen, R.; Metzger, M.C.; Eisenhardt, S.U.; Voss, P.J. Retrospective evaluation of diagnostic accuracy of free flap monitoring with the Cook-Swartz-Doppler probe in head and neck reconstruction. *J. Craniomaxillofac. Surg.* **2019**, *47*, 1973–1979. [CrossRef] [PubMed]

33. Yoshino, K.; Nara, S.; Endo, M.; Kamata, N. Intraoral free flap monitoring with a laser Doppler flowmeter. *Microsurgery* **1996**, *17*, 337–340. [CrossRef]
34. Mucke, T.; Hapfelmeier, A.; Schmidt, L.H.; Fichter, A.M.; Kanatas, A.; Wolff, K.D.; Ritschl, L.M. A comparative analysis using flowmeter, laser-Doppler l spectrophotometry, and indocyanine green-videoangiography for detection of vascular stenosis in free flaps. *Sci. Rep.* **2020**, *10*, 939. [CrossRef]
35. Holzle, F.; Loeffelbein, D.J.; Nolte, D.; Wolff, K.D. Free flap monitoring using simultaneous non-invasive laser Doppler flowmetry and tissue spectrophotometry. *J. Craniomaxillofac. Surg.* **2006**, *34*, 25–33. [CrossRef]
36. Kulcke, A.; Holmer, A.; Wahl, P.; Siemers, F.; Wild, T.; Daeschlein, G. A compact hyperspectral camera for measurement of perfusion parameters in medicine. *Biomed. Tech. Eng.* **2018**, *63*, 519–527. [CrossRef]
37. Kohler, L.H.; Kohler, H.; Kohler, S.; Langer, S.; Nuwayhid, R.; Gockel, I.; Spindler, N.; Osterhoff, G. Hyperspectral Imaging (HSI) as a new diagnostic tool in free flap monitoring for soft tissue reconstruction: A proof of concept study. *BMC Surg* **2021**, *21*, 222. [CrossRef] [PubMed]
38. Keller, A. A new diagnostic algorithm for early prediction of vascular compromise in 208 microsurgical flaps using tissue oxygen saturation measurements. *Ann. Plast. Surg.* **2009**, *62*, 538–543. [CrossRef]
39. Barberio, M.; Longo, F.; Fiorillo, C.; Seeliger, B.; Mascagni, P.; Agnus, V.; Lindner, V.; Geny, B.; Charles, A.L.; Gockel, I.; et al. HYPerspectral Enhanced Reality (HYPER): A physiology-based surgical guidance tool. *Surg. Endosc.* **2020**, *34*, 1736–1744. [CrossRef] [PubMed]
40. Barberio, M.; Felli, E.; Pizzicannella, M.; Agnus, V.; Al-Taher, M.; Seyller, E.; Moulla, Y.; Jansen-Winkeln, B.; Gockel, I.; Marescaux, J.; et al. Quantitative serosal and mucosal optical imaging perfusion assessment in gastric conduits for esophageal surgery: An experimental study in enhanced reality. *Surg. Endosc.* **2021**, *35*, 5827–5835. [CrossRef]
41. Chin, M.S.; Chappell, A.G.; Giatsidis, G.; Perry, D.J.; Lujan-Hernandez, J.; Haddad, A.; Matsumine, H.; Orgill, D.P.; Lalikos, J.F. Hyperspectral Imaging Provides Early Prediction of Random Axial Flap Necrosis in a Preclinical Model. *Plast. Reconstr. Surg.* **2017**, *139*, 1285e–1290e. [CrossRef] [PubMed]
42. Halicek, M.; Dormer, J.D.; Little, J.V.; Chen, A.Y.; Myers, L.; Sumer, B.D.; Fei, B. Hyperspectral Imaging of Head and Neck Squamous Cell Carcinoma for Cancer Margin Detection in Surgical Specimens from 102 Patients Using Deep Learning. *Cancers* **2019**, *11*, 1367. [CrossRef] [PubMed]
43. Thiem, D.G.E.; Romer, P.; Gielisch, M.; Al-Nawas, B.; Schluter, M.; Plass, B.; Kammerer, P.W. Hyperspectral imaging and artificial intelligence to detect oral malignancy-part 1-automated tissue classification of oral muscle, fat and mucosa using a light-weight 6-layer deep neural network. *Head Face Med.* **2021**, *17*, 38. [CrossRef] [PubMed]

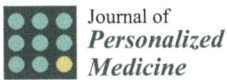

Article

# Personalized Reconstruction of Genital Defects in Complicated Wounds with Vertical Rectus Abdominis Myocutaneous Flaps including Urethral Neo-Orifice

Raymund E. Horch *, Ingo Ludolph, Andreas Arkudas and Aijia Cai

Department of Plastic and Hand Surgery and Laboratory for Tissue Engineering and Regenerative Medicine, University Hospital Erlangen, Friedrich Alexander University Erlangen-Nuernberg FAU, 91054 Erlangen, Germany; ingo.ludolph@uk-erlangen.de (I.L.); andreas.arkudas@uk-erlangen.de (A.A.); aijia.cai@uk-erlangen.de (A.C.)
* Correspondence: raymund.horch@uk-erlangen.de; Tel.: +49-9131-85-33296; Fax: +49-9131-85-39327

**Abstract:** Non-healing extensive wounds in the perineal region can lead to severe soft tissue infections and disastrous complications, which are not manageable with conservative measures. Specifically in recurrent or advanced pelvic malignancies, irradiation often leads to extensive scarring and wound breakdown, resulting in significant soft tissue defects during surgical tumor excision. Among several surgical options to reconstruct the perineum, the transpelvic vertical rectus abdominis myocutaneous (VRAM) flap has proven to be one of the most reliable methods. Specific modifications of this flap allow an individualized procedure depending on the patient's needs. We modified this technique to include the urethral orifice into the skin paddle of VRAM flaps in three patients as a novel option to circumvent urinary diversion and maintain an acceptable quality of life.

**Keywords:** perineal reconstruction; VRAM flap; neourethra; urethral reconstruction

## 1. Introduction

Perineal, genital and vulvar or scrotal defects often occur after infections or cancer treatment, and are difficult to handle by conservative measures. As for the former, Fournier gangrene, a necrotizing fasciitis of the perineum and external genitals, is a life-threatening disease, which mainly affects male patients. Its main treatment includes aggressive debridement, resulting in extensive soft tissue defects in the perineal region [1]. As for the latter, irradiated relapsing vulva, anal or rectal cancer can lead to severe soft tissue infections and disastrous wounds that significantly impede the patient´s quality of life. In current modern oncological concepts of far advanced cases of pelvic malignancies, chemoradiotherapy is an established therapy. It may provide temporary symptomatic relief; however, it can deteriorate existing wounds [2–7]. Neoadjuvant radiotherapy can lead to wound breakdown, urinary and sexual problems, as well as postoperative bowel dysfunction [8]. Furthermore, exposition of the pelvic floor after pelvic exenteration often creates a risk of intestinal fistulas, and prior irradiation increases this risk [9].

The usefulness of a transpelvic vertical rectus abdominis myocutaneous (VRAM) flap has been extensively demonstrated as a method of choice to revascularize irradiated pelvic floor defects and to reconstruct the vagina [6,10–14]. From our experiences with more than 300 patients receiving VRAM flaps for pelvic, perineal and vaginal reconstruction, we previously published the reconstruction of postoncological perineal and vaginal defects in 142 female patients [12]. The more seldom extrapelvic route of VRAM flap transfer has been described in cases where laparotomy is not necessary for tumor resection [15]. In the case of perineal defects due to Fournier gangrene, the VRAM flap has only been used for extensive defects due to its bulkiness [16,17].

The majority of patients with pelvic malignancies who undergo exenteration need urinary diversion, e.g., in the form of an ileocolonic reservoir [18]. However, this often comes

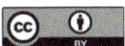

with complications such as ureteral strictures, pyelonephritis, difficulty in catheterization, or urinary stones [19]. Health-related quality of life is known to be negatively affected by a urostomy, leading to less participation in recreational activities and avoidance of social relationships [20].

We report on the extension of the surgical algorithm in reconstruction of complicated perineal wounds with VRAM flaps, utilizing an extrapelvic or transpelvic route combined with the creation of a neo-urethral orifice into the skin paddle of the VRAM flap in three patients. With this novel method, one can circumvent urinary diversion and maintain a better quality of life.

## 2. Patients and Methods

### 2.1. Technique of Surgery

The technique of harvesting of the VRAM flap and its translocation to the perineal area in an intrapelvic manner has been described in detail [10,21,22]. Briefly, a vertically oriented abdominal skin island is planned according to the (prospective) defect size in the perineal area and placed over the rectus muscle, preferably the right one. After the skin island is incised down to the anterior rectus sheath, the rectus muscle is raised from top to bottom after ligation of the superior epigastric vessels. During this procedure, the posterior rectus sheath is left intact and the skin island remains connected to the underlying muscle. The inferior epigastric vessels are visualized and dissected down to the external iliac vessels.

In the case of pelvic exenteration, a transpelvic translocation of the VRAM flap is used, and the attachment of the rectus abdominis muscle to the pubic bone is released, giving care to preserve the vascular pedicle by leaving the pyramidal component of the muscle insertion. Depending on the area to be reconstructed, the flap is then rotated at 180 degrees either into the pelvic cavity so that the skin paddle closes the defect with the proximal part facing the sacrum or it is transposed into the defect via a wide subcutaneous tunnel. By splitting a part of the skin paddle, a neovaginal orifice can be created if necessary.

When the urethra is maintained with a sufficient stump as in this series, a urethral orifice is created in the middle of the skin flap. The prospective location of the neourethra is marked on the skin paddle and the rectus muscle is carefully incised, preserving the epigastric vessels. The incision is continued through the skin paddle. A urinary catheter is pulled through the created orifice and placed into the remaining urethra. After the VRAM flap is sutured into the defect site, the bulky fat tissue of the skin island overlying the new orifice is carefully removed so that the urethral tissue can be sutured to the overlying skin with absorbable sutures.

An extrapelvic route can be used in cases where there is no need to occlude any dead space in the pelvis as is presented in this series. In this case, attachment of the rectus abdominis muscle to the pubic bone is left intact and a subcutaneous tunnel is created between the rectus muscle and the tissue of the pubic region until the defect site is reached. The muscle is carefully pulled through the subcutaneous tunnel, giving care not to stress the vascular pedicle. The neourethra can be reconstructed in case of a sufficient remaining urethral stump, as described above (Figure 1).

In both cases, the rectus sheath is reconstructed with an alloplastic mesh and the abdominal skin can be directly closed [22]. If necessary, indocyanine green angiography can be used to confirm adequate flap perfusion at the end of the surgery [23,24].

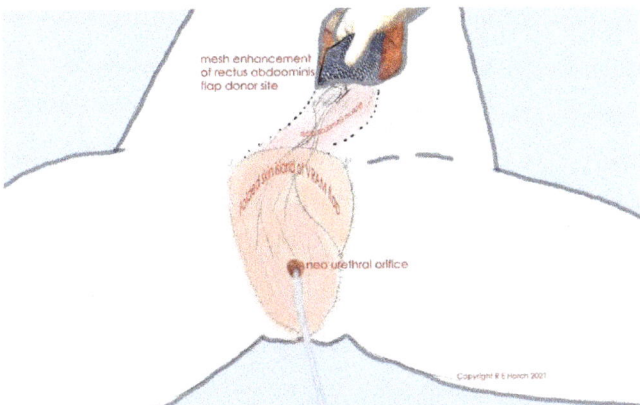

**Figure 1.** Schematic illustration of folded skin island of VRAM flap and neourethral orifice as well as of rectus abdominis muscle, tunneled subcutaneously. The flap donor site is closed with alloplastic mesh.

*2.2. Case 1*

A 67-year-old female patient with recurrent melanoma of the vulva had undergone prior skinning vulvectomy, inguinal lymphadenectomy, radiotherapy, and chemotherapy. She further developed liver metastasis and chronic pain of the vulva, impeding sitting. A necrotic tumor, measuring 6 cm could be inspected in the vaginal introitus. An interdisciplinary surgical procedure was performed with the gynecologists, which included radical vulvectomy, bilateral colpectomy, resection of the distal urethral, which was also infiltrated by the tumor. The resulting defect was reconstructed with an extrapelvic VRAM flap with a $30 \times 12$ cm$^2$ big skin paddle. Because intraoperative frozen sections of the resection margin of the distal urethra were tumor-free, a reconstruction of the remaining urethra was performed. For this purpose, a urinary catheter was tunneled through the middle of the VRAM flap, protecting the vascular pedicle, and inserted into the bladder through the remaining urethra. During the postoperative course, the VRAM flap healed without any complications, and the urinary catheter remained in the flap until the patient was discharged. A cystoscopy before discharge revealed no abnormalities. The patient received adjuvant chemotherapy in the Department of Dermatology and succumbed half a year later due to progressive multiple metastases, but expressed a comparatively good quality of life in terms of the defect reconstruction and the possibility to urinate through the neo-orifice.

*2.3. Case 2*

A 79-year-old female patient with recurrent vulva carcinoma had undergone multiple tumor excisions, lymphadenectomy, and radiotherapy. Another tumor recurrence eventually led to colpectomy, partial urethral resection, and brachytherapy. Half a year later, she was diagnosed with another recurrence, occupying the whole right labia. Furthermore, the rectum was infiltrated by the tumor. An interdisciplinary surgical procedure was performed with the gynecologists and the general surgeons, which involved a radical vulvectomy and excision of the rectum, respectively. Parts of the remaining urethra were also excised and analyzed via intraoperative frozen sections, which showed no signs of tumor infiltration. The resulting defect was reconstructed with a transpelvic VRAM flap with a $21 \times 7$ cm$^2$ big skin paddle according to the defect size. A neourethra was created with the remaining parts of the urethra as described above. A urinary catheter was inserted through the neourethra in the VRAM flap and into the remaining urethra. The VRAM flap healed without any complications and the patient succumbed one month later due to the progressive tumor disease.

## 2.4. Case 3

A 68-year-old male patient with a history of dilated cardiomyopathy, atrial fibrillation, hypertension, diabetes, and obesity developed Fournier gangrene after left epididymitis, which led to radical debridement of the perineal region, including left orchiectomy and penectomy (Figure 2).

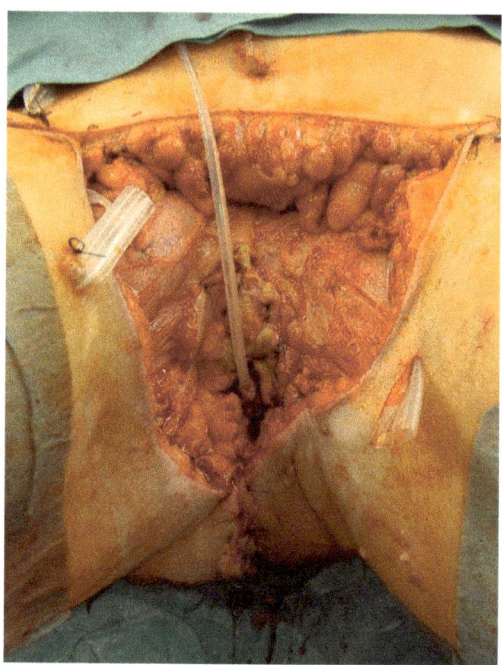

**Figure 2.** Extensive defect after radical debridement including penectomy for Fournier gangrene in a 68-year-old male patient. Urinary catheter is inserted into the remaining urethra.

He received a suprapubic cystostomy and a diverting colostomy. After the wound was conditioned via vacuum-assisted closure (Figure 3), reconstruction of the extensive wound was performed via an extrapelvic VRAM flap (Figure 1).

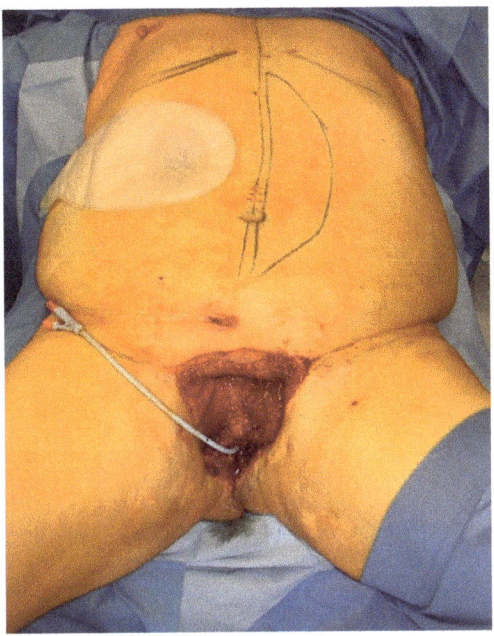

**Figure 3.** After adequate debridement, defect reconstruction was planned with an extrapelvic VRAM flap from the left abdomen. Skin paddle is marked.

A urinary catheter was tunneled through the middle of the VRAM flap, protecting the vascular pedicle, and inserted into the bladder through the remaining proximal urethra, measuring 2 cm (Figure 4). Afterwards, the flap was sutured into the defect and showed adequate perfusion (Figure 5).

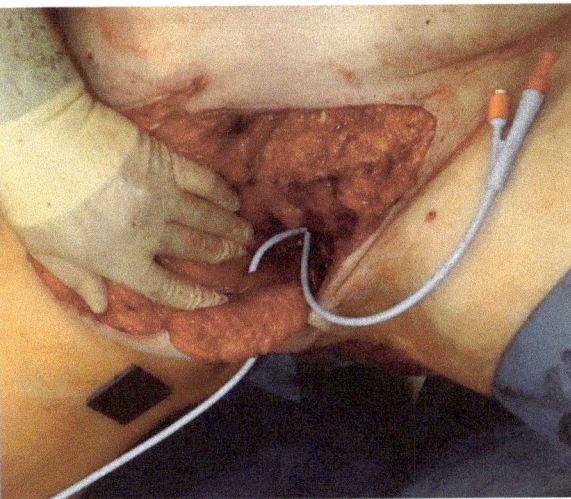

**Figure 4.** The VRAM flap was tunneled subcutaneously in an extrapelvic route to be placed into the perineal defect. A urinary catheter was tunneled through the middle of the VRAM flap and into the bladder through the remaining urethra. The old urinary catheter is still in place.

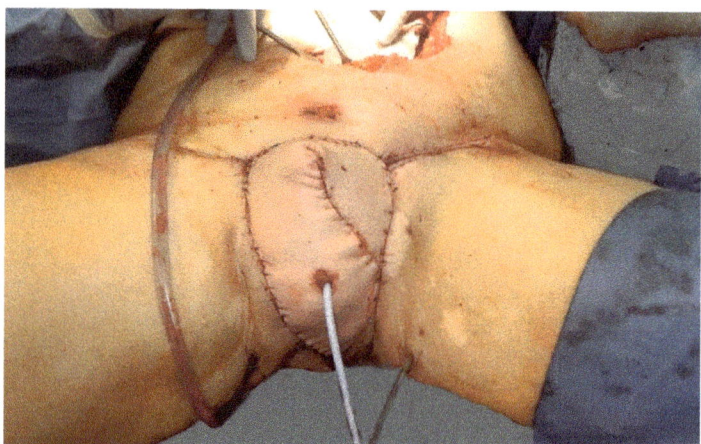

**Figure 5.** Immediate postoperative results after flap inset and reconstruction of the neourethra.

A few days later, the patient developed a hematoma under the flap, making surgical revision necessary. After hemostasis, the resulting wound was partially left open due to excessive swelling of the flap. Vacuum-assisted closure was applied and when swelling was reduced after several days, the defect was partially closed and partially reconstructed with a split-thickness skin graft. The patient developed renal insufficiency, which was managed by fluid resuscitation. A symptomatic pleural effusion was drained adequately. The further postoperative course was then uneventful and both the flap and the skin graft healed properly. The patient developed melanoma of his eye a few years later, leading to enucleation of his right eye. He paid regular visits to the urological department for changing his urinary catheter and was satisfied with the neo-orifice in the VRAM flap that he felt as an approvement compared to his intermediate previous situation.

## 3. Discussion

The VRAM flap has been a valuable tool for pelvic floor reconstruction in conjunction with oncological surgery of pelvic malignancies [6,10,12,21,22]. Gentileschi et al. have alternatively propagated the use of anterior lateral thigh (ALT) perforator flaps for reconstruction after vulvar cancer extirpative surgery due to a lower donor site morbidity [25]. There are certainly several reconstructive options to deal with defects in this context [21]. The VRAM flap is particularly suitable for cases of simultaneous reconstruction after tumor resection through an open laparotomy. In cases of secondary reconstruction, where a laparotomy is not indicated, alternative flaps can be used. However, there may be some limitations to harvesting a pedicled flap from the thigh when neoadjuvant extensive irradiation of the groin or thigh has been performed and lymphatic backflow in the extremity is compromised, resulting in donor site complication [26]. In the case of pelvic exenteration dead space, Gentileschi et al. harvested vastus lateralis muscle with the ALT flap [25]. Similar to standard bowel diversions through a rectus muscle, the vastus lateralis muscle may act as an additional buffer unlike a fasciocutaneous flap. Thus, we believe in the benefits of well-perfused muscle as can be found in a (transpelvic) VRAM flap to reconstruct irradiated perineal, vaginal, and/or gluteal regions. We were able to show an enormous improvement of both wound healing and quality of life in female patients with advanced or relapsing rectal, anal, or vaginal cancer. Patients did not report significant impairment in terms of sexual function as is commonly the case after abdominoperineal excision or low anterior excision and neoadjuvant radiotherapy as part of rectal cancer treatment [8,12]. Obviously, VRAM flap reconstruction leads to a lower complication rate after radical pelvic exenteration than in patients without a flap reconstruction, even though the extent of resection is usually larger and cancer disease is more advanced in those patients receiving radical pelvic exenteration. In addition, pelvic floor repair with a transpelvic VRAM flap reduces the number of perineal herniations when compared to primarily closed patients without flaps [27]. Modifications of the flap include splitting the distal portion longitudinally to produce "tongue" flaps to resurface vaginal and anal surfaces and creation of a neovaginal orifice through the central portion [15,28]. To our knowledge, creation of a neourethra by suturing the remaining stump to the surrounding tissue of the skin island has not been described as a modification of the VRAM flap so far.

Bregendahl et al. were able to show urinary dysfunction is also common in women after treatment for rectal cancer, especially after preoperative radiotherapy [8]. However, other malignancies such as vulvar cancer also necessitate (partial) urethral resection in the case of tumor infiltration, which might cause urinary tract dysfunction [29]. Reports on urethral reconstruction are scarce. Franchi et al. created a urethral neomeatus with vaginal mucosa in cases of partial urethrectomy [29]. However, in cases of radical pelvic exenteration, this option is not available. In male patients, the radial forearm free flap is the gold standard for reconstruction of the penis as well as the neourethra after penectomy or in terms of gender assigning surgery [30]. Phalloplasty with a radial forearm free flap has even been reported in a case after penectomy for Fournier gangrene. The reconstruction was successful even though the patient presented with comorbidities typical for those patients experiencing Fournier gangrene [31]. However, in the acute setting when the patient is in need of a safe and reliable reconstruction of an extensive defect, microsurgical procedures are not an option in those multimorbid patients. Fournier gangrene is a rapidly progressive necrotizing fasciitis of the genital and perineal tissues with a high mortality rate. Initial treatment includes radical surgical debridement of the affected tissues, broad spectrum antibiotics, and cardiopulmonary support [1,16,32]. After wounds have stabilized, reconstruction is needed, preferably with a technically simple and safe method. Loose wound approximation or split thickness skin grafts are only feasible in small or superficial wounds [1]. An extensive wound as described in our patient (Case 3) necessitates a flap coverage. Fasciocutaneous flaps as the pudendal thigh flap provide good cosmetic outcome and intact sensation [1]. For its bulkiness, the VRAM flap has rarely been used because it does not mimic the normal scrotum in appearance [17]. However, in defects as presented in our case where a penectomy was necessary, the VRAM flap is a safe and reliable option to reconstruct the whole defect area in the morbid patient. The VRAM flap is traditionally delivered in a transpelvic manner, using an intraperitoneal route. In cases where laparotomy is not used for tumor resection, an extrapelvic route is preferred [15]. This is also the case for tumors limited to the anterior part of the pelvis as described in our first case of recurrent melanoma of the vulva without rectal infiltration or in our third case of extensive genital and perineal defects after radical debridement, including penectomy due to Fournier's gangrene.

The limitations of this study include the short follow-up period of our first two cases due to the palliative situation. The first patient succumbed to her metastasized end-stage melanoma disease approximately 6 months after she was discharged from the gynecological department. We do not know if voiding without the urinary catheter was possible, but 2 months after the surgery, a cystoscopy could be performed easily through the neourethra. Cystoscopic findings and histological specimens of the remaining urethra did not reveal any pathologies. As described previously, long term observations of vaginal reconstructions with the VRAM flap showed that although the abdominal skin of the flap island is not primarily accommodated to the moist milieu of the vagina, the skin island seems to adapt to the new surrounding conditions even when the whole vagina was reconstructed with two flaps [33]. All in all, our study population was characterized by high morbidity and we were not able to quantify health-related quality of life with validated scores. However, all patients reported a subjective improvement of quality of life at follow-up visits, which were short for the majority of patients. The only alive patient with a potentially longer follow-up had multiple comorbidities typical for those suffering from Fournier gangrene and was diagnosed with melanoma a few years later. Documentations from his latest visits to the Department of Urology suggest regular changes of his urinary catheter. Removal of the catheter was not desired by the patient probably due to comfort reasons and because voiding without a penis might have imposed a great psychological challenge to the patient. A phalloplasty has not been desired by the patient so far. To evaluate the benefits of this modified technique of perineal and urethral VRAM flap reconstruction, a long-term follow-up of a set of younger and healthier patients would be necessary. However, Nigriny et al. reported on a case of perineal reconstruction with an extrapelvic VRAM flap and creation of a neovaginal and urethral orifice similar to our technique in a 54-year-old woman with anal squamous cell carcinoma. After a follow-up of 38 months, she maintained urinary continence. This case supports the viability of our technique [15].

When weighed against the gain in quality of life, the VRAM flap reconstruction is a readily available and safe tool to optimize the outcome even in palliative and multimorbid cases. All patients in this series described a subjective significant improvement in their quality of life by this repair technique. Taking the negative impact of a urostomy into account, one should always consider the reconstruction of a neourethra if possible in conjunction with a perineal VRAM flap reconstruction [20].

## 4. Conclusions

The VRAM flap is not only a safe and reliable reconstructive option for perineal defects following abdominoperineal excision—with or without vaginal wall resection—but also for extensive perineal defects after Fournier gangrene. In the latter case, an extrapelvic route is preferred. Modifications of the VRAM flap and further personalization of the surgical approach allow for a neourethral reconstruction in the case of available remaining urethral tissue. Whenever possible, this technique should be applied to ensure that future urinary continence may be maintained. This can add enormous improvements to the quality of life of those patients.

**Author Contributions:** Conceptualization: R.E.H., methodology: R.E.H., formal analysis: R.E.H., A.C., I.L. and A.A., supervision: R.E.H., visualization: R.E.H., writing—original draft preparation: A.C. and R.E.H., writing—review and editing: I.L., A.A., A.C. and R.E.H., visualization: A.C. and R.E.H. All authors have read and agreed to the published version of the manuscript.

**Funding:** The research received no external funding.

**Institutional Review Board Statement:** Ethical review and approval were waived for this study due to the retrospective and descriptive character of this study. Written informed consent for participation was not required for this study in accordance with the national legislation and the institutional requirements because there are no potentially identifiable images or data included in this article.

**Informed Consent Statement:** Ethical review and approval were waived for this study due to the retrospective and descriptive character of this study. Written informed consent for participation was not required for this study in accordance with the national legislation and the institutional requirements because there are no potentially identifiable images or data included in this article.

**Data Availability Statement:** The data presented in the study are available on reasonable request from the corresponding author. The data are not publicly available due to ethical reasons.

**Acknowledgments:** The authors want to thank The Manfred Roth Stiftung, Forschungsstiftung Universitätsklinikum Erlangen of the Friedrich-Alexander University Erlangen-Nürnberg (FAU), Boya Marshall and Hans Peter Mall for their continuing support of scientific research of the Department of Plastic and Hand Surgery of the University Hospital Erlangen of the Friedrich Alexander University Erlangen-Nuernberg FAU.

**Conflicts of Interest:** The authors declare no conflict of interest.

## References

1. Karian, L.S.; Chung, S.Y.; Lee, E.S. Reconstruction of Defects After Fournier Gangrene: A Systematic Review. *Eplasty* **2015**, *15*, e18.
2. Wong, A.A.; Delclos, M.E.; Wolff, R.A.; Evans, D.B.; Abbruzzese, J.L.; Tamm, E.P.; Xiong, H.Q.; Ho, L.; Crane, C.H. Radiation dose considerations in the palliative treatment of locally advanced adenocarcinoma of the pancreas. *Am. J. Clin. Oncol.* **2005**, *28*, 227–233. [CrossRef] [PubMed]
3. Wong, C.S.; Cummings, B.J.; Brierley, J.D.; Catton, C.N.; McLean, M.; Catton, P.; Hao, Y. Treatment of locally recurrent rectal carcinoma—Results and prognostic factors. *Int. J. Radiat. Oncol. Biol. Phys.* **1998**, *40*, 427–435. [CrossRef]
4. Sugiyama, T.; Yakushiji, M.; Noda, K.; Ikeda, M.; Kudoh, R.; Yajima, A.; Tomoda, Y.; Terashima, Y.; Takeuchi, S.; Hiura, M.; et al. Phase II study of irinotecan and cisplatin as first-line chemotherapy in advanced or recurrent cervical cancer. *Oncology* **2000**, *58*, 31–37. [CrossRef] [PubMed]
5. Gerard, J.P.; Romestaing, P.; Chapet, O. Radiotherapy alone in the curative treatment of rectal carcinoma. *Lancet Oncol.* **2003**, *4*, 158–166. [CrossRef]
6. Brodbeck, R.; Horch, R.E.; Arkudas, A.; Beier, J.P. Plastic and Reconstructive Surgery in the Treatment of Oncological Perineal and Genital Defects. *Front. Oncol.* **2015**, *5*, 212. [CrossRef] [PubMed]
7. Beier, J.P.; Croner, R.S.; Lang, W.; Arkudas, A.; Schmitz, M.; Gohl, J.; Hohenberger, W.; Horch, R.E. Avoidance of complications in oncological surgery of the pelvic region: Combined oncosurgical and plastic reconstruction measures. *Chirurg* **2015**, *86*, 242–250. [CrossRef] [PubMed]
8. Bregendahl, S.; Emmertsen, K.J.; Lindegaard, J.C.; Laurberg, S. Urinary and sexual dysfunction in women after resection with and without preoperative radiotherapy for rectal cancer: A population-based cross-sectional study. *Colorectal. Dis.* **2015**, *17*, 26–37. [CrossRef] [PubMed]
9. Jakowatz, J.G.; Porudominsky, D.; Riihimaki, D.U.; Kemeny, M.; Kokal, W.A.; Braly, P.S.; Terz, J.J.; Beatty, J.D. Complications of pelvic exenteration. *Arch. Surg.* **1985**, *120*, 1261–1265. [CrossRef] [PubMed]
10. Horch, R.E.; Hohenberger, W.; Eweida, A.; Kneser, U.; Weber, K.; Arkudas, A.; Merkel, S.; Gohl, J.; Beier, J.P. A hundred patients with vertical rectus abdominis myocutaneous (VRAM) flap for pelvic reconstruction after total pelvic exenteration. *Int. J. Colorectal. Dis.* **2014**, *29*, 813–823. [CrossRef] [PubMed]
11. Krautz, C.; Weber, K.; Croner, R.; Denz, A.; Maak, M.; Horch, R.E.; Grutzmann, R. Cylindric Abdominoperineal Rectum Exstirpation with Partial Vulvar and Vaginal Resection as well as Perineal and Vaginal Defect Reconstruction by a Vertical Rectus Abdominis Myocutaneous (VRAM) Flap. *Zentralbl. Chir.* **2017**, *142*, 543–547. [CrossRef] [PubMed]
12. Horch, R.E.; Ludolph, I.; Cai, A.; Weber, K.; Grutzmann, R.; Arkudas, A. Interdisciplinary Surgical Approaches in Vaginal and Perineal Reconstruction of Advanced Rectal and Anal Female Cancer Patients. *Front. Oncol.* **2020**, *10*, 719. [CrossRef] [PubMed]
13. Berger, J.L.; Westin, S.N.; Fellman, B.; Rallapali, V.; Frumovitz, M.; Ramirez, P.T.; Sood, A.K.; Soliman, P.T. Modified vertical rectus abdominis myocutaneous flap vaginal reconstruction: An analysis of surgical outcomes. *Gynecol. Oncol.* **2012**, *125*, 252–255. [CrossRef] [PubMed]
14. O'Connell, C.; Mirhashemi, R.; Kassira, N.; Lambrou, N.; McDonald, W.S. Formation of functional neovagina with vertical rectus abdominis musculocutaneous (VRAM) flap after total pelvic exenteration. *Ann. Plast. Surg.* **2005**, *55*, 470–473. [CrossRef] [PubMed]
15. Nigriny, J.F.; Wu, P.; Butler, C.E. Perineal reconstruction with an extrapelvic vertical rectus abdominis myocutaneous flap. *Int. J. Gynecol. Cancer* **2010**, *20*, 1609–1612. [CrossRef]
16. Insua-Pereira, I.; Ferreira, P.C.; Teixeira, S.; Barreiro, D.; Silva, A. Fournier's gangrene: A review of reconstructive options. *Cent. Eur. J. Urol* **2020**, *73*, 74–79. [CrossRef]
17. Tan, B.K.; Tan, K.C.; Khoo, A.K. Total scrotal reconstruction after Fournier's gangrene—A case report using rectus abdominis myocutaneous flap. *Ann. Acad. Med. Singap.* **1996**, *25*, 890–892. [PubMed]
18. Mirhashemi, R.; Averette, H.E.; Lambrou, N.; Penalver, M.A.; Mendez, L.; Ghurani, G.; Salom, E. Vaginal reconstruction at the time of pelvic exenteration: A surgical and psychosexual analysis of techniques. *Gynecol. Oncol.* **2002**, *87*, 39–45. [CrossRef]
19. Penalver, M.A.; Angioli, R.; Mirhashemi, R.; Malik, R. Management of early and late complications of ileocolonic continent urinary reservoir (Miami pouch). *Gynecol. Oncol.* **1998**, *69*, 185–191. [CrossRef] [PubMed]
20. Pazar, B.; Yava, A.; Basal, S. Health-related quality of life in persons living with a urostomy. *J. Wound Ostomy Cont. Nurs.* **2015**, *42*, 264–270. [CrossRef] [PubMed]
21. Horch, R.E.; Ludolph, I.; Arkudas, A. Reconstruction of oncological defects of the perianal region. *Chirurg* **2021**. [CrossRef]
22. Schellerer, V.S.; Bartholomé, L.; Langheinrich, M.C.; Grützmann, R.; Horch, R.E.; Merkel, S.; Weber, K. Donor Site Morbidity of Patients Receiving Vertical Rectus Abdominis Myocutaneous Flap for Perineal, Vaginal or Inguinal Reconstruction. *World J. Surg.* **2021**, *45*, 132–140. [CrossRef] [PubMed]
23. Ludolph, I.; Arkudas, A.; Schmitz, M.; Boos, A.M.; Taeger, C.D.; Rother, U.; Horch, R.E.; Beier, J.P. Cracking the perfusion code? Laser-assisted Indocyanine Green angiography and combined laser Doppler spectrophotometry for intraoperative evaluation of tissue perfusion in autologous breast reconstruction with DIEP or ms-TRAM flaps. *J. Plast Reconstr. Aesthet. Surg.* **2016**, *69*, 1382–1388. [CrossRef] [PubMed]
24. Ludolph, I.; Horch, R.E.; Arkudas, A.; Schmitz, M. Enhancing Safety in Reconstructive Microsurgery Using Intraoperative Indocyanine Green Angiography. *Front. Surg.* **2019**, *6*, 39. [CrossRef]

25. Gentileschi, S.; Servillo, M.; Garganese, G.; Simona, F.; Scambia, G.; Salgarello, M. Versatility of pedicled anterolateral thigh flap in gynecologic reconstruction after vulvar cancer extirpative surgery. *Microsurgery* **2017**, *37*, 516–524. [CrossRef] [PubMed]
26. Fuzzard, S.K.; Mah, E.; Choong, P.F.M.; Grinsell, D. Lymphoedema rates in pedicled anterolateral thigh flaps for coverage of irradiated groin defects. *ANZ J. Surg.* **2020**, *90*, 135–138. [CrossRef] [PubMed]
27. Lefevre, J.H.; Parc, Y.; Kerneis, S.; Shields, C.; Touboul, E.; Chaouat, M.; Tiret, E. Abdomino-perineal resection for anal cancer: Impact of a vertical rectus abdominis myocutaneus flap on survival, recurrence, morbidity, and wound healing. *Ann. Surg.* **2009**, *250*, 707–711. [CrossRef] [PubMed]
28. Hui, K.; Zhang, F.; Pickus, E.; Rodriguez, L.F.; Teng, N.; Lineaweaver, W.C. Modification of the vertical rectus abdominis musculocutaneous (VRAM) flap for functional reconstruction of complex vulvoperineal defects. *Ann. Plast. Surg.* **2003**, *51*, 556–560. [CrossRef]
29. Franchi, M.; Uccella, S.; Zorzato, P.C.; Dalle Carbonare, A.; Garzon, S.; Lagana, A.S.; Casarin, J.; Ghezzi, F. Vaginal flap for urethral neomeatus reconstruction after radical surgery for vulvar cancer: A retrospective cohort analysis. *Int. J. Gynecol. Cancer* **2019**, *29*, 1098–1104. [CrossRef] [PubMed]
30. Dabernig, J.; Shelley, O.P.; Cuccia, G.; Schaff, J. Urethral reconstruction using the radial forearm free flap: Experience in oncologic cases and gender reassignment. *Eur. Urol* **2007**, *52*, 547–553. [CrossRef]
31. Hoang, D.; Goel, P.; Chen, V.W.; Carey, J. Phalloplasty Following Penectomy for Fournier's Gangrene at a Tertiary Care Center. *Cureus* **2018**, *10*, e3698. [CrossRef] [PubMed]
32. Horch, R.E. Fournier-Gangrän. *Chirurg* **2008**, *79*, 1080–1081. [CrossRef]
33. Horch, R.E.; Gitsch, G.; Schultze-Seemann, W. Bilateral pedicled myocutaneous vertical rectus abdominus muscle flaps to close vesicovaginal and pouch-vaginal fistulas with simultaneous vaginal and perineal reconstruction in irradiated pelvic wounds. *Urology* **2002**, *60*, 502–507. [CrossRef]

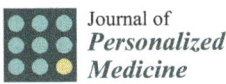

Article

# Posttraumatic Lymphedema after Open Fractures of the Lower Extremity—A Retrospective Cohort Analysis

Johannes Maximilian Wagner [1], Victoria Grolewski [1], Felix Reinkemeier [1], Marius Drysch [1], Sonja Verena Schmidt [1], Mehran Dadras [1], Julika Huber [1], Christoph Wallner [1], Alexander Sogorski [1], Maxi von Glinski [1], Thomas A. Schildhauer [2], Marcus Lehnhardt [1] and Björn Behr [1,*]

[1] Department of Plastic Surgery, BG-University Hospital Bergmannsheil, 44789 Bochum, Germany;
max.jay.wagner@gmail.com (J.M.W.); strohvictoria@gmail.com (V.G.);
Felix.Reinkemeier@ruhr-uni-bochum.de (F.R.); Marius.Drysch@ruhr-uni-bochum.de (M.D.);
sva.schmidt@yahoo.de (S.V.S.); mdadras@outlook.com (M.D.); julika.huber@hotmail.com (J.H.);
c.wallner88@gmail.com (C.W.); alexander.sogorski@gmx.de (A.S.);
maxi.vonglinski@bergmannsheil.de (M.v.G.); marcus.lehnhardt@rub.de (M.L.)
[2] Department of Traumatology and Orthopedic Surgery, BG-University Hospital Bergmannsheil, 44789 Bochum, Germany; thomas.schildhauer@bergmannsheil.de
* Correspondence: bjorn.behr@rub.de; Tel.: +49-2343443; Fax: +49-2346379

**Abstract:** Secondary lymphedema is a very common clinical issue with millions of patients suffering from pain, recurrent skin infections, and the constant need for a decongestive therapy. Well-established as a consequence of oncologic procedures, secondary lymphedema is also a well-known phenomenon after trauma. However, precise epidemiological data of lymphedema progress upon severe extremity injuries are still missing. In the present work, we analyzed a patient cohort of 94 individuals who suffered open fractures of the lower extremity and soft tissue injury, of 2nd and 3rd grade according to Tscherne classification, between 2013 and 2019. Typical symptoms of lymphedema have been obtained via interviews and patient medical records in a retrospective cohort analysis. Of all patients, 55% showed symptoms of secondary lymphedema and 14% reported recurrent skin infections, indicating severe lymphedema. Furthermore, comparing patients with and without lymphedema, additional parameters, such as obesity, total number of surgeries, infections, and compartment syndrome, related to lymphedema progress could be identified. According to these data, posttraumatic secondary lymphedema has a highly underestimated clinical prevalence. Further prospective studies are needed to validate this first observation and to identify high-risk groups in order to improve patient's health care.

**Keywords:** posttraumatic lymphedema; long bone fractures; soft tissue injury; lower extremity

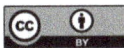

## 1. Introduction

Lymphedema is a localized fluid collection within the interstitium caused by insufficient lymphatic drainage, and is a progressive disease, being favored by two aspects: increased hydrostatic pressure, consequently pressing out more fluid into the interstitium and furthermore increased oncotic pressure, as lymph fluid is rich in protein [1]. Another contributing factor of lymphedema progression is recurrent infections of the skin. Lymph fluid is an ideal breeding ground for bacteria and even small skin lesions can lead to severe erysipelas. A rare but serious consequence after recurrent infections is lymphangiosarcoma [1–3]. According to its etiology, lymphedema can be classified as primary or secondary. Primary lymphedema is very rare and mostly caused by an innate dysfunction of lymph vessels. Most patients suffer from secondary lymphedema after tumor resection, radiation, infection, or overweight [1,3,4]. The most common cause of secondary lymphedema posed here is tumor resection. In particular, patients after cervical, axillary, or inguinal lymphadenectomy have a high risk of developing lymphedema [5].

Diagnosis of lymphedema is mostly based on clinical criteria (volumetry, circumferential measurements) and the presence of predispositional factors, such as malignant diseases or trauma. Additionally, ultrasound, CT, MRI, and especially near-infrared-fluorescence angiography are important tools to gain further clinical information about the severity and progress of lymphedema [6]. Important differential diagnoses of lymphedema are lipedema, chronical venous insufficiency, drug-induced edema, or hypoalbuminemia.

A quite underestimated cause of secondary lymphedema is trauma. Patients suffer from secondary lymphedema especially after open or closed fractures of the long bones [7]. The accompanying lymphedema in the acute phase of bone and wound healing often leads to delayed wound healing and wound infections, requiring complex and prolonged treatments.

However, precise data of the prevalence of posttraumatic lymphedema are still missing. In the present study, we evaluated the prevalence of lymphedema in a patient cohort who suffered open fractures of the lower leg or thigh between 2013 and 2019, in a single institution. Furthermore, this work aimed to assess the prevalence of posttraumatic lymphedema in this patient cohort, and thereby identify patients who have a high risk of secondary lymphedema progress.

## 2. Materials and Methods

The study was conducted according to the guidelines of the Declaration of Helsinki, and approved by the Institutional Review Board of Ruhr University Bochum. In this work we performed a retrospective cohort study in order to assess the prevalence of posttraumatic lymphedema after open fractures of the lower leg or thigh, and to further identify risk factors of the occurrence of posttraumatic lymphedema. In total, 200 patients which suffered from open long bone fractures of the lower extremity with soft tissue injuries of grade 2 and 3 according to Tscherne, and were treated between 2013 and 2019 in a single institution were identified and contacted personally via telephone and asked about prolonged swelling of the injured extremity, need for compression garments, manual lymph drainage, pain, and recurrent skin infections.

Soft tissue injury of patients was classified according to ICD-10, adapted from Tscherne and Oestern classification.

Moreover, clinical, demographic, and outcome data were assessed from medical records. In total, 106 of these patients could not be contacted successfully and had to be excluded from the analyzed patient cohort.

The prevalence of lymphedema was defined by the existence of at least a prolonged swelling and the constant need for a decongestive therapy. Furthermore, references for a secondary lymphedema had to be found within the medical records, which were based on a prolonged swelling of the affected limb, the occurrence of pitting edema, or stemmer sign.

### 2.1. Patients

Inclusion criteria for this study were long bone fractures (femur, tibia, fibula) of the thigh and lower leg combined with soft tissue injuries grade 2 and 3, according to Tscherne classification, receiving open reduction, and fixation in a single institution between 2013 and 2019.

### 2.2. Statistics

Data are shown as means (range) or median. Patients were subdivided into two groups according to the occurrence of lymphedema and non-lymphedema. Pearson's chi-square test and Fisher's exact test was used for categorial variables (when expected value of any cell was below 5, Fisher's exact test was used instead of chi-square test). For continuous variables, independent t-test was used. $p$-value below 0.05 was considered statistically significant.

## 3. Results

A total of 70 men and 24 women who suffered from open long bone fractures and 2–3° soft tissue injury between 2013 and 2019 were contacted personally via telephone. According to specific symptoms and additional information based on their medical records, a secondary lymphedema could be found in 52 (55%) of these 94 patients. Thirteen of these patients (14%) reported recurrent skin infections, indicating a severe lymphedema of the injured extremity.

Patient related characteristics are shown in Table 1. Although about three times more men than women existed in the analyzed patient cohort, no gender specific differences between the lymphedema and non-lymphedema group could be noted.

Table 1. Patient characteristics.

|  | All Patients $n = 94$ (%) | Patients with Lymphedema $n = 52$ (%) | Patients without Lymphedema $n = 42$ (%) | $p$-Value (Comparison) |
|---|---|---|---|---|
| Age mean (median) | 48.6 (16–84) | 48.48 (17–84) | 48.92 (16–80) | 0.904 |
| >40 | 30 (31.9) | 14 (26.9) | 16 (38.1) | 0.248 |
| 40–65 | 47 (50.0) | 32 (61.5) | 15 (35.7) | **0.013** |
| >65 | 17 (18.1) | 6 (11.5) | 11 (26.2) | 0.067 |
| Sex |  |  |  |  |
| Male | 70 (74.5) | 42 (80.8) | 28 (66.7) | 0.119 |
| Female | 24 (25.5) | 10 (19.2) | 14 (33.3) |  |
| Obesity (BMI > 30 kg/m$^2$) | 12 (10.6) | 10 (19.2) | 2 (4.8) | **0.035** |
| Diabetes mellitus type 2 | 10 (10.6) | 6 (11.5) | 4 (9.5) | 0.106 |
| Arterial hypertension | 29 (30.9) | 16 (30.8) | 13 (31.0) | 0.309 |
| Pain | 46 (48.9) | 33 (63.5) | 13 (30.9) | **0.001** |

The mean age of all patients included was 48.6 years (16–84 years). The mean age of patients with lymphedema (48.48 years) did not differ from patients without lymphedema (48.92 years, $p = 0.904$). Interestingly, when comparing different age groups in detail, a significantly increased number of patients in the lymphedema group were noted between 40 and 65 years (61.5% vs. 35.7%, $p = 0.013$).

Furthermore, significantly more patients with severe obesity (BMI > 30 kg/m$^2$) (BMI upon trauma) suffered from posttraumatic lymphedema (19.2% vs. 4.8%, $p = 0.035$). No differences between both groups could be found concerning pre-existing conditions, such as arterial hypertension and diabetes mellitus type 2. Of great interest was the fact that significantly more patients with lymphedema (63.5%) suffered from pain in the injured extremity than patients without lymphedema (30.9%, $p = 0.001$).

As there were few differences in patient characteristics related to the occurrence of posttraumatic lymphedema, we wondered if characteristics of the trauma itself, treatment, and complications could be helpful to find distinct variables related to lymphedema.

Trauma related characteristics are presented in Table 2.

Table 2. Trauma characteristics.

| | All Patients n = 94 (%) | Patients with Lymphedema n = 52 (%) | Patients without Lymphedema n = 42 (%) | p-Value (Comparison) |
|---|---|---|---|---|
| Trauma | | | | |
| Contusion | 27 (28.7) | 13 (25.0) | 14 (33.3) | 0.375 |
| Traffic accident | 40 (42.6) | 28 (53.9) | 12 (28.6) | **0.013** |
| Fall | 27 (28.7) | 11 (21.1) | 16 (28.1) | 0.071 |
| Soft tissue injury (Tscherne) | | | | |
| 2nd grade | 34 | 17 (32.7) | 17 (40.5) | 0.362 |
| 3rd grade | 60 | 35 (67.3) | 25 (59.5) | 0.435 |
| Fractured long bone | | | | |
| Femur | 7 (7.4) | 5 (9.6) | 2 (4.8) | 0.372 |
| Tibia | 92 (97.9) | 50 (96.2) | 42 (1.0) | 0.199 |
| Fibula | 26 (27.7) | 14 (26.9) | 12 (28.6) | 0.859 |
| Total number of surgeries | | | | |
| 1 | 7 (7.4) | 0 (0) | 7 (16.7) | **0.003** |
| 2 | 7 (7.4) | 1 (1.9) | 6 (14.3) | **0.042** |
| 3 | 18 (19.1) | 10 (19.2) | 8 (19.0) | 0.982 |
| 4 | 10 (10.6) | 6 (11.5) | 4 (9.5) | 0.753 |
| 5 or more | 52 (55.3) | 35 (67.3) | 17 (40.5) | **0.009** |
| Multiple fractures | 57 (60.6) | 35 (67.3) | 22 (52.4) | 0.141 |
| Vascular trauma | 7 (7.4) | 6 (11.5) | 1 (2.4) | 0.099 |
| Polytrauma | 13 (13.8) | 8 (15.4) | 5 (11.9) | 0.138 |
| Infection (soft tissue, bone) | 32 (34.0) | 23 (44.2) | 9 (21.4) | **0.02** |
| Compartment syndrome | 12 (12.8) | 10 (19.2) | 2 (4.8) | **0.035** |
| Skin graft | 44 (46.8) | 30 (57.7) | 14 (33.3) | **0.018** |
| Local, pedicled, free flaps | 40 (42.6) | 28 (53.8) | 12 (28.6) | **0.014** |

The vast majority of all patients suffered fractures of the tibia (97.9%), while femur fractures could only be noted in 7.4%. Furthermore, a slight majority of 67.3% of lymphedema patients showed multiple fractures of the lower extremity, however, compared to non-lymphedema group (52.4%), no statistical difference became evident ($p = 0.141$).

Comparing different mechanisms of injury in our patient cohort, we categorized contusion, traffic accident, and fall. Interestingly, a significantly increased number of patients in the lymphedema group (53.9%) sustained a traffic accident compared to trauma patients without lymphedema (28.6%, $p = 0.013$). Soft tissue injury, according to Tscherne classification (Table 3), was evenly distributed in lymphedema and non-lymphedema group.

Table 3. Classification of open fractures according to Tscherne and Oestern 1982.

| Grade | Soft Tissue Injury |
|---|---|
| 1 | minimal skin laceration |
| 2 | skin laceration, circumferential contusions, moderate contamination |
| 3 | extensive: major vascular and or nerve damage, compartment syndrome |
| 4 | subtotal and complete amputations |

Interestingly, vascular trauma and polytrauma patients were not significantly enhanced in the lymphedema group ($p = 0.099$; $p = 0.138$), although a distinct trend could be noted in vascular trauma patients developing a lymphedema.

Having analyzed trauma characteristics of the patients, we were further interested in treatment and complications as important indicators for lymphedema progress. Subsequently, we matched total number of surgeries, which indirectly exhibited the severity of trauma and soft tissue injury. Interestingly, only 1.9% of lymphedema patients required one or two surgeries, while 31% of non-lymphedema patients could be successfully treated with this small number of interventions. Most lymphedema patients needed five or more surgical interventions (67.3%), while this quantity was significantly smaller in non-lymphedema patients (40.5%, $p = 0.009$). Furthermore, significantly heightened number of lymphedema patients required skin grafts (57.7%, $p = 0.018$) or flap tissue reconstruction (53.8%, $p = 0.014$).

Finally, infections of soft tissue or bone, as well as the occurrence of a compartment syndrome of the lower leg seemed to be related to lymphedema development in trauma patients ($p = 0.020$; $p = 0.035$).

## 4. Discussion

Although posttraumatic lymphedema is a well-known problem of orthopedic surgery, there is still a lack of precise epidemiological data in current literature. First descriptions on the occurrence of secondary lymphedema after trauma to the affected limb can be found in Italian and Russian literature in the 1960s [8,9].

In the present study, we analyzed 94 patients suffering from traumatic fractures and 2° and 3° soft tissue injury of the lower limb who were treated at a single institution between 2013 and 2019. Although these patients are believed to be at high risk of developing secondary lymphedema [7], the data presented here indicate that the occurrence of posttraumatic lymphedema is a highly underestimated issue. More than half of the analyzed patients showed typical symptoms of a secondary lymphedema of the injured limb. This prevalence number is comparable to other patients who are at a high risk of secondary lymphedema, for example breast cancer patients after complete axillary lymph node dissection with a prevalence of 20–50% [6]. As already mentioned previously, relevant literature providing epidemiological data is still rare. Only few studies reported about the occurrence of this highly relevant issue in trauma patients. For example, Pereira et al. performed SCIP lymphatic vessel transfer in patients with secondary lymphedema after trauma, and furthermore were able to surgically prevent development of secondary lymphedema after soft tissue injury in a small patient cohort [10,11]. However, no information was given about the prevalence of secondary lymphedema. Furthermore, successful treatment of prolonged hand lymphedema after trauma was reported in two young woman by vascularized lymph node transfer [12]. A rare but very serious complication of a prolonged lymphedema, the occurrence of an angiosarcoma, has been reported by Trattner et al. as a consequence of posttraumatic lymphedema [13].

While there is certain evidence for the appearance of a posttraumatic lymphedema, it can only be speculated about the underlying pathomechanism. Interestingly, Szczesny et al. reported about dilatated lymph vessels and lymph nodes during the follow-up of patients with lower extremity fractures and assumed an ongoing inflammatory process, contributing to the development of a secondary lymphedema after trauma [14]. An obvious explanation in our case series would be the disruption and lack of proper regeneration of the lymphatic system at the injury site.

After defining the prevalence of posttraumatic lymphedema in this particular patient cohort, which is demonstrably at high risk, we were interested in further patient or trauma related properties that could be used to define high-risk groups.

Interestingly, only limited findings could be concluded from patient characteristics. While obesity seems to contribute to lymphedema progress in this context, patients' age only had little impact. Although significant differences could be detected in the age group of 40 years to 65 years, we assume this result to be biased by an increased severity of trauma within this group. Moreover, we propose that the severity of trauma is directly related to occurrence of lymphedema. However, which parameters should be taken into account for this purpose? We assumed that the grade of soft tissue injury directly affects the incidence of posttraumatic lymphedema, which could be concluded from oncologic studies, examining the occurrence of secondary lymphedema after extremity sarcoma resection. According to Wu et al., patients with large tumors at the medial thigh have the highest risk of secondary lymphedema after tumor resection [15].

To our surprise, soft tissue injury classification according to Tscherne did not show significant differences in the occurrence of a lymphedema, and therefore seemed not to be suitable, similar to the assessment of multiple fractures or polytrauma.

The most sensitive parameter which could be identified in the data analysis was the number of total surgeries. Only one patient requiring two surgeries developed a lymphedema, while 31% of patients in the non-lymphedema group with one or two surgical interventions was free of lymphedema symptoms. The authors assume the number of surgeries to be a sensitive parameter for trauma severity, as patients with highly traumatized soft tissue often require multiple surgeries.

We provide first data reporting the prevalence of secondary posttraumatic lymphedema. However, these data are preliminary and need to be further validated by prospective studies. Furthermore, classification of soft tissue injury has been performed by different surgeons, which could have caused a possible bias and has to be taken into account when interpreting these data.

Further limitations of this work concern the retrospective lymphedema assessment based on telephone interviews and the corresponding medical records.

## 5. Conclusions

The analysis of this patient cohort suffering from lower extremity fractures and soft tissue injury did reveal a very high prevalence of secondary lymphedema, even multiple years after trauma. The results of this study suggest that the appearance of a posttraumatic lymphedema seems to be a highly underestimated clinical issue. Although the first interesting parameters for identification of high-risk groups could be identified, further studies are mandatory to identify patient cohorts who are at highest risk of lymphedema development. This may help to reduce the burden of chronic lymphedema for these patients or could even help to prevent the occurrence or enable early interventions to decrease symptoms.

**Author Contributions:** Conceptualization, B.B. and J.M.W.; data curation, J.M.W., V.G. and M.L.; formal analysis, S.V.S. and J.H.; investigation, J.M.W., M.D. (Mehran Dadras) and A.S.; methodology, C.W.; project administration, J.M.W., T.A.S., M.L. and B.B.; writing—original draft, M.D. (Marius Drysch), J.M.W. and B.B.; writing—review and editing, F.R., M.v.G. and T.A.S. All authors have read and agreed to the published version of the manuscript.

**Funding:** This research received no external funding.

**Institutional Review Board Statement:** The study was conducted according to the guidelines of the Declaration of Helsinki, and approved by the Institutional Ethics Committee of Ruhr University Bochum (19-6772).

**Informed Consent Statement:** Informed consent was obtained from all subjects involved in the study.

**Data Availability Statement:** Data sharing is not applicable to this article.

**Conflicts of Interest:** The authors declare no conflict of interest.

## References

1. Warren, A.G.; Brorson, H.; Borud, L.J.; Slavin, S.A. Lymphedema: A comprehensive review. *Ann. Plast. Surg.* **2007**, *59*, 464–472. [CrossRef] [PubMed]
2. Nagase, T.; Gonda, K.; Inoue, K.; Higashino, T.; Fukuda, N.; Gorai, K.; Mihara, M.; Nakanishi, M.; Koshima, I. Treatment of lymphedema with lymphaticovenular anastomoses. *Int. J. Clin. Oncol.* **2005**, *10*, 304–310. [CrossRef] [PubMed]

3. Grada, A.A.; Phillips, T.J. Lymphedema: Diagnostic workup and management. *J. Am. Acad. Dermatol.* **2017**, *77*, 995–1006. [CrossRef] [PubMed]
4. Yamamoto, T.; Iida, T.; Yoshimatsu, H.; Fuse, Y.; Hayashi, A.; Yamamoto, N. Lymph Flow Restoration after Tissue Replantation and Transfer: Importance of Lymph Axiality and Possibility of Lymph Flow Reconstruction without Lymph Node Transfer or Lymphatic Anastomosis. *Plast. Reconstr. Surg.* **2018**, *142*, 796–804. [CrossRef] [PubMed]
5. Rockson, S.G.; Rivera, K.K. Estimating the population burden of lymphedema. *Ann. N. Y. Acad. Sci.* **2008**, *1131*, 147–154. [CrossRef] [PubMed]
6. Garza, R., 3rd; Skoracki, R.; Hock, K.; Povoski, S.P. A comprehensive overview on the surgical management of secondary lymphedema of the upper and lower extremities related to prior oncologic therapies. *BMC Cancer* **2017**, *17*, 468. [CrossRef] [PubMed]
7. Hirsch, T.; Wahl, U. Practical Approaches for Post-Operative and Post-Traumatic Lymphoedemas. *Zent. Chir.* **2017**, *142*, 287–296.
8. Gorshkov, S.Z. Post-traumatic elephantiasis of the lower extremities. *Vestn. Khirurgii Grek.* **1967**, *99*, 118–120.
9. Wedenissow, U. Pathogenetic and therapeutic notes on post-traumatic lymphedema of the extremities. *G. Ital. Chir.* **1960**, *16*, 759–766. [PubMed]
10. Pereira, N.; Cambara, Á.; Kufeke, M.; Roa, R. Prevention and Treatment of Posttraumatic Lymphedema by Soft Tissue Reconstruction With Lymphatic Vessels Free Flap: An Observational Study. *Ann. Plast. Surg.* **2021**, *86*, 434–439. [CrossRef] [PubMed]
11. Pereira, N.; Cámbara, Á.; Kufeke, M.; Roa, R. Post-traumatic lymphedema treatment with superficial circumflex iliac artery perforator lymphatic free flap: A case report. *Microsurgery* **2019**, *39*, 354–359. [CrossRef] [PubMed]
12. Becker, C.; Arrivé, L.; Mangiameli, G.; Pricopi, C.; Randrianambinina, F.; Le Pimpec-Barthes, F. Post-traumatic massive hand lymphedema fully cured by vascularized lymph node flap transfer. *SICOT-J* **2018**, *4*, 53. [CrossRef] [PubMed]
13. Trattner, A.; Shamai-Lubovitz, O.; Segal, R.; Zelikovski, A. Stewart-Treves angiosarcoma of arm and ipsilateral breast in post-traumatic lymphedema. *Lymphology* **1996**, *29*, 57–59. [PubMed]
14. Szczesny, G.; Olszewski, W.L. The pathomechanism of posttraumatic edema of the lower limbs: II–Changes in the lymphatic system. *J. Trauma* **2003**, *55*, 350–354. [CrossRef] [PubMed]
15. Wu, P.; Elswick, S.M.; Arkhavan, A.; Molinar, V.E.; Mohan, A.T.; Curiel, D.; Sim, F.H.; Martinez-Jorge, J.; Saint-Cyr, M. Risk Factors for Lymphedema after Thigh Sarcoma Resection and Reconstruction. *Plast. Reconstr. Surg. Glob. Open* **2020**, *8*, e2912. [CrossRef] [PubMed]

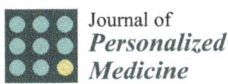

Article

# Thermal, Hyperspectral, and Laser Doppler Imaging: Non-Invasive Tools for Detection of the Deep Inferior Epigastric Artery Perforators—A Prospective Comparison Study

Sebastian P. Nischwitz [1,2,*], Hanna Luze [1,2], Marlies Schellnegger [2,3], Simon J. Gatterer [4], Alexandru-Cristian Tuca [1], Raimund Winter [1] and Lars-Peter Kamolz [1,2]

[1] Division of Plastic, Aesthetic and Reconstructive Surgery, Department of Surgery, Medical University of Graz, 8036 Graz, Austria; hanna.luze@joanneum.at (H.L.); alexandru.tuca@medunigraz.at (A.-C.T.); r.winter@medunigraz.at (R.W.); lars.kamolz@medunigraz.at (L.-P.K.)
[2] COREMED—Cooperative Centre for Regenerative Medicine, JOANNEUM RESEARCH Forschungsgesellschaft mbH, 8010 Graz, Austria; marlies.schellnegger@joanneum.at
[3] Division of Macroscopic and Clinical Anatomy, Medical University of Graz, 8036 Graz, Austria
[4] Medical University of Graz, 8036 Graz, Austria; simon.gatterer@stud.medunigraz.at
\* Correspondence: sebastian.nischwitz@joanneum.at

**Abstract:** Perforator flaps have become one of the leading procedures in microsurgical tissue transfer. Individual defects require a tailored approach to guarantee the most effective treatment. A thorough understanding of the individual vascular anatomy and the location of prominent perforators is of utmost importance and usually requires invasive angiography or at least acoustic Doppler exploration. In this study, we aimed at evaluating different non-invasive imaging modalities as possible alternatives for perforator location detection. After a cooling phase, we performed thermal, hyperspectral and Laser Doppler imaging and visually evaluated a possible detection of the perforator for a period of five minutes with an image taken every minute. We identified the most prominent perforator of the deep inferior epigastric artery by handheld acoustic Doppler in 18 patients. The detected perforator locations were then correlated. Eighteen participants were assessed with six images each per imaging method. We could show a positive match for 94.44%, 38.89%, and 0% of patients and 92.59%, 25.93%, and 0% of images for the methods respectively compared to the handheld acoustic Doppler. Sex, age, abdominal girth, and BMI showed no correlation with a possible visual detection of the perforator in the images. Therefore, thermal imaging can yield valuable supporting data in the individualized procedure planning. Future larger cohort studies are required to better assess the full potential of modern handheld thermal imaging devices.

**Keywords:** perforator flaps; flap imaging; microsurgery; DIEP; thermal imaging; hyperspectral imaging; laser Doppler

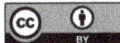

## 1. Introduction

Skin defects secondary to chronic wounds, traumatic or oncological conditions require effective closure. Depending on the patient's prerequisites and the extent of the defect and the involved tissues, a tailored approach needs to be derived for every such defect. One of the main techniques of reconstruction is the use of perforator flaps which have gained tremendous popularity in recent decades and were adopted into widespread fields of application throughout plastic and reconstructive surgery. A perforator flap is used for microsurgical tissue transfer of tissue(s) that are supplied by a single perforating artery and concomitant veins that derive from a deep vascular system and pierce (perforate) the underlying fascia or muscle. One of the most viable perforator flaps is the deep inferior epigastric perforator (DIEP) flap, which is located on the lower abdomen and mostly used for breast reconstruction due to its relatively voluminous constitution [1]. A profound understanding of the individual vascular anatomy is a necessary requirement for proper surgery planning, optimal surgical procedures, and successful outcome [2,3]. Despite known anatomical landmarks, individual features often necessitate preoperative imaging, especially with the DIEP flap, given its branched vascular anatomy and the often-pronounced thickness of the adipose layer [4–6]. Particularly the use of delicate perforators of a few millimeters' diameter calls for a diligent individualized approach; insufficient understanding of the precise location of a perforator may jeopardize the entire procedure [7]. Perforator mapping has not only been demonstrated to increase safety, but to reduce morbidity, hospital length of stay and duration of surgery [5].

Depending on the respective institution, several perforator detection methods are in use, with CT- or MR-angiography (CT-A, MR-A) being the gold standard that could be complemented with new techniques [5,8–11]. Critics of these techniques describe several limitations thereof, e.g., radiation exposure (CT-A), need for an intravenous contrast agent, or imprecise transferability from a digital image rendered on a screen to the actual patient [12]. Generally accepted alternatives include duplex sonography or handheld acoustic Doppler [13–15]. In addition to CT-A, MR-A or duplex sonography, the preoperative perforator detection is frequently conducted using a handheld Doppler device at our institution. The handheld Doppler is preferred by many surgeons in clinical practice, given its widespread availability, its portability and low cost, while being able to locate perforators pre-, intra- and postoperatively [16]. It is straightforward to use and said to be the most commonly used perforator detection device [14]. Yet, some authors doubt its performance [17]: Like the color-coded Doppler ultrasound, the handheld Doppler requires training and is highly user-dependent, leading to reduced reliability, especially in small caliber vessels [18–20]. Moreover, its feedback is solely provided by an acoustic signal rather than a visible image that could indicate caliber and spatial orientation of the vessel. According to our own and the experience of other institutions, the handheld Doppler is a reliable tool for perforator detection with appropriate training [21]. Yet, a non-invasive, user-independent device with direct spatial correlation to the patient would be a valuable addition to the armamentarium of plastic and reconstructive surgeons.

The recent, diversified use of modern imaging devices for perforator detection and variable availabilities of devices [22–25] triggered the idea of comparing mobile smartphone-based thermal imaging (TI), hyperspectral imaging (HS) and Laser Doppler (LD) after a brief application of a cooling pack to the handheld Doppler. TI has been described as a quick and easy method warranting further investigation to assess thermal perforators in previous studies [9]. HS is a more recent technology assessing perfusion and oxygenation of tissues in different skin depths (up to 6 mm) [26,27]. This technique allows differentiation between better and lesser perfused areas, allowing for the indirect localization of a perforator [20]. LD is used routinely in burn surgery to assess tissue perfusion and, therefore, burn depth [28]. Furthermore, it is used to assess the perfusion of different perforator flaps [29].

This study's aim was to increase evidence and to identify the most suitable non-invasive, portable imaging device for an individualized perforator identification approach.

## 2. Materials and Methods

The study was approved by the ethics committee at the Medical University Graz, Austria (31-477 ex 18/19). Written informed consent was obtained from all individual participants included in the study. All procedures performed were in accordance with the ethical standards of the institutional and/or national research committee and with the 1964 Helsinki declaration and its later amendments.

*2.1. Detection Devices*

TI: Non-invasive TI was performed with the FLIR One® Pro for iOS Attachment for iOS Smartphones. (FLIR Systems, Inc., Wilsonville, OR, USA). Temperature differences of up to 0.07 °C can be detected by this device, enabling a distinction between the blood flow in the perforator and the surrounding "cooled" tissue. Detailed specifications are available on the manufacturer's homepage [30]. Imaging acquisition was further processed with the FLIR One® App.

HS: The TIVITA® Wound (500–1000nm, Diaspective Vision GmbH, Am Salzhaff-Pepelow, Germany) was used for HS imaging. This technology uses the remission of light of different wavelengths of illuminated tissues to assess parameters like perfusion, oxygen saturation, and hemoglobin content. There is no direct contact between the device and the patient, and the results are visualized by color-coded images on a computer. Detailed specifications of the device are available on the manufacturer's homepage [31].

LD: LD is a non-invasive imaging technique whose working principle is the Doppler shift of laser light that is backscattered by moving red blood cells in the cutaneous microcirculation [32]. The detection of the Doppler shift by optical heterodyning allows for rendering of an image, in a technique that can be considered analogous to the acoustic Doppler [33]. The moorLDLS-BI LaserDoppler (785 nm, Moor Instruments Ltd., Axminster UK) was used for LD imaging, and detailed specifications are available on the manufacturer's homepage [34].

*2.2. Study Design & Patient Collective*

The study was designed as a prospective, monocentric comparison study. The study collective consisted of 18 patients that were treated for any reason requiring inpatient treatment at our institution (Division of Plastic, Aesthetic & Reconstructive Surgery). Inclusion criteria were: (1) inpatient stay at our department, (2) individual willing to participate in this study, (3) between 18 and 80 years old. Patients that (1) had any prior surgery in their abdominal region, (2) showed scars on their abdomen, (3) suffered from any known disease compromising micro-circulation (like diabetes mellitus or peripheral arterial obliterative disease) or (4) received steroid or other immunosuppressive therapy were excluded from the study. We chose to further exclude patients with planned DIEP surgery to not increase burden on those patients.

The patient collective of 18 patients was divided into three groups with six patients each. Each participant's abdominal area was investigated with each of the three devices, with the group determining the sequence of the different acquisition methods to avoid possible bias by repeated measurements. Group 1's order was TI, LD, HS; group 2's order was HS, TI, LD; group 3's order was LD, HS, TI. The group allocation was chosen merely on patients' age to reach a homogeneous age distribution amongst the groups. Due to the low case numbers, we chose not to randomize patients.

*2.3. Study Course*

Prior to any study-related activity, the participants were informed in detail, and written informed consent was obtained. Sex, age, Body-Mass-Index (BMI) and abdominal girth (rounded to the full cm) were assessed. The region of interest (ROI) was defined as a square of $10 \times 10$ cm spanning from the umbilicus downwards around the midline. This ROI was chosen based on clinical experience and easy reproducibility. The ROI was identified and screened for a perforator with the acoustic handheld Doppler.

The ROI was cooled for 20 min with a commercially available cool pack that had been stored in a temperature-monitored fridge at 5 °C for at least 20 h, to diminish perfusion of the abdominal skin. The cool pack was then removed and the respective image acquisition method was employed every 60 s for a total of 5 min to evaluate changes in detection rate over time since cessation of cooling. The subsequent image acquisition methods were employed following a break of 60 min in the same manner. We therefore acquired 6 images per patient per imaging method, resulting in 324 images overall. The study course for group 1 is depicted in Figure 1.

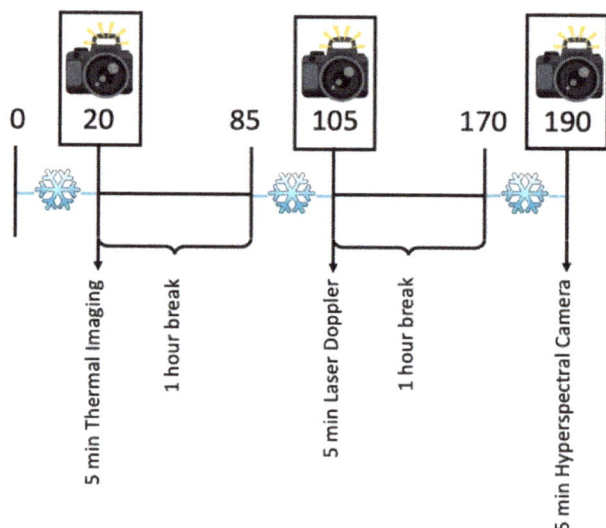

**Figure 1.** Exemplary study course for group 1. After 20 min of cooling, thermal imaging was performed minutely for five minutes. After an hour break the same process was repeated with laser Doppler and hyperspectral imaging after another hour break.

After completion of image acquisition, two investigators who are plastic surgery residents experienced in the use of the pencil Doppler, identified the most prominent perforator in the area independent of each other, which would most likely be chosen were a procedure to be conducted. If concordance could not be reached, both identified perforators were used as further reference. Perforators outside the ROI were not considered.

*2.4. Image Analysis*

The TI, HS and LD images were then screened for a possible perforator ("warmer" area in TI, "more perfused" are in HS and LD). The identification of a perforator location on TI, HS and LD images was conducted by two different investigators that were blinded to the pencil Doppler assessment. The identification was at the discretion of the investigators, given the lack of predefined requirements for a perforator in these image acquisition methods in the literature. The ROI in the images was divided into 16 equal squares (4 × 4). Then, perforator locations in TI, HS and LD images on one side, and the locations of pencil Doppler identification were compared and matched. A positive correlation (true positive) was assigned to the image if the perforator's location in the ROI matched. Any image with a visible perforator that was distinctly more prominent than the reference perforator was declared false positive. Several visible perforators were seen as true positive, if at least one reference perforator was included as well. If no perforator was seen at all, pictures were classified as true negative (if no perforator had been detected by pencil Doppler) or false negative if a perforator had been identified by pencil Doppler. First, patients have been evaluated for their availability of a positive match, but ultimately, since the aim was to investigate a possible detection over time since cessation of cooling, images have been evaluated rather than patients.

*2.5. Statistical Analysis*

Normality testing was not performed given the small sample size and the expected low power thereof [35]. Data is presented using medians and 25th and 75th percentile. Specificity, sensitivity, wrong positive and negative rates were calculated using cross-tabulation. Differences between the groups were determined using One-Way ANOVA. Spearman correlation coefficient was used to determine correlation between biometric parameters and a successful match to investigate a possible bias. The level of significance was set to $p < 0.05$. Prism 9.0.2 (GraphPad Software, LLC., San Diego, CA, USA) was used for statistical analysis.

## 3. Results

A total of 18 patients were investigated in three different groups (group 1: subject 01-06, group 2: subject 07–12, group 3: subject 13–18). The groups showed no significant difference in sex, ($p = 0.34$), age ($p = 0.76$), BMI ($p = 0.30$) or abdominal girth ($p = 0.27$). The participants' specifics are displayed in Table 1.

**Table 1.** Participants' characteristics. The order of the imaging was determined by the group. Group 1: Subject 01–06. Group 2: Subject 07–12. Group 3: Subject 13–18. BMI = Body Mass Index. m.d. = missing data.

| Subject ID | Sex | Age [years] | BMI [kg/m$^2$] | Abdominal Girth [cm] | Perforator Detection |
|---|---|---|---|---|---|
| 01 | Male | 36 | m.d. | m.d. | Left |
| 02 | Male | 30 | 22.86 | 78 | Right |
| 03 | Male | 58 | 29.30 | 111 | Right |
| 04 | Male | 41 | 32.53 | 108 | Left |
| 05 | Male | 65 | m.d. | m.d. | Left |
| 06 | Female | 71 | 27.89 | 92 | Left + Right |
| 07 | Female | 28 | 23.88 | 82 | Left + Right |
| 08 | Female | 22 | 19.13 | 68 | Left |
| 09 | Female | 52 | 23.44 | 70 | Left + Right |
| 10 | Male | 41 | 31.56 | 102 | Left |
| 11 | Male | 61 | 22.21 | 92 | Left + Right |
| 12 | Male | 62 | 23.66 | 93 | Left |
| 13 | Male | 24 | 25.98 | 92 | Left |
| 14 | Female | 24 | 20.44 | 70 | Left |
| 15 | Male | 49 | 32.77 | 132 | Right |
| 16 | Female | 45 | 34.72 | 110 | Left |
| 17 | Male | 60 | 26.47 | 100 | Left + Right |
| 18 | Male | 60 | 25.08 | 98 | Left + Right |
| Total/median (25th, 75th percentile) | 66.6% Male 33.3% Female | 47.00 (29.50, 60.25) | 25.53 (23.01, 31.00) | 92.50 (79.00, 106.50) | 9 Left, 3 Right 6 Left + Right |

### 3.1. Perforator Detection

In all 18 participants, at least one perforator was detected by pencil Doppler. Nine participants showed perforators on the left side, three on the right, and six on both sides with two reference perforators.

In total, 324 images were taken with TI, HS and LD (108 each). In 128 images, a match was observed (39.51%). One participant (5.56%) showed no match at all, independent of the imaging method. No correlation was seen between a possible match (true positive) and any of the parameters mentioned above ($p > 0.05$). There was no correlation between the imaging sequence (group) and a possible detection ($p > 0.05$). Table 2 and Figure 2 summarize the detection of the perforators.

**Table 2.** True positive images per patient. Group 1: Subject 01–06. Group 2: Subject 07–12. Group 3: Scheme 13. TI = Thermal Imaging, HS = Hyperspectral Imaging, LD = Laser Doppler Imaging.

| Subject ID | TI | HS | LD |
|---|---|---|---|
| 01 | 6 | 0 | 0 |
| 02 | 6 | 0 | 0 |
| 03 | 6 | 3/6 | 0 |
| 04 | 6 | 2/6 | 0 |
| 05 | 6 | 3/6 | 0 |
| 06 | 4/6 | 0 | 0 |
| 07 | 6 | 0 | 0 |
| 08 | 6 | 0 | 0 |
| 09 | 6 | 0 | 0 |
| 10 | 0 | 0 | 0 |
| 11 | 6 | 0 | 0 |
| 12 | 6 | 6 | 0 |
| 13 | 6 | 2/6 | 0 |
| 14 | 6 | 0 | 0 |
| 15 | 6 | 0 | 0 |
| 16 | 6 | 6 | 0 |
| 17 | 6 | 0 | 0 |
| 18 | 6 | 6 | 0 |
| Total | 100/108 | 28/108 | 0/108 |

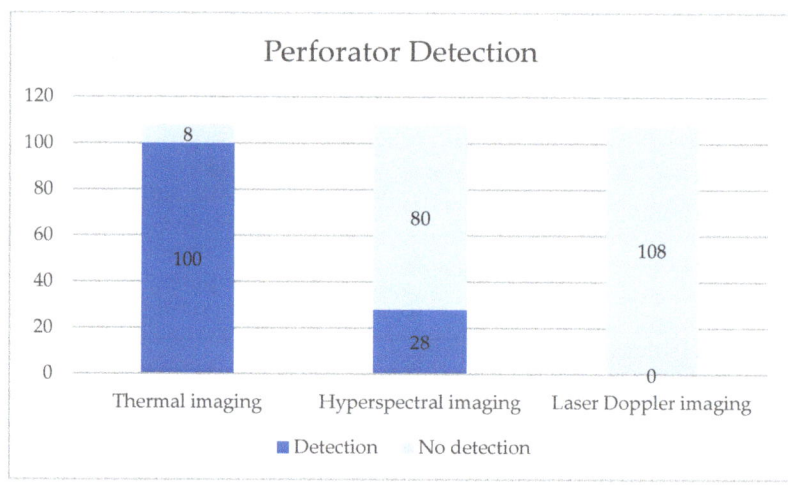

**Figure 2.** Summary of the detection results of the three imaging methods.

### 3.2. TI Detection

On a patient level, 17 of 18 patients showed a positive match (true positive) resulting in a sensitivity of 94.44%. One-hundred of 108 images showed a matching perforator resulting in a sensitivity of 92.59%. All six images of 16 patients showed a positive match. One patient's images started to match after two minutes and one patient's images showed no perforator at all. The false negative rate is therefore 5.56 (1/18 patients) or 7.41% (8/108 images). No false positive (0%) perforator has been detected. Since no true negative could be detected (no patient without a perforator in the handheld Doppler), specificity cannot be indicated. The temporal aspect did not significantly influence the detection rate, since in all but one patient's images the perforator could be seen immediately after the cooling as well as 5 min later. Figure 3 shows an exemplary TI image with a detected perforator.

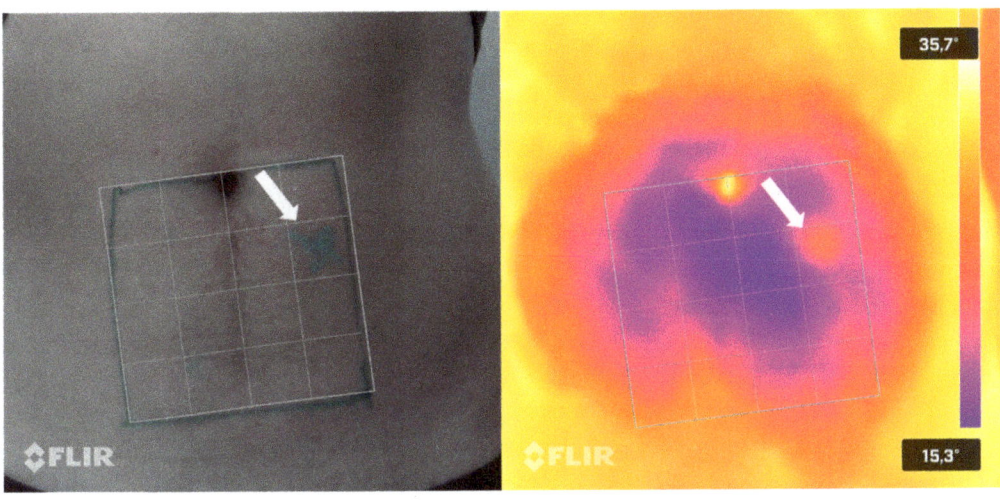

**Figure 3.** Exemplary depiction of a marked perforator (**A**) and the corresponding perforator in the TI (infrared) image (**B**).

*3.3. HS Detection*

On a patient level, 7 of 18 patients showed at least on positive match, resulting in a sensitivity of 38.89%. Twenty-eight of 108 images showed a matching perforator resulting in a sensitivity of 25.93%. Three patients' images showed the reference perforator in all six images, in two patients the perforator was seen for two minutes (3/6 images) and in two patients for one minute (2/6 images). Eleven patients showed no matching perforator at all, yielding a false negative rate of 61.11% (11/18 patients) or 74.07% (80/108 images). No false positive perforator has been detected. Since no true negative had been detected (no patient without a perforator in the handheld Doppler), specificity cannot be indicated. Figure 4 shows an exemplary HS image with a matching perforator.

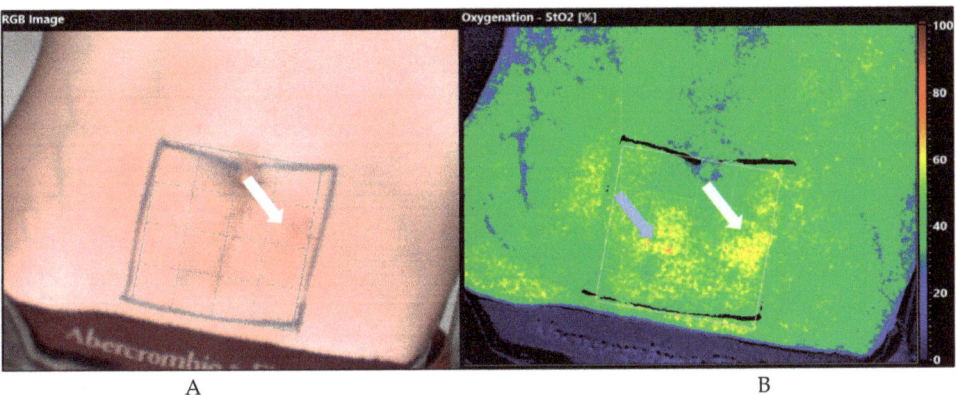

**Figure 4.** Exemplary depiction of a marked perforator (**A**) and the corresponding perforator in the HS (Oxygenation StO$_2$) image (**B**). The mark has been removed and is visible palely to not interfere with the HS imaging. The grey arrow shows another possible perforator that had not been referenced with the pencil Doppler; it was not distinctly more prominent than the reference perforator.

*3.4. LD Detection*

None of the 108 images allowed the detection of the reference perforator yielding a sensitivity of 0% in this setup. Since no true negative has been detected (no patient without a perforator in the handheld Doppler), specificity cannot be indicated. Figure 5 shows an LD image of an abdomen, where no perforator was detected.

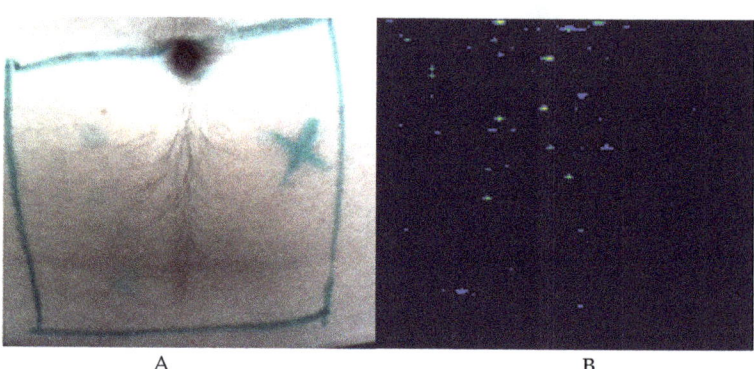

**Figure 5.** Exemplary depiction of a marked perforator (**A**) and the corresponding LD image (**B**), where no perforator was detectable.

## 4. Discussion

Our study investigated the usability of non-invasive, portable imaging devices compared to the handheld Doppler to support an individualized approach in abdominal perforator detection as used in the DIEP flap. We could demonstrate a sensitivity of 94.44%, 38.89% and 0% for TI, HS and LD in this study setup respectively.

While all three methods are used in different clinical indications to assess skin perfusion to some extent, the acquired results yielded different outcomes: TI is a rather new technology indicating a surface's temperature by a smartphone-compatible plug-in. In our study, we could reach a sensitivity of 94.44% when compared to the handheld pencil Doppler device. These results are very promising and quite similar to the ones obtained in other studies with a sensitivity of 86.2% and a specificity of 80% [36], but could not reach the sensitivity of 100% and the specificity of 98% postulated by Pereira et al. who compared the FLIR One to a CT angiography in 20 patients with 38 anterior-lateral-thigh (ALT) flap regions. These rates, however, strongly depend on the methods of evaluation and the standard compared to. In our study setup, image acquisition followed a 20 min period of cooling. This setup was chosen to show the dynamic reperfusion of the abdominal skin to identify the "competing" perforators as proposed by Weum et al. and Muntean et Achimas-Cadariu [37,38]. Other study groups have published TI perforator studies with limited (air fan on the bare abdomen for two minutes) [39] or no cooling at all [23], reaching a sensitivity of 100% and 67% respectively, compared to their standard (intraoperative visualization and pencil Doppler). Both study groups used an older TI device with different specifications. As indicated by de Weerd et al. [40] the "cold challenge" was not reported as uncomfortable by any patient in our study either, and might prove helpful in identifying a more efficient perforator having pushed through the cold earlier than the competitors. We could, however, not reach our goal of completely inhibiting the abdominal skin perfusion entirely using our cold challenge to visualize the dynamics of reperfusion, as perforators in all but one participant were seen immediately after removal of the ice pack. Therefore, our results show a high diagnostic value of the FLIR One TI, which at least complements the preoperative perforator imaging. We observed no correlation of sex, age, BMI, abdominal girth with a possible perforator detection, therefore implying a universal applicability in most patients. TI is a promising and individualized alternative in case CT angiography is unavailable or contraindicated (e.g., allergy to contrast agent) or a lack of experience with the handheld Doppler device to at least support the latter. However, future larger scale studies are necessary to substantiate these findings. TI can be manually calibrated prior to its use to adapt to the surrounding temperatures. Furthermore, it impressed with its ease-to-use requiring close to no training at all, while being cost efficient (currently retails at 229.99$ at the FLIR One homepage) and readily available. The fact that it is used in a no touch, non-invasive technique that can be performed basically anywhere additionally underscores its versatility. Amongst others, its medical applications are the evaluation of burn depth [41–43], detection of postoperative infections [44] or intra- or postoperative free flap monitoring [45,46], but it also allows the assessment of specific research interests [47].

The results of the HS imaging could not reach the accuracy of TI. A sensitivity of 38.89% on a patient level, and 25.93% on an image level is surprisingly low in contrast to the only other HS perforator detection study we could retrieve from the literature: Goetze et al. achieved a sensitivity of 97% when comparing HS to color-coded ultrasound in the detection of ALT flap sites [20]. In two of our study participants the detected perforator was seen for one, and in two participants for two minutes after the 20-min cooling period, before becoming indistinguishable from the surrounding tissue. Goetze et al. used a cooling protocol of three minutes with another three minutes of reperfusion without cooling, in which the images were acquired and showed the highest concordance after three minutes of cooling and after one minute of reperfusion. This might suggest that cooling is indeed necessary for a proper perforator detection, but the timing remains to be investigated. However, it appears that our cooling protocol might have been too long for most of the perforators to be detected. Other parameters like body temperature and blood pressure might also influence a detection and should be evaluated as confounding factors in future assessments. Possibly, another reason for these highly deviating results might be the fact that a different HS device was used, having other focal points within the included software package. Another downside we experienced compared to TI was the unwieldy design of the HS camera and the need for a dark surrounding environment. The HS camera requires a desktop computer and is therefore attached to a trolley, resulting in a bulky device, limiting ease of transport from A to B. Retailing at several thousand Euros, the device requires significant investment. While we could not reproduce the promising results of Goetze et al. in our study and are unable to recommend the device for perforator detection with the described cooling protocol, it has been demonstrated to be of significant value *following* surgical anastomosis for perfusion monitoring and to detect underperfused areas within the flap in other studies [48,49]. Some authors postulate it to be even more effective than the gold standard for flap monitoring, clinical assessment and handheld Doppler [50,51]. Similar aspects are valid for LD imaging. As we did not detect a single perforator using LD in our study, we deem it not suitable for perforator detection in conjunction with our cooling protocol. Significant asset cost, bulky device and training requirements are similarly valid for LD and for HS imaging devices. Just like HS, the value of LD does not lie in the detection of perforators, but the detection of perfusion changes, therefore being a valuable tool for flap monitoring *after* surgery [52–54].

*Limitations & Outlook*

One of this study's limitations is that we have assessed the perforators in a limited number of patients who were not scheduled for flap surgery; therefore, we had no visual confirmation of the perforator to serve as control. Furthermore, the low number of participants in the three groups could possibly conceal an influence of the repeated measurements and is a limitation for meaningful statistical analysis; due to the low case number, we also decided not to analyze the influence of co-morbidities and medication on possible detection. Since no true negatives and false positives were detected, the validation of the devices in our study is also limited. Our study population consisted of only 33.3% females; even though we did not demonstrate a correlation between gender and possible detection, DIEP flaps are usually performed in females. Hence, the gender distribution should be listed as a limitation as well. Another major limitation is the fact, that the detection of a perforator was at the subjective discretion of investigators. We were not able to retrieve predefined requirements for a perforator to be objectively evaluated as "positive" in these imaging methods from the literature. To reduce the impact of this limitation, we had two independent investigators assess the images who were blinded to the handheld Doppler. Additionally, a possible bias cannot be excluded due to human error. Another limitation is our study setup that included a 20-min cooling period prior to the imaging, which might have had an influence on the sensitivity of the devices. Physical parameters like blood pressure and body temperature, which we did not assess, should also be evaluated in future assessments to detect possible correlations. Since we defined a ROI below the umbilicus, it is possible to have missed matching perforators outside of the ROI, and of course, to have misinterpreted findings. Lastly, since the devices have their imaging focus in different depths (surface vs. mm), results should be considered complementary and not competitively.

Future studies should focus on different cooling strategies/protocols, and the question whether these are actually necessary for perforator detection with TI. They should be designed as prospective case-control-studies with larger patient cohorts.

## 5. Conclusions

In conclusion, we conducted this study to assess non-invasive, portable imaging tools as to their ability to detect perforators. We demonstrated a high value of TI for perforator detection, being almost as effective as the handheld Doppler device, which is in frequent use in our institution. To obtain the best possible outcome after surgery, an individualized approach should be derived. This approach should not only take into consideration the individual patient, but also the treating physician, institution and everyone else in patient care. Individual patients requiring a sophisticated reconstruction with a perforator flap should be planned as individually and personalized as possible. Therefore, perforator detection by TI can be a valid alternative in a patient with an allergy to contrast agents, or a surgeon not sufficiently experienced with the handheld Doppler. Postoperative flap monitoring could be performed by HS or LD, both of which are not as suitable for perforator detection, according to our results. A combination of available tools/devices should be used that is most appropriate, with each device being justified given the respective indication [33] to guarantee the most beneficial possible for the patient.

**Author Contributions:** Conceptualization, S.P.N. and L.-P.K.; methodology, H.L.; validation, S.P.N., R.W. and L.-P.K.; formal analysis, A.-C.T., R.W. and L.-P.K.; investigation, S.P.N., S.J.G. and M.S.; resources, L.-P.K.; data curation, S.J.G., A.-C.T., H.L. and S.P.N.; writing—original draft preparation, S.P.N.; writing—review and editing, H.L., A.-C.T., M.S., S.J.G., R.W. and L.-P.K.; visualization, H.L. and M.S.; supervision, L.-P.K.; project administration, H.L., M.S.; funding acquisition, L.-P.K. and S.P.N. All authors have read and agreed to the published version of the manuscript.

**Funding:** This research received no external funding.

**Institutional Review Board Statement:** The study was conducted according to the guidelines of the Declaration of Helsinki, and approved by the Ethics Committee of Medical University Graz, Austria (protocol code 31-477 ex 18/19, 27 August 2019).

**Informed Consent Statement:** Informed consent was obtained from all subjects involved in the study.

**Data Availability Statement:** Detailed data supporting the results are available at the authors.

**Acknowledgments:** We would like to thank Robert Zrim and team for his English editing.

**Conflicts of Interest:** The authors declare no conflict of interest.

## References

1. Lee, B.T.; Agarwal, J.P.; Ascherman, J.A.; Caterson, S.A.; Gray, D.D.; Hollenbeck, S.T.; Khan, S.A.; Loeding, L.D.; Mahabir, R.C.; Miller, A.S.; et al. Evidence-Based Clinical Practice Guideline: Autologous Breast Reconstruction with DIEP or Pedicled TRAM Abdominal Flaps. *Plast. Reconstr. Surg.* **2017**, *140*, 651e–664e. [CrossRef]
2. Renzulli, M.; Clemente, A.; Brocchi, S.; Gelati, C.; Zanotti, S.; Pizzi, C.; Tassone, D.; Cappabianca, S.; Cipriani, R.; Golfieri, R. Preoperative Computed Tomography Assessment for a Deep Inferior Epigastric Perforator (DIEP) Flap: A New Easy Technique from the Bologna Experience. *Acta Radiol.* **2020**. [CrossRef]
3. Chaput, B.; Meresse, T.; Bekara, F.; Grolleau, J.; Gangloff, D.; Gandolfi, S.; Herlin, C. Lower Limb Perforator Flaps: Current Concept. *Ann. Chir. Plast. Esthet.* **2020**, *65*, 496–516. [CrossRef] [PubMed]
4. Cina, A.; Barone-Adesi, L.; Rinaldi, P.; Cipriani, A.; Salgarello, M.; Masetti, R.; Bonomo, L. Planning Deep Inferior Epigastric Perforator Flaps for Breast Reconstruction: A Comparison between Multidetector Computed Tomography and Magnetic Resonance Angiography. *Eur. Radiol.* **2013**, *23*, 2333–2343. [CrossRef] [PubMed]
5. Wade, R.G.; Watford, J.; Wormald, J.C.R.; Bramhall, R.J.; Figus, A. Perforator Mapping Reduces the Operative Time of DIEP Flap Breast Reconstruction: A Systematic Review and Meta-Analysis of Preoperative Ultrasound, Computed Tomography and Magnetic Resonance Angiography. *J. Plast. Reconstr. Aesthetic Surg.* **2018**, *71*, 468–477. [CrossRef]
6. D'angelo, A.; Cina, A.; Macrì, G.; Belli, P.; Mercogliano, S.; Barbieri, P.; Grippo, C.; Franceschini, G.; D'archi, S.; Mason, E.J.; et al. Conventional Ct versus Dedicated Ct Angiography in Diep Flap Planning: A Feasibility Study. *J. Pers. Med.* **2021**, *11*, 277. [CrossRef]
7. Rozen, W.M.; Ashton, M.W.; Taylor, G.I. Reviewing the vascular supply of the anterior abdominal wall: Redefining anatomy for increasingly refined surgery. *Clin. Anat.* **2008**, *21*, 89–98. [CrossRef]
8. Kiely, J.; Kumar, M.; Wade, R.G. The Accuracy of Different Modalities of Perforator Mapping for Unilateral DIEP Flap Breast Reconstruction: A Systematic Review and Meta-Analysis. *J. Plast. Reconstr. Aesthetic Surg.* **2021**, *74*, 945–956. [CrossRef]
9. Pereira, N.; Valenzuela, D.; Mangelsdorff, G.; Kufeke, M.; Roa, R. Detection of Perforators for Free Flap Planning Using Smartphone Thermal Imaging: A Concordance Study with Computed Tomographic Angiography in 120 Perforators. *Plast. Reconstr. Surg.* **2018**, *141*, 787–792. [CrossRef]
10. Kagen, A.C.; Hossain, R.; Dayan, E.; Maddula, S.; Samson, W.; Dayan, J.; Smith, M.L. Modern Perforator Flap Imaging with High-Resolution Blood Pool MR Angiography. *Radiographics* **2015**, *35*, 901–915. [CrossRef]
11. Schmauss, D.; Beier, J.P.; Eisenhardt, S.U.; Horch, R.E.; Momeni, A.; Rab, M.; Rieck, B.; Rieger, U.; Schaefer, D.J.; Schmidt, V.J.; et al. The „safe" Flap—Preoperative Perforator-Mapping and Intraoperative Perfusion Assessment to Reduce Flap-Associated Morbidity Statement of the German Speaking Working Group for Microsurgery of the Peripheral Nerves and Vessels. *Handchir. Mikrochir. Plast. Chir.* **2019**, *51*, 410–417. [CrossRef]
12. Chubb, D.; Rozen, W.M.; Whitaker, I.S.; Ashton, M.W. Images in Plastic Surgery: Digital Thermographic Photography ("thermal Imaging") for Preoperative Perforator Mapping. *Ann. Plast. Surg.* **2011**, *66*, 324–325. [CrossRef]
13. Daigeler, A.; Schubert, C.; Hirsch, T.; Behr, B.; Lehnhardt, M. Colour Duplex Sonography and "Power-Duplex" in Perforator Surgery—Improvement of Patients Safety by Efficient Planning. *Handchir. Mikrochir. Plast. Chir.* **2018**, *50*, 101–110. [CrossRef] [PubMed]
14. Ono, S.; Ohi, H.; Ogawa, R. Propeller Flaps: Imaging in Propeller Flap Surgery. *Semin. Plast. Surg.* **2020**, *34*, 145. [CrossRef] [PubMed]
15. Khan, U.D.; Miller, J.G. Reliability of Handheld Doppler in Planning Local Perforator-Based Flaps for Extremities. *Aesthetic Plast. Surg.* **2007**, *31*, 521–525. [CrossRef] [PubMed]
16. Taylor, G.; Doyle, M.; McCarten, G. The Doppler Probe for Planning Flaps: Anatomical Study and Clinical Applications. *Br. J. Plast. Surg.* **1990**, *43*, 1–16. [CrossRef]
17. Stekelenburg, C.M.; Sonneveld, P.M.D.G.; Bouman, M.B.; van der Wal, M.B.A.; Knol, D.L.; de Vet, H.C.W.; van Zuijlen, P.P.M. The Hand Held Doppler Device for the Detection of Perforators in Reconstructive Surgery: What You Hear Is Not Always What You Get. *Burns* **2014**, *40*, 1702–1706. [CrossRef]
18. Ono, S.; Hayashi, H.; Ohi, H.; Ogawa, R. Imaging Studies for Preoperative Planning of Perforator Flaps: An Overview. *Clin. Plast. Surg.* **2017**, *44*, 21–30. [CrossRef]
19. Unger, M.; Markfort, M.; Halama, D.; Chalopin, C. Automatic Detection of Perforator Vessels Using Infrared Thermography in Reconstructive Surgery. *Int. J. Comput. Assist. Radiol. Surg.* **2019**, *14*, 501–507. [CrossRef]
20. Goetze, E.; Thiem, D.G.E.; Gielisch, M.W.; Kämmerer, P.W. Identification of Cutaneous Perforators for Microvascular Surgery Using Hyperspectral Technique—A Feasibility Study on the Antero-Lateral Thigh. *J. Cranio-Maxillofac. Surg.* **2020**, *48*, 1066–1073. [CrossRef]
21. Chaput, B.; Bertheuil, N.; Gandolfi, S.; Grolleau, J.L.; Herlin, C. Perforator Detection with a Hand-Held Doppler Device: Importance of the Learning Curve. *Burns* **2015**, *41*, 197. [CrossRef]
22. Sheena, Y.; Jennison, T.; Hardwicke, J.T.; Titley, O.G. Detection of Perforators Using Thermal Imaging. *Plast. Reconstr. Surg.* **2013**, *132*, 1603–1610. [CrossRef] [PubMed]
23. Tenorio, X.; Mahajan, A.L.; Elias, B.; van Riempst, J.S.; Wettstein, R.; Harder, Y.; Pittet, B. Locating Perforator Vessels by Dynamic Infrared Imaging and Flow Doppler with No Thermal Cold Challenge. *Ann. Plast. Surg.* **2011**, *67*, 143–146. [CrossRef] [PubMed]

24. Holmer, A.; Tetschke, F.; Marotz, J.; Malberg, H.; Markgraf, W.; Thiele, C.; Kulcke, A. Oxygenation and Perfusion Monitoring with a Hyperspectral Camera System for Chemical Based Tissue Analysis of Skin and Organs. *Physiol. Meas.* **2016**, *37*, 2064–2078. [CrossRef] [PubMed]
25. Xiao, W.; Li, K.; Kiu-Huen Ng, S.; Feng, S.; Zhou, H.; Nicoli, F.; Blondeel, P.; Zhang, Y. A Prospective Comparative Study of Color Doppler Ultrasound and Infrared Thermography in the Detection of Perforators for Anterolateral Thigh Flaps. *Ann. Plast. Surg.* **2020**, *84*, S190–S195. [CrossRef] [PubMed]
26. Holmer, A.; Marotz, J.; Wahl, P.; Dau, M.; Kämmerer, P.W. Hyperspectral Imaging in Perfusion and Wound Diagnostics-Methods and Algorithms for the Determination of Tissue Parameters. *Biomed. Tech.* **2018**, *63*, 587–594. [CrossRef] [PubMed]
27. Thiem, D.G.E.; Frick, R.W.; Goetze, E.; Gielisch, M.; Al-Nawas, B.; Kämmerer, P.W. Hyperspectral Analysis for Perioperative Perfusion Monitoring—A Clinical Feasibility Study on Free and Pedicled Flaps. *Clin. Oral Investig.* **2021**, *25*, 933–945. [CrossRef]
28. Shin, J.Y.; Yi, H.S. Diagnostic Accuracy of Laser Doppler Imaging in Burn Depth Assessment: Systematic Review and Meta-Analysis. *Burn. J. Int. Soc. Burn. Inj.* **2016**, *42*, 1369–1376. [CrossRef]
29. Tindholdt, T.; Saidian, S.; Tønseth, K. Microcirculatory Evaluation of Deep Inferior Epigastric Artery Perforator Flaps with Laser Doppler Perfusion Imaging in Breast Reconstruction. *J. Plast. Surg. hand Surg.* **2011**, *45*, 143–147. [CrossRef]
30. FLIR ONE. Pro Thermal Imaging Camera for Smartphones | Teledyne FLIR. Available online: https://www.flir.eu/products/flir-one-pro/ (accessed on 4 July 2021).
31. TIVITA®. Wound—Diaspective Vision. Available online: https://diaspective-vision.com/en/produkt/tivita-wound/ (accessed on 24 September 2021).
32. Oberg, P. Laser-Doppler Flowmetry. *Crit. Rev. Biomed. Eng.* **1990**, *18*, 125–163.
33. Hallock, G. Acoustic Doppler Sonography, Color Duplex Ultrasound, and Laser Doppler Flowmetry as Tools for Successful Autologous Breast Reconstruction. *Clin. Plast. Surg.* **2011**, *38*, 203–211. [CrossRef] [PubMed]
34. Laser Doppler Line Scanning—MoorLDLS-BI—Moor Instruments. Available online: https://www.moorclinical.com/products/imaging/line-imaging/ (accessed on 24 September 2021).
35. Öztuna, D.; Elhan, A.H.; Tüccar, E. Investigation of Four Different Normality Tests in Terms of Type 1 Error Rate and Power under Different Distributions. *Turk. J. Med. Sci.* **2006**, *36*, 171–176.
36. Rabbani, M.; Ilyas, A.; Rabbani, A.; Abidin, Z.; Tarar, M. Accuracy of Thermal Imaging Camera in Identification of Perforators. *J. Coll. Physicians Surg. Pak. JCPSP* **2020**, *30*, 512–515. [CrossRef] [PubMed]
37. Weum, S.; Lott, A.; de Weerd, L. Detection of Perforators Using Smartphone Thermal Imaging. *Plast. Reconstr. Surg.* **2016**, *138*, 938e–940e. [CrossRef] [PubMed]
38. Muntean, M.V.; Achimas-Cadariu, P.A. Detection of Perforators for Free Flap Planning Using Smartphone Thermal Imaging: A Concordance Study with Computed Tomographic Angiography in 120 Perforators. *Plast. Reconstr. Surg.* **2018**, *142*, 604E. [CrossRef] [PubMed]
39. De Weerd, L.; Weum, S.; Mercer, J.B. The Value of Dynamic Infrared Thermography (DIRT) in Perforator Selection and Planning of Free DIEP Flaps. *Ann. Plast. Surg.* **2009**, *63*, 274–279. [CrossRef] [PubMed]
40. De Weerd, L.; Weum, S.; Mercer, J.B. Locating Perforator Vessels by Dynamic Infrared Imaging and Flow Doppler with No Thermal Cold Challenge. *Ann. Plast. Surg.* **2014**, *72*, 261. [CrossRef] [PubMed]
41. Xue, E.Y.; Chandler, L.K.; Viviano, S.L.; Keith, J.D. Use of FLIR ONE Smartphone Thermography in Burn Wound Assessment. *Ann. Plast. Surg.* **2018**, *80*, S236–S238. [CrossRef] [PubMed]
42. Jaspers, M.E.H.; Carrière, M.E.; Meij-de Vries, A.; Klaessens, J.H.G.M.; van Zuijlen, P.P.M. The FLIR ONE Thermal Imager for the Assessment of Burn Wounds: Reliability and Validity Study. *Burns* **2017**, *43*, 1516–1523. [CrossRef]
43. Ganon, S.; Guédon, A.; Cassier, S.; Atlan, M. Contribution of Thermal Imaging in Determining the Depth of Pediatric Acute Burns. *Burns* **2020**, *46*, 1091–1099. [CrossRef]
44. Romanò, C.L.; Logoluso, N.; Dell'Oro, F.; Elia, A.; Drago, L. Telethermographic Findings after Uncomplicated and Septic Total Knee Replacement. *The Knee* **2012**, *19*, 193–197. [CrossRef] [PubMed]
45. Just, M.; Chalopin, C.; Unger, M.; Halama, D.; Neumuth, T.; Dietz, A.; Fischer, M. Monitoring of Microvascular Free Flaps Following Oropharyngeal Reconstruction Using Infrared Thermography: First Clinical Experiences. *Eur. Arch. Oto-Rhino-Laryngol.* **2015**, *273*, 2659–2667. [CrossRef] [PubMed]
46. Verstockt, J.; Thiessen, F.; Cloostermans, B.; Tjalma, W.; Steenackers, G. DIEP Flap Breast Reconstructions: Thermographic Assistance as a Possibility for Perforator Mapping and Improvement of DIEP Flap Quality. *Appl. Opt.* **2020**, *59*, E48. [CrossRef]
47. Nischwitz, S.P.; Luze, H.; Kamolz, L.P. Thermal Imaging via FLIR One—A Promising Tool in Clinical Burn Care and Research. *Burns* **2020**, *46*, 988–989. [CrossRef] [PubMed]
48. Heimes, D.; Becker, P.; Thiem, D.; Kuchen, R.; Kyyak, S.; Kämmerer, P. Is Hyperspectral Imaging Suitable for Assessing Collateral Circulation Prior Radial Forearm Free Flap Harvesting? Comparison of Hyperspectral Imaging and Conventional Allen's Test. *J. Pers. Med.* **2021**, *11*, 531. [CrossRef]
49. Schulz, T.; Marotz, J.; Stukenberg, A.; Reumuth, G.; Houschyar, K.; Siemers, F. Hyperspectral Imaging for Postoperative Flap Monitoring of Pedicled Flaps. *Handchir. Mikrochir. Plast. Chir. Organ Dtsch. Arb. Handchir. Organ Dtsch. Arb. Mikrochir. Peripher. Nerven Gefasse Organ V* **2020**, *52*, 316–324. [CrossRef]

50. Kohler, L.H.; Köhler, H.; Kohler, S.; Langer, S.; Nuwayhid, R.; Gockel, I.; Spindler, N.; Osterhoff, G. Hyperspectral Imaging (HSI) as a New Diagnostic Tool in Free Flap Monitoring for Soft Tissue Reconstruction: A Proof of Concept Study. *BMC Surgery* **2021**, *21*, 1–9. [CrossRef]
51. Smit, J.M.; Zeebregts, C.J.; Acosta, R.; Werker, P.M.N. Advancements in Free Flap Monitoring in the Last Decade: A Critical Review. *Plast. Reconstr. Surg.* **2010**, *125*, 177–185. [CrossRef]
52. Tindholdt, T.T.; Saidian, S.; Pripp, A.H.; Tønseth, K.A. Monitoring Microcirculatory Changes in the Deep Inferior Epigastric Artery Perforator Flap with Laser Doppler Perfusion Imaging. *Ann. Plast. Surg.* **2011**, *67*, 139–142. [CrossRef]
53. Van den Heuvel, M.G.W.; Mermans, J.F.; Ambergen, A.W.; van der Hulst, R.R.W.J. Perfusion of the Deep Inferior Epigastric Perforator Flap Measured by Laser Doppler Imager. *Ann. Plast. Surg.* **2011**, *66*, 648–653. [CrossRef]
54. Abdelrahman, M.; Jumabhoy, I.; Qiu, S.S.; Fufa, D.; Hsu, C.-C.; Lin, C.-H.; Lin, Y.-T.; Lin, C.-H. Perfusion Dynamics of the Medial Sural Artery Perforator (MSAP) Flap in Lower Extremity Reconstruction Using Laser Doppler Perfusion Imaging (LDPI): A Clinical Study. *J. Plast. Surg. Hand Surg.* **2019**, *54*, 112–119. [CrossRef] [PubMed]

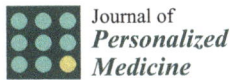

*Article*

# Preliminary Results of the "Capasquelet" Technique for Managing Femoral Bone Defects—Combining a Masquelet Induced Membrane and Capanna Vascularized Fibula with an Allograft

Alexis Combal [1], François Thuau [2], Alban Fouasson-Chailloux [3], Pierre-Paul Arrigoni [4], Marc Baud'huin [5], Franck Duteille [2] and Vincent Crenn [1,6,*]

1. Clinique Chirurgicale Orthopédique et Traumatologique, CHU de Nantes, University Hospital of Nantes, 44093 Nantes, France; alexis.combal@chu-nantes.fr
2. Service de Chirurgie Plastique et Reconstructrice, CHU de Nantes, University Hospital of Nantes, 44093 Nantes, France; francois.thuau@chu-nantes.fr (F.T.); franck.duteille@chu-nantes.fr (F.D.)
3. Service de Médecine Physique et de Réadaptation Locomotrice, CHU de Nantes, University Hospital of Nantes, 44093 Nantes, France; alban.fouassonchailloux@chu-nantes.fr
4. Service de Radiologie, CHU de Nantes, University Hospital of Nantes, 44093 Nantes, France; pierrepaul.arrigoni@chu-nantes.fr
5. Banque Multi-Tissus, CHU de Nantes, University Hospital of Nantes, 44093 Nantes, France; marc.baudhuin@chu-nantes.fr
6. INSERM U1238—Faculté de Médecine 1 rue Gaston Veil, 44035 Nantes, France
* Correspondence: vincent.crenn@chu-nantes.fr

**Abstract:** We describe the preliminary results of a novel two-stage reconstruction technique for extended femoral bone defects using an allograft in accordance with the Capanna technique with an embedded vascularized fibula graft in an induced membrane according to the Masquelet technique. We performed what we refer to as "Capasquelet" surgery in femoral diaphyseal bone loss of at least 10 cm. Four patients were operated on using this technique: two tumors and two traumatic bone defects in a septic context with a minimum follow up of one year. Consolidation on both sides, when achieved, occurred at 5.5 months (4–7), with full weight-bearing at 11 weeks (8–12). The functional scores were satisfactory with an EQ5D of 63.3 (45–75). The time to bone union and early weight-bearing with this combined technique are promising compared to the literature. The osteoinductive role of the induced membrane could play a positive role in the evolution of the graft. Longer follow up and a larger cohort are needed to better assess the implications. Nonetheless, this two-stage technique appears to have ample promise, especially in a septic context or in adjuvant radiotherapy in an oncological context.

**Keywords:** critical bone defect; vascularized fibula; Capanna technique; Masquelet induced membrane; intercalary reconstruction; bone tumor; ballistic trauma

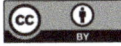

## 1. Introduction

Critical diaphyseal bone defects remain a surgical challenge, and several treatment methods have been described [1–6] (autograft, vascularized fibula, bone transport, diaphyseal endoprosthesis, etc.). The gold-standard indications are still a matter of debate, and the results are variable. Malignant bone tumors, with their specificities, such as chemotherapy and radiotherapy [7] or septic ballistic trauma, add complexity to this challenging management [7–10].

We describe a novel two-stage technique for reconstruction of extended femoral bone defects, combining the allograft technique with inlay of a vascularized fibula (i.e., "Capanna technique") [11] and the induced membrane technique (i.e., "Masquelet technique") [1,12]. We performed this innovative procedure in critical bone defects of at least 10 cm that were due to the fact of tumor pathology secondary to carcinologic resection or a traumatic event. The combination proposed by what we refer to as the "Capasquelet" technique provides several advantages: the biological chamber with the induced membrane prevents resorption of the graft and has an osteoinductive role [13–16]; it also limits septic risks, and it avoids a long one-stage surgery [17]. The vascularized fibula can be more than 20 cm in size, and it improves both intercalary allograft survival and bone union [18]; some of the autologous grafts are also impacted at the interfaces [19]. By combining these methods, the "Capasquelet" technique can pool these advantages: the contribution of a living graft through the vascularized fibula, associated with the primary mechanical strength of the allograft in an environment that encourages osteogenesis, and an autologous bone graft at the extremities.

This preliminary study describes this novel hybrid surgical technique. We assessed the bone healing, the time to full weight-bearing, and the complications in addition to conducting a functional score analysis.

## 2. Method

The Masquelet technique proposes a two-stage procedure combining induced membrane and cancellous autograft [12]. While the Capanna technique offers a hybrid reconstruction with a vascularized fibula embedded in an allograft [11]. With the "Capasquelet" procedure, we propose to combine these two methods. This two-stage surgery was performed on four patients in a similar manner. The time between the two surgical stages was decided on a case-by-case basis (17 weeks (8–24)). An angio-CT scan was systematically performed before the second stage to check the blood supply and to confirm the feasibility of performing the vascular anastomosis of the fibular graft.

*2.1. Surgical Technique*

2.1.1. The First Stage

The two patients with bone tumors underwent initial oncologic resection; the other patients had post-traumatic septic lesions that required debridement, irrigation, bacteriological sampling, and antibiotic therapy. The femur was prepared with a clear, clean cut in a healthy zone, if necessary, either transversally ($n = 3$) or in step-cut ($n = 1$). The aim of this first step was to model a cement spacer using high-viscosity Heraeus Palacos® R + G cement (Hanau, Germany); it has to fill the bone loss as fully as possible. We preferred to oversize it somewhat in width if the soft tissue coverage was not an issue, as it increases reconstruction space and facilitates induced membrane closure for the second stage. The spacer was needed to cover the bone–host interfaces as recommended in the Masquelet technique [12]. It was enhanced on a locked intramedullary nailing, positioned back and forth ($n = 3$) or on a plate ($n = 1$) (Figure 1).

2.1.2. Interstage Planification

The femoral allograft dimensions were determined to obtain a morphology that resembles that of the patient as much as possible; the diaphysis shaft width must allow the fibula to slide into it. We used cryopreserved allografts from the Nantes Multi-Tissue Bank, in compliance with the criteria of the French Agency of Biomedicine. The delay between the two stages depended on the indication and its requirements: the degree of tissue and skin healing or the antibiotic duration in trauma and adjuvant therapy planning in oncological situations.

2.1.3. The Second Stage

The length and the rotational axis had to be carefully determined before spacer removal. The vascularized fibula graft required microsurgical expertise for harvesting and vascular anastomoses. The fibula graft could be $\geq 4$ cm of the bone defect length. Graft harvesting could be undertaken from the contralateral limb by a second team with microsurgical skills in order to limit the operative time. The harvesting was performed with a tourniquet while ensuring that at least 8 cm [20] of the distal fibula was left in order to limit malleolar instability. A lateral surgical approach was used to raise the osseous flap. The fibula was mainly vascularized by an artery from the peroneal artery that entered the middle-third of the bone. The section must include this part of the bone. After identification of the artery, it was dissected to its origin from the tibio-fibular trunk [21,22].

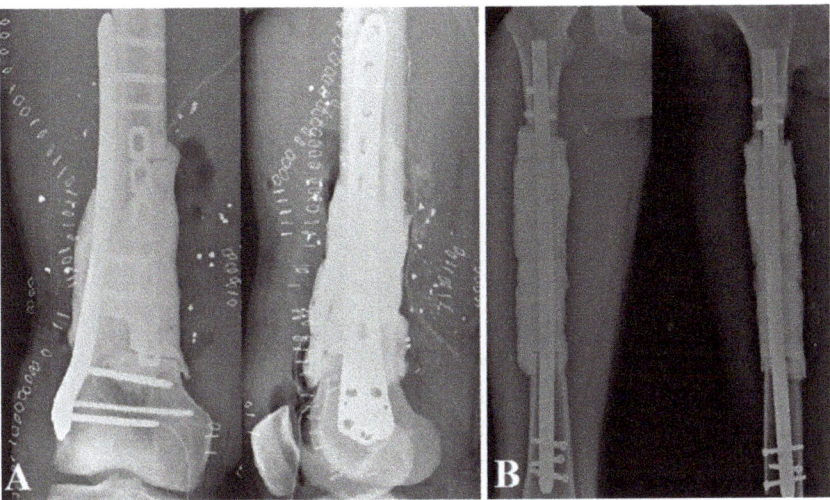

**Figure 1.** Postoperative X-ray AP and lateral view of the spacers: (**A**) a plate-enhanced spacer on a bone defect with step-cut in setting a septic ballistic trauma of the right distal femur (patient No. 4); (**B**) an intramedullary nail-enhanced spacer on a bone defect after an Ewing sarcoma resection.

The allograft was left for one hour in a warm physiological serum bath and then prepared with an oscillating saw in relation to the length of the bone defect; one team could be devoted to preparing the allograft (Figure 2). The microsurgical anastomosis was usually performed at the terminal branches of the profunda femoris artery or with an end-to-side anastomosis with the superficial femoral artery (Figure 2) [23].

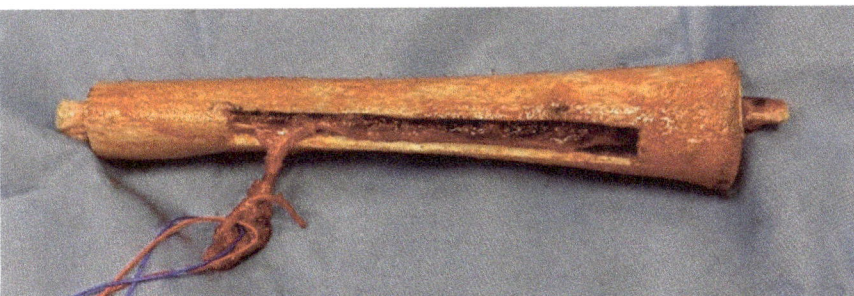

**Figure 2.** Vascularized fibula embedded in the femoral allograft before implantation. The allograft window makes vascular anastomosis possible. There was an extra 20 mm after each extremity of the fibula (patient No. 3).

The allograft was reamed to the diameter required ($\geq 2$ mm of the maximum diameter of the fibula). A bone window was created for the passage and preservation of the arteriovenous axis given the micro-anastomoses, oriented towards the vascular axis for anastomosis. The patient's femur was also reamed, and the reaming material was preserved to perform a complementary autologous bone graft at the interfaces.

The composite graft was then placed in the correct orientation, while taking into account the rotational axes. The fibula had to be well-positioned to obtain an equivalent proximal and distal overlap of approximately 2 cm.

Stabilization was achieved with a large LCP plate; the graft was held in place by at least two single cortical screws. Finally, compression was applied at both interfaces after the autologous graft bone from the reaming was added (Figure 3).

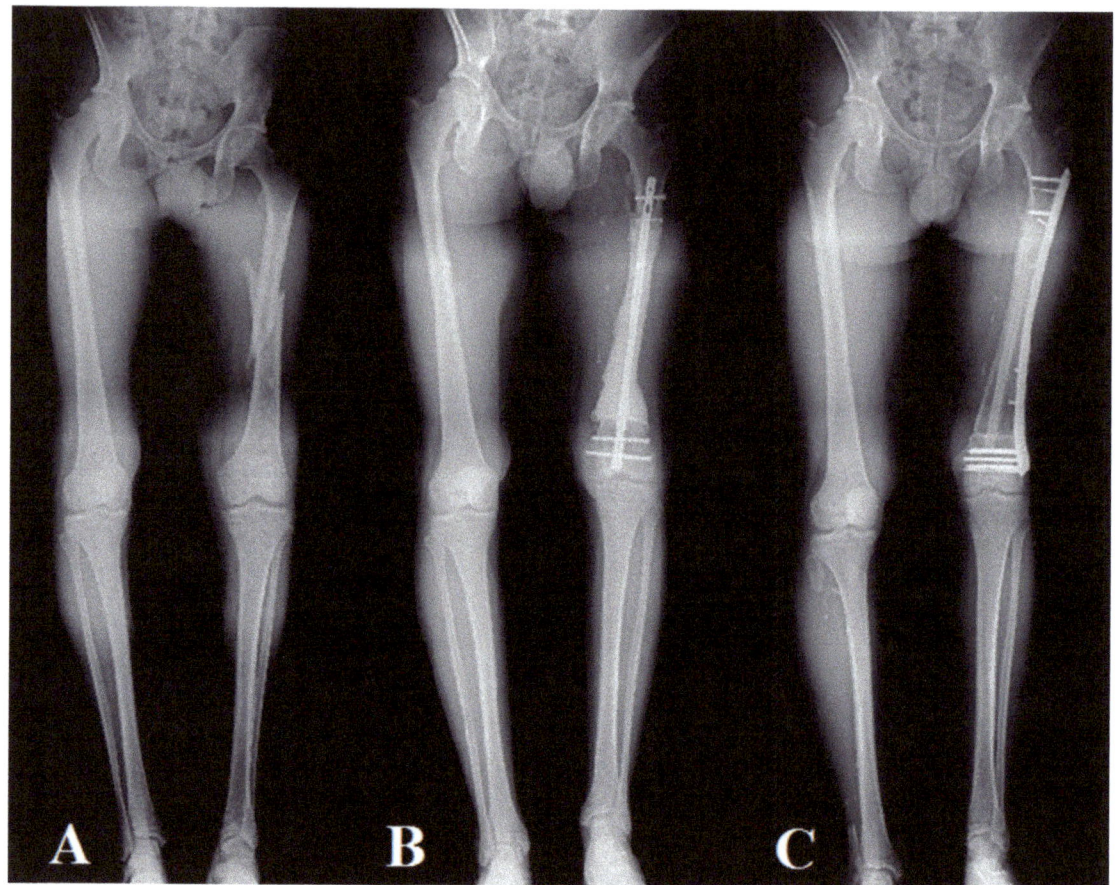

**Figure 3.** Progression of a Capasquelet technique reconstruction, using a pangonogram X-ray view, in a 28 year old patient with high-grade osteosarcoma (patient No. 2): (**A**) preoperative X-ray, fractured high-grade osteosarcoma with a length inequality of 80 mm; (**B**) postoperative X-ray of the 1st surgical stage after carcinologic resection and placement of the spacer on an intramedullary nail with a length inequality of 60 mm (post-T1 delay: 1 month); (**C**) postoperative X-ray at 1 year, residual lower limb inequality of 40 mm.

2.1.4. Postoperative Management

Early mobilization and progressive weight-bearing were allowed postoperatively. Strictly limited weight-bearing was prescribed for the first six weeks, with progressive full weight-bearing depending on the patient's pain and condition.

2.2. Data Collection and Analysis

We performed the "Capasquelet" technique on four patients with bone defects of at least 10 cm. Two tumors and two traumatic lesions were operated on between 2018 and

2020 with a minimum follow up of one year. We collected the following data for each case: age, gender, BMI, characteristics of the defect, and surgical and postoperative data. Bone consolidation was assessed radiologically (postoperative X-rays were performed at least every three months until union). This criterion was defined by cortical union of at least 75%, as determined on standard X-rays. If the assessment of union was inconclusive on conventional X-rays, the union was assessed using computed tomography (CT) [24]. Surgical intervention to facilitate union of osseous junctions in Henderson type 2 complications, at least six months after the primary surgery, was defined as non-union [25]. We selected the International Society of Limb Salvage (ISOLS) method to determine the degree of integration of the grafts [26]. The functional results were assessed using the EQ5D score (EQ5D is an instrument that evaluates the generic quality of life) [27].

## 3. Results

The mean age of the patients was 23.6 years (18–44), the mean length of the femoral bone defect was 150 mm (100–240), the length of the vascularized contralateral harvested fibula autograft was 220 mm (150–280), and the duration of the second stage surgical reconstruction was 520 min (464–580). No fibula donor site morbidity was noted (Table 1). The four patients did not have comorbidities or risk factors for vascularized graft failure, excluding oncologic status and treatment for patients 2 and 3.

Table 1. Summarized data for the four patients operated on using the Capasquelet technique. IMN: Intramedullary nail, T1: first stage, T2: second stage, RTA: road traffic accident, DOD: dead of disease, * Patient refused radiological follow up, with only clinical follow up.

| Patient No. | 1 | 2 | 3 | 4 |
|---|---|---|---|---|
| Epidemiology data | | | | |
| Gender | Female | Male | Male | Male |
| Age (years) | 44 | 28 | 18 | 24 |
| BMI (kg/m$^2$) | 24.5 | 22.3 | 20.5 | 24.9 |
| Etiology | Traumatic (RTA) | Osteosarcoma | Ewing Tumor | Traumatic (Ballistic) |
| Length Bone Loss (mm) | 100 | 220 | 180 | 110 (Step-cut) |
| Follow up (months) | 36 | 22 | 14 | 12 |
| Surgical data | | | | |
| First-stage associated surgery | Preparation | Resection R0 | Resection R0 | Sepsis treatment |
| Spacer stabilization | IMN | IMN | IMN | Plate |
| Total operative time (T1; T2) (minutes) | 716 (136; 580) | 774 (295; 479) | 656 (192; 464) | 793 (235; 558) |
| Fibula graft length (mm) | 150 | 280 | 220 | 160 |
| Graft stabilization | Plate | Plate | Plate | Platex2 |
| Delay T1 and T2 (weeks) | 8 | 22 | 24 | 12 |
| Postoperative data | | | | |
| Complications | Hematoma | No | Material failure | No |
| Delay surgical revision (weeks) | 3 (after T2) | | 28 (after T2) | |
| Type of surgery | Hematoma evacuation | | Fixation revision | |
| Time for consolidation (months) | 4 | 7 | DOD | No X-ray * |
| ISOLS score at three months (%) | 86.7 | 73.3 | 75.6 | |
| ISOLS score at six months (%) | 95.6 | 95.6 | 68.9 | |
| Functional results | | | | |
| Full weight-bearing (weeks) | 12 | 12 | 12 | 8 |
| EQ5D | 70 | 75 | DOD | 45 |

The average time between the two stages was 17 weeks (8–24). Bone union of both interfaces (defined as bridging bone across three of the four cortices evaluated at each junction in the biplane radiographs or CT scan fusion) was achieved at 5.5 months (4–7), except for one irradiated area with a patient who died of their disease. Full weight-bearing was possible at 11 weeks (8–12) in the cohort. Revision surgery was performed for one patient at three weeks for evacuation of a hematoma. Another was performed for stabilization revision (Henderson type 3) on an irradiated area; this patient died of his disease and could not achieve full bone healing due to the pronounced deterioration in their general condition. The functional scores were satisfactory with an EQ5D of 63.3 (45–75) (Figure 4). Patient No. 4 did not obtain postoperative X-rays or CT scans due to the fact of socio-financial difficulties but achieved full weight-bearing at 2 months, with no revision surgery, and was evaluated clinically.

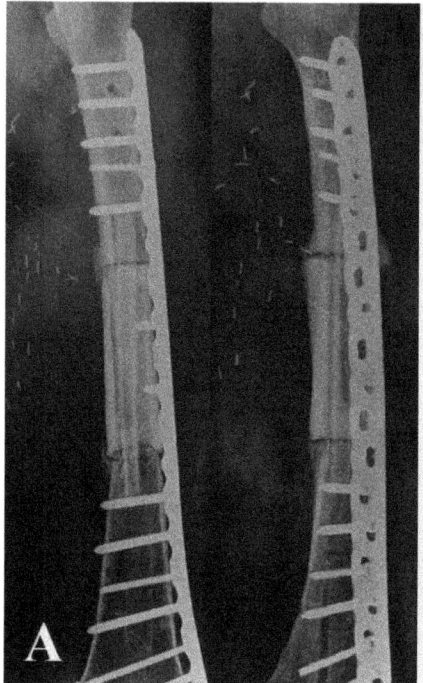
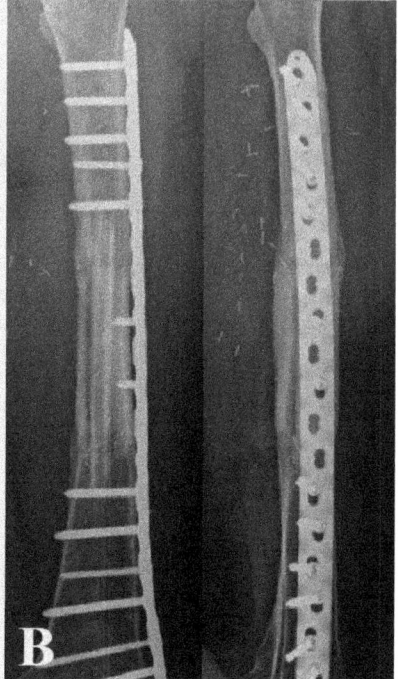

**Figure 4.** (**A**) Control X-rays for patient No. 1 at 3 months postoperatively; (**B**) control X-rays for patient No. 1 at 10 months postoperatively.

## 4. Discussion

The preliminary results of this innovative surgical technique are encouraging, with bone consolidation being achieved within a short time, thereby allowing early full weight-bearing.

We obtained a 5.5-month (4–7) radiological bone healing time for patients with radiological follow up. This appears to be slightly better than with an isolated Capanna technique, which generally requires from six to twelve months for efficient consolidation to be obtained [4,28,29]. It also seems slightly better than an isolated Masquelet technique, which obtains full union in 4–18 months, usually on smaller tibia defects [30].

Full weight-bearing was achieved early (11 weeks (8–12)), with physiotherapy involving progressive weight-bearing, which was allowed postoperatively, while keeping the patient's pain in mind. We assumed that fibula fusion, seen on CT scans but not necessarily on standard X-rays, may have facilitated this process. Bone healing was observed earlier on the first postoperative CT scan than on standard X-rays; CT scans performed earlier in the follow-up could have revealed better fusion times in our patients.

The "Capasquelet" can be considered a method of choice for bone defects extending into the femur, particularly in complex cases requiring two-stage management; it might also be proposed in tibial resections. In the literature, the combination of several types of techniques appears to result in fewer complications, thus providing a cumulative advantage, and in tumor cases, it avoids long and harrowing one-stage surgeries [29,31–35]. Obtaining an osteoinductive membrane promotes bone consolidation and management of septic contexts. This osteoinductive membrane needs to be preserved for the second stage, and it should only be incised and not excised [36]. The placement of an allograft and a vascularized fibula in this induced membrane after cement removal is straightforward, with an easy workspace preserving reconstruction placement. It may allow primary (allograft compression) and secondary mechanical stability (fibula fusion) (Figure 5).

In the context of tumor resection in the case of Ewing's sarcoma (with residual viable cells or inadequate margins), it made adjuvant radiotherapy a theoretical possibility without the risk of radiation-mediated destruction of the graft. Indeed, irradiation's pejorative effect on bone is well described, as it causes deterioration by interfering with the trabecular architecture through increased osteoclast activity and decreased osteoblast activity [37]. With our, we might prevent the hybrid graft from these adverse events. However, the recipient bone was still subjected to irradiation, and we noted that the proximal interface did not consolidate with patient No. 3. This might be linked to irradiated recipient's bone status, as well as due to the adverse oncological progression associated with chemotherapy and deterioration of the health status in this case.

Nonetheless, the "Capasquelet" technique also allows progressive correction of the limb length discrepancy in the first and second stages, as in the case of patient No. 2 who had a pathological fracture with recovery of 2 cm of leg discrepancy in the first stage and 2 cm in the second stage, resulting in a total correction of 4 cm. We noted two sequences of bone stability, the first obtained thanks to the allograft stabilized with a 4.5 mm LCP lateral plate, which allowed for early initiation of rehabilitation sessions and progressive weight-bearing; in the second, the vascularized fibula was able to osseointegrate as could be seen on the CT scan.

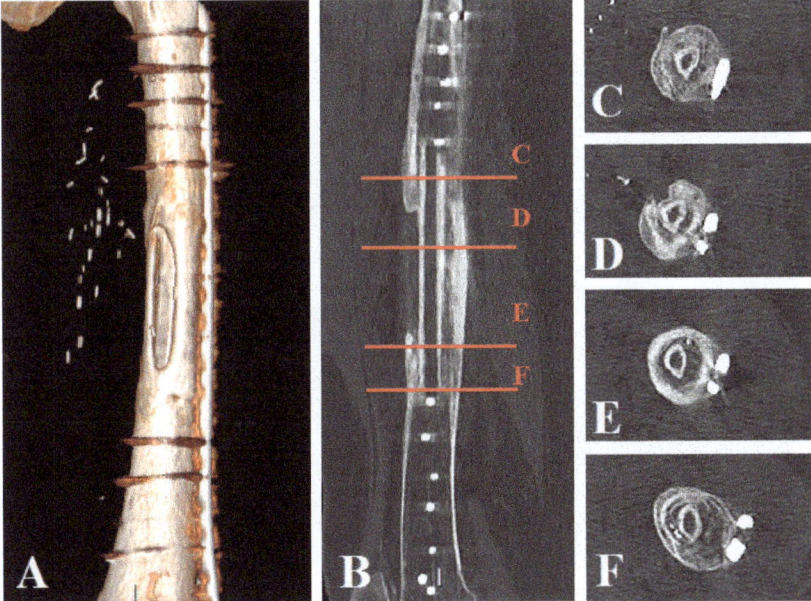

**Figure 5.** Patient No. 1 CT scan control at 14 months postoperatively: (**A**) CT scan 3D reconstruction of the healed allograft; (**B**) sagittal plane view with axial view level representation: (**C–F**) (**C**) axial view of the proximal host femur with the healed fibula graft, (**D,E**) axial views of the healed fibula graft in the allograft, (**F**) axial view of the distal host femur with the healed fibula graft.

Nonetheless, with our limited follow up (as this is a new technique), these results need to be viewed with a degree of caution. Moreover, the small size of our cohort, which was mainly the result of the rarity of the indication for a two-stage reconstruction in large femoral bone defects, also needs to be taken into account. These preliminary results are of interest as, in our practice, this combination makes progressive weight-bearing possible, with full weight-bearing occurring at 3 months in complex situations, which also allows for early re-education. However, it is essential to note that this two-stage technique results in morbidity associated with the fibular harvest [38], and it requires microsurgical skills and access to a femoral allograft bank facility. The operating times involved in the two stages must also be taken into account.

## 5. Conclusions

The mean time to union in the biological reconstruction of extended bone defects varies and depends on the technique used, ranging from four to over twelve months, and full weight-bearing rarely occurs before four to six months [12,39–42]. With our method, the osteoinductive role played by the induced membrane can exert a positive impact on the bone healing of the graft, with fast allograft and fibula union, early weight-bearing, and a satisfactory functional score. This technique appears to be suitable for restoration of bone length in pathological fractures but also for preserving a hybrid graft from radiation therapy or in complex trauma cases, which are most often septic. Mid- and long-term follow up needs to be evaluated on a larger cohort with a focus on fibula behavior, allograft resorption, and functional results. Nonetheless, to our knowledge, the "Capasquelet" technique that we report here is the first to assess the combination of two main techniques for massive bone defect management, namely, the Capanna and the Masquelet techniques [11,12]. Therefore, despite its complexity, in light of the promising preliminary results with bone healing, the "Capasquelet" hybrid technique may represent a new tool for surgeons to treat critical bone defects after tumor resection or trauma in a septic context.

**Author Contributions:** Conceptualization, F.D. and V.C.; methodology, A.C., F.D. and V.C.; surgeries, F.D. and V.C.; investigation and data curation, A.C., F.T., P.-P.A. and V.C.; writing—original draft preparation, A.C. and V.C.; writing—review and editing, A.C., F.T., A.F.-C., P.-P.A., M.B., F.D. and V.C.; supervision, F.D. and V.C. All authors have read and agreed to the published version of the manuscript.

**Funding:** This research received no external funding.

**Institutional Review Board Statement:** The institutional review board approved the protocol. According to French legislation on anonymized data retrospective studies (articles L.1121-1 paragraph 1 and R1121-2, Public Health Code), Nantes University Hospital confirmed that approval of the ethics committee was not needed due to the non-interventional nature of the study; no ethics committee approval was necessary at the time the study was started. The database was anonymized, and all patients provided their verbal consent and received an information document.

**Informed Consent Statement:** Informed consent was obtained from all of the subjects involved in the study.

**Data Availability Statement:** The data sets generated and/or analyzed during the current study are available from the corresponding author upon reasonable request.

**Acknowledgments:** We would like to thank Peggy Ageneau and Julianne Berchoud for their support in the administrative proceedings.

**Conflicts of Interest:** The authors have no conflict of interest to declare.

## References

1. Zekry, K.M.; Yamamoto, N.; Hayashi, K.; Takeuchi, A.; Alkhooly, A.Z.A.; Abd-Elfattah, A.S.; Elsaid, A.N.S.; Ahmed, A.R.; Tsuchiya, H. Reconstruction of Intercalary Bone Defect after Resection of Malignant Bone Tumor. *J. Orthop. Surg. (Hong Kong)* **2019**, *27*. [CrossRef]
2. Rajasekaran, R.B.; Jayaramaraju, D.; Venkataramani, H.; Agraharam, D.; Shanmuganathan, R.S.; Shanmuganathan, R. Successful Reconstruction of a Post-Traumatic Defect of 16 cm of the Distal Femur by Modified Capanna's Technique (Vascularised Free Fibula Combined with Allograft)—A Case Report and Technical Note. *Trauma Case Rep.* **2018**, *17*, 29–32. [CrossRef] [PubMed]
3. Fuchs, B.; Ossendorf, C.; Leerapun, T.; Sim, F.H. Intercalary Segmental Reconstruction after Bone Tumor Resection. *Eur. J. Surg. Oncol.* **2008**, *34*, 1271–1276. [CrossRef] [PubMed]
4. Panagopoulos, G.N.; Mavrogenis, A.F.; Mauffrey, C.; Lesenský, J.; Angelini, A.; Megaloikonomos, P.D.; Igoumenou, V.G.; Papanastassiou, J.; Savvidou, O.; Ruggieri, P.; et al. Intercalary Reconstructions after Bone Tumor Resections: A Review of Treatments. *Eur. J. Orthop. Surg. Traumatol.* **2017**, *27*, 737–746. [CrossRef] [PubMed]
5. Vidal, L.; Kampleitner, C.; Brennan, M.Á.; Hoornaert, A.; Layrolle, P. Reconstruction of Large Skeletal Defects: Current Clinical Therapeutic Strategies and Future Directions Using 3D Printing. *Front. Bioeng. Biotechnol.* **2020**, *8*, 61. [CrossRef]
6. Brunet, O.; Anract, P.; Bouabid, S.; Babinet, A.; Dumaine, V.; Toméno, B.; Biau, D. Intercalary Defects Reconstruction of the Femur and Tibia after Primary Malignant Bone Tumour Resection. A Series of 13 Cases. *Orthop. Traumatol. Surg. Res.* **2011**, *97*, 512–519. [CrossRef]
7. San Julian Aranguren, M.; Leyes, M.; Mora, G.; Cañadell, J. Consolidation of Massive Bone Allografts in Limb-Preserving Operations for Bone Tumours. *Int. Orthop.* **1995**, *19*, 377–382. [CrossRef]
8. Frisoni, T.; Cevolani, L.; Giorgini, A.; Dozza, B.; Donati, D.M. Factors Affecting Outcome of Massive Intercalary Bone Allografts in the Treatment of Tumours of the Femur. *J. Bone Joint Surg. Br.* **2012**, *94-B*, 836–841. [CrossRef]
9. Hornicek, F.J.; Gebhardt, M.C.; Tomford, W.W.; Sorger, J.I.; Zavatta, M.; Menzner, J.P.; Mankin, H.J. Factors Affecting Nonunion of the Allograft-Host Junction. *Clin. Orthop Relat Res.* **2001**, *382*, 87–98. [CrossRef]
10. Li, J.; Chen, G.; Lu, Y.; Zhu, H.; Ji, C.; Wang, Z. Factors Influencing Osseous Union Following Surgical Treatment of Bone Tumors with Use of the Capanna Technique. *J. Bone Joint Surg.* **2019**, *101*, 2036–2043. [CrossRef]
11. Capanna, R.; Campanacci, D.A.; Belot, N.; Beltrami, G.; Manfrini, M.; Innocenti, M.; Ceruso, M. A New Reconstructive Technique for Intercalary Defects of Long Bones: The Association of Massive Allograft with Vascularized Fibular Autograft. Long-Term Results and Comparison with Alternative Techniques. *Orthop. Clin. N. Am.* **2007**, *38*, 51–60. [CrossRef]
12. Karger, C.; Kishi, T.; Schneider, L.; Fitoussi, F.; Masquelet, A.-C. French Society of Orthopaedic Surgery and Traumatology (SoFCOT) Treatment of Posttraumatic Bone Defects by the Induced Membrane Technique. *Orthop. Traumatol. Surg. Res.* **2012**, *98*, 97–102. [CrossRef] [PubMed]
13. Masquelet, A.C.; Fitoussi, F.; Begue, T.; Muller, G.P. [Reconstruction of the long bones by the induced membrane and spongy autograft]. *Ann. Chir. Plast. Esthet.* **2000**, *45*, 346–353.
14. Masquelet, A.C. Muscle Reconstruction in Reconstructive Surgery: Soft Tissue Repair and Long Bone Reconstruction. *Langenbeck's Arch. Surg.* **2003**, *388*, 344–346. [CrossRef] [PubMed]
15. Pelissier, P.; Masquelet, A.C.; Bareille, R.; Pelissier, S.M.; Amedee, J. Induced Membranes Secrete Growth Factors Including Vascular and Osteoinductive Factors and Could Stimulate Bone Regeneration. *J. Orthop. Res.* **2004**, *22*, 73–79. [CrossRef]
16. Cuthbert, R.J.; Churchman, S.M.; Tan, H.B.; McGonagle, D.; Jones, E.; Giannoudis, P.V. Induced Periosteum a Complex Cellular Scaffold for the Treatment of Large Bone Defects. *Bone* **2013**, *57*, 484–492. [CrossRef]
17. Masquelet, A.C. La technique de la membrane induite dans les reconstructions osseuses segmentaires: Développement et perspectives. *Bull. Acad. Natl. Méd.* **2017**, *201*, 439–453. [CrossRef]
18. Masson, E. Fibula Vascularisée. Techniques, Indications en Orthopédie et Traumatologie. Available online: https://www.em-consulte.com/article/20991/fibula-vascularisee-techniques-indications-en-orth (accessed on 30 January 2021).
19. Dréano, T.P.; Lecestre, P.; Levadoux, M.; Masquelet, A.C.; Poitout, D.; Polle, G.; Rigal, F.; Roussignol, X.; Tripon, P. Traumatic Bone Loss of the Diaphysis, Table Ronde Sous la Direction de Xavier ROUSSIGNOL. 2005. Available online: https://soo.com.fr/download/media/f0e/13d/156-com.pdf (accessed on 30 June 2021).
20. Ganel, A.; Yaffe, B. Ankle Instability of the Donor Site Following Removal of Vascularized Fibula Bone Graft. *Ann. Plast. Surg.* **1990**, *24*, 7–9. [CrossRef] [PubMed]
21. Gilbert, A. Surgical Technique. Vascularized Transfer of the the Fibular Shaft. *J. Microsurg.* **1979**, *1*, 100.
22. Bumbasirevic, M.; Stevanovic, M.; Bumbasirevic, V.; Lesic, A.; Atkinson, H.D.E. Free Vascularised Fibular Grafts in Orthopaedics. *Int. Orthop.* **2014**, *38*, 1277–1282. [CrossRef]
23. Yajima, H.; Tamai, S.; Mizumoto, S.; Ono, H. Vascularised Fibular Grafts for Reconstruction of the Femur. *J. Bone Joint Surg. Br.* **1993**, *75*, 123–128. [CrossRef]
24. Sanders, P.T.J.; Spierings, J.F.; Albergo, J.I.; Bus, M.P.A.; Fiocco, M.; Farfalli, G.L.; van de Sande, M.A.J.; Aponte-Tinao, L.A.; Dijkstra, P.D.S. Long-Term Clinical Outcomes of Intercalary Allograft Reconstruction for Lower-Extremity Bone Tumors. *JBJS* **2020**, *102*, 1042–1049. [CrossRef]
25. Henderson, E.R.; Groundland, J.S.; Pala, E.; Dennis, J.A.; Wooten, R.; Cheong, D.; Windhager, R.; Kotz, R.I.; Mercuri, M.; Funovics, P.T.; et al. Failure Mode Classification for Tumor Endoprostheses: Retrospective Review of Five Institutions and a Literature Review. *J. Bone Joint Surg.* **2011**, *93*, 418–429. [CrossRef]

26. Ahmed, A.; Manabe, J.; Kawaguchi, N.; Matsumoto, S.; Matsushita, Y. Radiographic Analysis of Pasteurized Autologous Bone Graft. *Skeletal Radiol.* **2003**, *32*, 454–461. [CrossRef]
27. Devlin, N.J.; Brooks, R. EQ-5D and the EuroQol Group: Past, Present and Future. *Appl. Health Econ. Health Policy* **2017**, *15*, 127–137. [CrossRef] [PubMed]
28. Campanacci, D.A.; Totti, F.; Puccini, S.; Beltrami, G.; Scoccianti, G.; Delcroix, L.; Innocenti, M.; Capanna, R. Intercalary Reconstruction of Femur after Tumour Resection: Is a Vascularized Fibular Autograft plus Allograft a Long-Lasting Solution? *Bone Joint J.* **2018**, *100-B*, 378–386. [CrossRef] [PubMed]
29. Ogura, K.; Miyamoto, S.; Sakuraba, M.; Fujiwara, T.; Chuman, H.; Kawai, A. Intercalary Reconstruction after Wide Resection of Malignant Bone Tumors of the Lower Extremity Using a Composite Graft with a Devitalized Autograft and a Vascularized Fibula. *Sarcoma* **2015**, *2015*, 861575. [CrossRef]
30. Masquelet, A.; Kanakaris, N.K.; Obert, L.; Stafford, P.; Giannoudis, P.V. Bone Repair Using the Masquelet Technique. *JBJS* **2019**, *101*, 1024–1036. [CrossRef] [PubMed]
31. Errani, C.; Ceruso, M.; Donati, D.M.; Manfrini, M. Microsurgical Reconstruction with Vascularized Fibula and Massive Bone Allograft for Bone Tumors. *Eur. J. Orthop. Surg. Traumatol.* **2019**, *29*, 307–311. [CrossRef] [PubMed]
32. Muratori, F.; Totti, F.; D'Arienzo, A.; Scorianz, M.; Scoccianti, G.; Beltrami, G.; Campo, F.R.; Citarelli, C.; Capanna, R.; Campanacci, D.A. Biological Intercalary Reconstruction with Bone Grafts After Joint-Sparing Resection of the Lower Limb: Is This an Effective and Durable Solution for Joint Preservation? *Surg. Technol. Int.* **2018**, *32*, 345–346.
33. Bakri, K.; Stans, A.A.; Mardini, S.; Moran, S.L. Combined Massive Allograft and Intramedullary Vascularized Fibula Transfer: The Capanna Technique for Lower-Limb Reconstruction. *Semin. Plast Surg.* **2008**, *22*, 234–241. [CrossRef] [PubMed]
34. Pazourek, L.; Tomáš, T.; Mahdal, M.; Janíček, P.; Černý, J.; Ondrůšek, Š. [Use of Solid Intercalary Allografts for Reconstruction Following the Resection of Primary Bone Tumors]. *Acta Chir. Orthop. Traumatol. Cech.* **2018**, *85*, 171–178. [PubMed]
35. Houdek, M.T.; Wagner, E.R.; Stans, A.A.; Shin, A.Y.; Bishop, A.T.; Sim, F.H.; Moran, S.L. What Is the Outcome of Allograft and Intramedullary Free Fibula (Capanna Technique) in Pediatric and Adolescent Patients With Bone Tumors? *Clin. Orthop. Relat. Res.* **2016**, *474*, 660–668. [CrossRef] [PubMed]
36. Yin, Q.; Sun, Z.; Gu, S. [Progress of Masquelet technique to repair bone defect]. *Zhongguo Xiu Fu Chong Jian Wai Ke Za Zhi* **2013**, *27*, 1273–1276. [PubMed]
37. Costa, S.; Reagan, M.R. Therapeutic Irradiation: Consequences for Bone and Bone Marrow Adipose Tissue. *Front. Endocrinol.* **2019**, *10*, 587. [CrossRef]
38. Ling, X.F.; Peng, X. What Is the Price to Pay for a Free Fibula Flap? A Systematic Review of Donor-Site Morbidity Following Free Fibula Flap Surgery. *Plast. Reconstr. Surg.* **2012**, *129*, 657–674. [CrossRef]
39. Jones, C.W.; Shatrov, J.; Jagiello, J.M.; Millington, S.; Hong, A.; Boyle, R.; Stalley, P.D. Clinical, Functional and Radiological Outcomes of Extracorporeal Irradiation in Limb Salvage Surgery for Bone Tumours. *Bone Joint J.* **2017**, *99*, 1681–1688. [CrossRef]
40. Liu, Q.; He, H.; Duan, Z.; Zeng, H.; Yuan, Y.; Wang, Z.; Luo, W. Intercalary Allograft to Reconstruct Large-Segment Diaphysis Defects After Resection of Lower Extremity Malignant Bone Tumor. *Cancer Manag. Res.* **2020**, *12*, 4299–4308. [CrossRef]
41. Jayaramaraju, D.; Venkataramani, H.; Rajasekaran, R.B.; Agraharam, D.; Sabapathy, S.R.; Rajasekaran, S. Modified Capanna's Technique (Vascularized Free Fibula Combined with Allograft) as a Single-Stage Procedure in Post-Traumatic Long-Segment Defects of the Lower End of the Femur: Outcome Analysis of a Series of 19 Patients with an Average Gap of 14 Cm. *Indian J. Plast. Surg.* **2019**, *52*, 296–303. [CrossRef]
42. Zaretski, A.; Amir, A.; Meller, I.; Leshem, D.; Kollender, Y.; Barnea, Y.; Bickels, J.; Shpitzer, T.; Ad-El, D.; Gur, E. Free Fibula Long Bone Reconstruction in Orthopedic Oncology: A Surgical Algorithm for Reconstructive Options. *Plast. Reconstr. Surg.* **2004**, *113*, 1989–2000. [CrossRef]

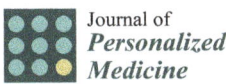

*Article*

# Is Hyperspectral Imaging Suitable for Assessing Collateral Circulation Prior Radial Forearm Free Flap Harvesting? Comparison of Hyperspectral Imaging and Conventional Allen's Test

Diana Heimes [1,*,†], Philipp Becker [2,†], Daniel G. E. Thiem [1], Robert Kuchen [3], Solomiya Kyyak [1] and Peer W. Kämmerer [1]

1. Department of Oral–and Maxillofacial and Plastic Surgery, University Medical Center Mainz, Augustusplatz 2, 55131 Mainz, Germany; daniel.thiem@uni-mainz.de (D.G.E.T.); Solomiya.kyyak@unimedizin-mainz.de (S.K.); peer.kaemmerer@unimedizin-mainz.de (P.W.K.)
2. Department of Oral and Maxillofacial Surgery, Federal Armed Forces Hospital, Rübenacher Straße 170, 56072 Koblenz, Germany; Becker-ph@web.de
3. Institute for Medical Statistics, Epidemiology and Informatics, University Medical Center of the Johannes-Gutenberg-University Mainz, 55131 Mainz, Germany; robert.kuchen@uni-mainz.de
\* Correspondence: diana.heimes@icloud.com
† These authors contributed equally.

**Abstract:** (1) Background: This cross-sectional study aims to compare a new and non-invasive approach using hyperspectral imaging (HSI) with the conventional modified Allen's test (MAT) for the assessment of collateral perfusion prior to radial forearm free flap harvest in healthy adults. (2) HSI of the right hand of 114 patients was recorded. Here, three recordings were carried out: (I) basic status (perfusion), (II) after occlusion of ulnar and radial artery (occlusion) and (III) after releasing the ulnar artery (reperfusion). At all recordings, tissue oxygenation/superficial perfusion ($StO_2$ (0–100%); 0–1 mm depth), tissue hemoglobin index (THI (0–100)) and near infrared perfusion index/deep perfusion (NIR (0–100); 0–4 mm depth) were assessed. A modified Allen's test (control) was conducted and compared with the HSI-results. (3) Results: Statistically significant differences between perfusion (I) and artery occlusion (II) and between artery occlusion (II) and reperfusion (III) could be observed within the population with a non-pathological MAT (each <0.001). Significant correlations were observed for the difference between perfusion and reperfusion in THI and the height of the MAT ($p < 0.05$). Within the population with a MAT >8 s, an impairment in reperfusion was shown (each $p < 0.05$) and the difference between perfusion and reperfusion exhibited a strong correlation to the height of the MAT (each $p < 0.01$). (4) Conclusions: The results indicate a reliable differentiation between perfusion and occlusion by HSI. Therefore, HSI could be a useful tool for verification of the correct performance of the MAT as well as to confirm the final diagnosis, as it provides an objective, reproducible method whose results strongly correlate with those obtained by MAT. What is more, it can be easily applied by non-medical personnel.

**Keywords:** hyperspectral imaging; Allen's test; radial forearm free flap; microvascular surgery; microsurgery; reconstructive surgery; perfusion monitoring; flap imaging

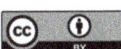

## 1. Introduction

The "Chinese flap", the fascio-cutaneous radial forearm free flap (RFFF) was first described in 1981 by Yang et al. [1,2]. It is used for diverse reconstruction purposes with a survival rate of 97% [3,4]; the popularity of its use has increased due to its pliability and thinness, the ease of flap raising using a two-team approach, a consistent anatomy, and the long and high-caliber vascular pedicle [1–3]. As the flap is vascularized by a segment of the radial artery that needs to be removed during the surgery, it is essential to ensure an adequate perfusion of the whole hand by the ulnar artery alone. Though, radial artery occlusion is a common complication with frequencies ranging from 1–33% [5]. Here, the Allen's test, a simple bedside test is traditionally used as a preoperative assessment ahead of RFFF harvest. Its validity depends on the degree of arterial compression applied by the examiner, as well as the subjective evaluation of the reperfusion and a potential error by the hyperextension of the hand [3,6]. Furthermore, there are technical differences in the test procedure as well as the cut-off point for reperfusion (the shorter the cut-off time, the more sensitive and less specific Allen's test is [7]). In addition, Allen's test requires the cooperation of the patient for its correct performance and does not give information about the vascular anatomy [8]. As acute ischemia of the hand after flap raising has been reported, even after satisfactory Allen's test results, further measurement methods have been evaluated to minimize the risk of such ischemic complications [3,4,6]. Here, arteriography is a very precise but also highly invasive method for assessing the vascular anatomy and perfusion of the donor hand. Color flow duplex scanning and doppler ultrasound are noninvasive options that require experience and rely on a subjective interpretation [3]. Besides, transcutaneous pulse oximetry has been shown to correlate with arterial doppler waveforms and therefore provides an objective means of monitoring of potential ischemic complications [9].

Hyperspectral imaging (HSI) is an imaging modality for medical applications and has been tested for the determination of perfusion parameters for diabetic foot and skin ulcer [10–13], tissue perfusion measurement and wound analysis [14,15] as well as flap monitoring [16]. TIVITA™ (Diaspective Vision, Pepelow, Germany) is a new, contact-free HSI system for the assessment of tissue oxygenation and perfusion. It is an internal pushbroom imaging spectrograph (CMOS camera) and acquires a three-dimensional HyperCube with spatial (x, y; resolution 0.1 mm/pixel at 50 cm distance) and spectral (λ; resolution 5 nm) dimensions [17]. Every point in a row (x-axis) is analyzed in parallel; the row is moved along the y-axis and the spectral dimension (λ) is generated [18,19]. The system detects hemoglobin and its derivates oxyhemoglobin, deoxyhemoglobin and water [20]. Optical remission spectroscopy in the visible and near infrared range (400–1000 nm) allows contact-free acquisition of information about tissue properties, such as tissue oxygenation/superficial perfusion ($StO_2$ (0–100%); 0–1 mm depth), tissue hemoglobin index (THI (0–100)), near infrared perfusion index/deep perfusion (NIR (0–100); 0–4 mm depth) and tissue water index (TWI (0–100)) without influencing the tissue (Figure 1).

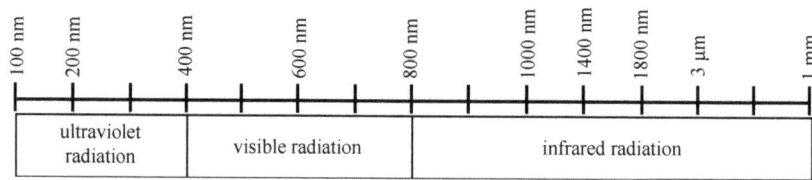

**Figure 1.** Wavelengths of different types of light. The hyperspectral camera processes visual light with a wavelength from 380 to 740 nm and light in the near infrared range from 750 to 1000 nm.

$StO_2$ reflects the percentage of hemoglobin oxygen saturation in the capillary area of the tissue microcirculation and shows changes in tissue oxygenation. Thus, $StO_2$ represents the tissue oxygen saturation, which is mainly due to the blood volume in the venous part (75%) of the microcirculation after the oxygen has been released to the surrounding tissue. The parameter NIR perfusion (near infrared) describes the quality of the blood flow, which is determined by the relative oxygen saturation of the hemoglobin and the relative hemoglobin content in the microcirculatory system in deeper tissue layers of 4 to 6 mm. This parameter can be used to identify undersupplied tissue areas in deeper layers. The color scale ranges from red (high perfusion) to blue (low perfusion). THI describes the existing hemoglobin distribution in the superficial microcirculatory system.

By this means, index parameter problems with the arterial supply or the venous drainage can be recognized. The color scale ranges from red (high hemoglobin content) to blue (low hemoglobin content). As an index value, TWI describes the relative water content in the tissue area under consideration [21]. The tissue is irradiated with white light and the remitted light is detected; scattering and absorption by tissue structures depends on the wavelength [13,19] and light penetration depth is approximately 0.8 mm (500 nm) to 2.6 mm (1000 nm). The method has previously been described by Klucke et al. [17].

In the need of an objective, reliable and investigator-independent method to evaluate the vascular perfusion of the donor hand, this cross-sectional study aims to compare a new and non-invasive approach using HSI with the conventional Allen's test for the assessment of collateral perfusion prior to RFFF harvest in healthy adults. The findings obtained in this study will be used to set limits for the evaluation of hyperspectral data, in order to facilitate interpretation and perioperative assessment.

## 2. Materials and Methods

*2.1. Patients*

The patients included within this study were picked randomly and independently of their medical history as part of the preoperative assessment ahead of surgery. All patients had a modified Allen's test and a TIVITA™ (Diaspective Vision, Pepelow, Germany) scan as part of the assessment. The study was approved by the local ethic committee of Rhineland-Palatinate (registration number: 2020-15022_1) and was conducted in accordance with the protocol and in compliance with moral, ethical and scientific principles governing clinical research as set out in the Declaration of Helsinki of 1975 as revised in 1983.

*2.2. Methods*

All tests were performed by the same surgeon to avoid interobserver variability.

2.2.1. Allen's Test

Modified Allen's test (MAT) was carried out as previously described by Habib et al. and Abdullakutty et al. (the patient makes a fist for 30 s, while pressure is applied on the ulnar and radial artery to occlude them. The patient opens the fist, and the ulnar artery is selectively released) [7,22]. An 8 s cut-off point was used to discriminate between positive test and results without pathological findings [7,23,24]. A longer period to arterial refill indicated a vascular anomaly potentially resulting in ischemia after radial artery harvest.

A time period of 9 s and above until reperfusion was evaluated as positive and therefore pathological; tests with reperfusion times of 0–8 s were considered negative and therefore non-pathological.

2.2.2. HSI Imaging

The TIVITA™ Tissue System (Diaspective Vision, Pepelow, Germany) is an HSI system consisting of a hyperspectral camera, a lens, an illumination unit, a medical cart, a box-computer and the integrated TIVITA™ Suite basic software. The light source is arranged around the camera lens and consists of six halogen spots (20 W each). The standard measurement distance is 50 cm, represented by two indicator light points in an overlapped position. The patient was asked to place the hand flat on a table with the palm up. The central point for all measurements was the middle of the palm. After HSI images are recorded over 10 s, additional 8 s are needed to compute a RGD (red, green and blue) true colour image and additional four pseudo-colour images, representing the physiologic parameters. The camera-specific software package (TIVITA™ Suite) was used to quantify the generated information [20]. Three circular shaped regions of interest (ROI) that contain the mean value of the spectral and spatial information per pixel were manually positioned. The ROI were: in the middle of the palm (40 pixel), the proximal phalanx of the thump (15 pixel) and the proximal phalanx of the index finger (15 pixel). The software automatically calculated the average values for each perfusion parameter (StO$_2$, THI, NPI and TWI). Afterwards, a mean of the three measurements was calculated (Figure 2).

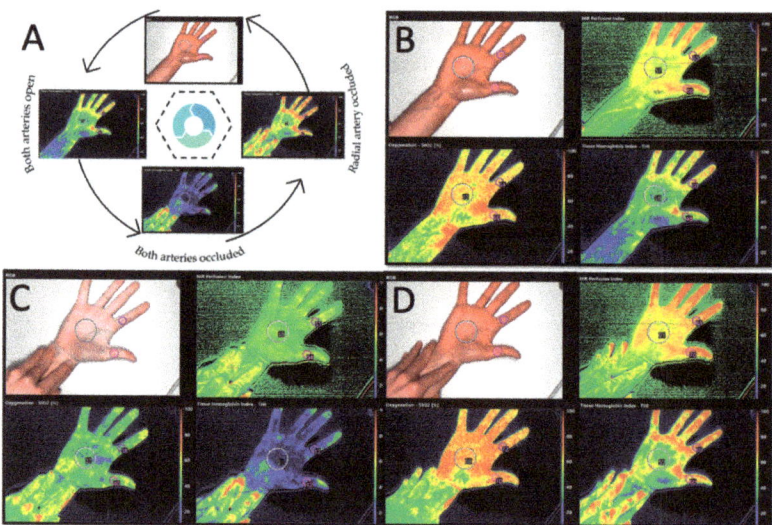

**Figure 2.** (**A**) Course of the experiment. First, a baseline measurement was taken (time point I, both arteries open), then both, the radial and the ulnar artery were occluded (time point II) and at time point III, the ulnar artery was released. Hyperspectral images were taken at all three time points throughout the course of the experiment as part of the hyperspectral accompanied MAT. In (**B**) the baseline measurement is displayed showing the NIR perfusion index, oxygenation and tissue hemoglobin index. Three circular shaped regions of interest (ROI) were manually positioned. (**C**) After occlusion of the ulnar and radial artery, the hand obviously turns pale. The values for NIR perfusion index decrease from 57 to 49 in the middle of the palm indicated by a less red and more green color of the hand. The same applies for the tissue oxygenation showing many red spots before occlusion and a green and blue color after occlusion of the vessels (StO$_2$ decrease from 63% to 37%). Changes in THI are most obvious indicated by a color change from green to dark blue (THI decrease from 38 to 5). (**D**) shows the measurements after release of the ulnar artery in a healthy participant. The return to perfusion is indicated by the red and green colors in all pictures. After reperfusion, there is a slight hyperemia of the hand, which is evidenced by the increase in the measured values (NIR1: 57 and NIR3:61; StO$_2$1: 63% and StO$_2$3: 68%; THI1: 38 and THI3:50).

The measurement was performed in a dark room with constant temperature. (I) First, a basis recording was conducted in order to show the individual hands' perfusion (perfusion). (II) Then, MAT was carried out by occluding both the radial and the ulnar artery (occlusion). This was followed by a HSI measurement. (III) To verify the hand perfusion by the ulnar artery only, the radial artery stayed occluded while releasing the ulnar artery (reperfusion). Here, HSI-image acquisition for reperfusion started 1 s after release of the ulnar artery. For each time point the mean values of the following parameters were recorded: (StO$_2$ (0–100%)), tissue hemoglobin index (THI (0–100)), near infrared perfusion index/deep perfusion (NIR (0–100)) and tissue water index (TWI (0–100)).

### 2.3. Statistics

In their review concerning the reliability and validity of the modified Allen's test, Romeu-Bordas and Ballesteros-Pena listed a total of 9 studies that were included in the review. While the number of analyzed patients ranged from 42 to 150 (mean 81.88), the number of analyzed hands was on average 104.

Case number calculation (according to [25]):

$$n = K * \frac{[(R+1) - p_2 * (R^2+1)]}{[p_2 + (1-R)^2]} \quad (1)$$

The calculation is based on the study by Grambow et al. [26] and the measured differences in tissue oxygen content, which were found to be significantly different.

$$n = 7.85 * \frac{[(0.757+1) - 0.7 * (0.757^2+1)]}{[0.7 + (1-0.757)^2]} = 124.578 \quad (2)$$

Considering the previous studies and the sample size calculation, the numbers of cases were averaged, resulting in a total necessary volume of 114 patients.

In order to test the assumption that the measured values follow a normal distribution, a Kolmogorov–Smirnov and a Shapiro–Wilk test were previously performed. Correlation analyses were performed using Pearson and Spearman test. Furthermore, Wilcoxon tests were used in order to assess whether the population mean ranks differ between related samples (non-parametric statistical hypothesis test). To measure the strength of the relationship between two variables in the statistical population, the effect size was calculated according to the following formula:

$$r = \left|\frac{Z}{\sqrt{n}}\right| \quad (3)$$

The following definitions were used:

$$0.1 \leq r < 0.3 \sim \text{weak effect}$$

$$0.3 \leq r < 0.5 \sim \text{medium effect}$$

$$r \geq 0.5 \sim \text{strong effect}$$

Values are displayed as mean and standard deviation; where appropriate confidency intervals are given. Moreover, in addition to the measured values, a fictive value was calculated to reflect the return-to-normal perfusion. This was done as follwos:

$$RTP = 100 - \left(\frac{TP3}{TP1} * 100\right) \quad (4)$$

with $RTP$ and $TP$ denoting return to perfusion time point, respectively. Statistical analyses were performed using SPSS version 24 for Windows (IBM, Armonk, NY, USA); A $p$-value $\leq 0.05$ was termed significant.

## 3. Results

A total of 114 patients were included within this study, all of whom had a modified Allen's test and an HSI-scan as part of the assessment. The results were categorized into two groups according to the results of the MAT. Non-pathological results were those with a time to reperfusion of less than 9 s; if it took 9 or more seconds, the MAT was considered pathological.

*3.1. Population with a Non-Pathological Modified Allen's Test*

Allen's Test

Here, 100 patients were included. Mean time to arterial refill was 4.12 s (SD = 1.903 s; 95% CI:3.74–4.50 s). The values were not normally distributed (Figure 3).

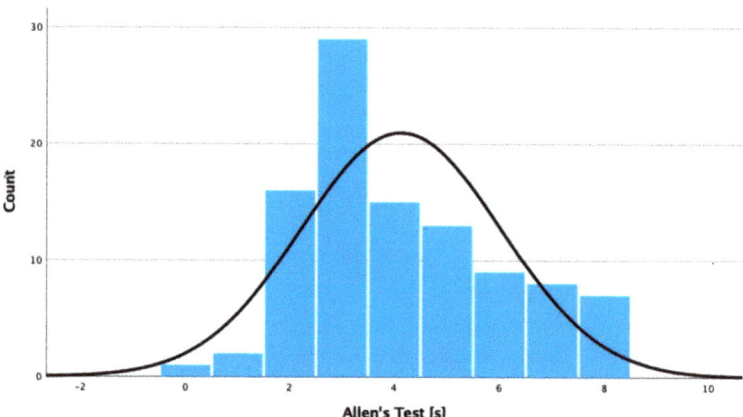

**Figure 3.** Boxplot diagram of the values obtained from the population with a non-pathological modified Allen's test.

*3.2. Hyperspectral Imaging*
3.2.1. Tissue Oxygenation ($StO_2$)

The Shapiro–Wilk test was not able to reject the hypothesis that measured values at every time point were normally distributed. At time point I, mean $StO_2$ was 51.34% (SD = 7.972%; 95% CI:49.76–52.92%). After vessel occlusion (II), mean $StO_2$ decreased to 40.56% (SD = 6.929%; 95% CI: 39.19–41.93%) and after releasing the ulnar artery (III), $StO_2$-values increased again up to 50.42% (SD = 8.117%; 95% CI: 38.81–52.03%) (Figures 4 and 5). Pearson and Spearman test showed a statistically significant correlation between the different time points (each $p < 0.001$). Whereas mean ranks differed significantly between related samples time points I and II as well as between II and III (each $p < 0.001$), the values between time point I and III did not differ significantly ($p = 0.06$). This indicates a strong effect within the compared groups that showed significantly different mean ranks (r each >0.5) and a weak effect for group comparison I and III (r = 0.133).

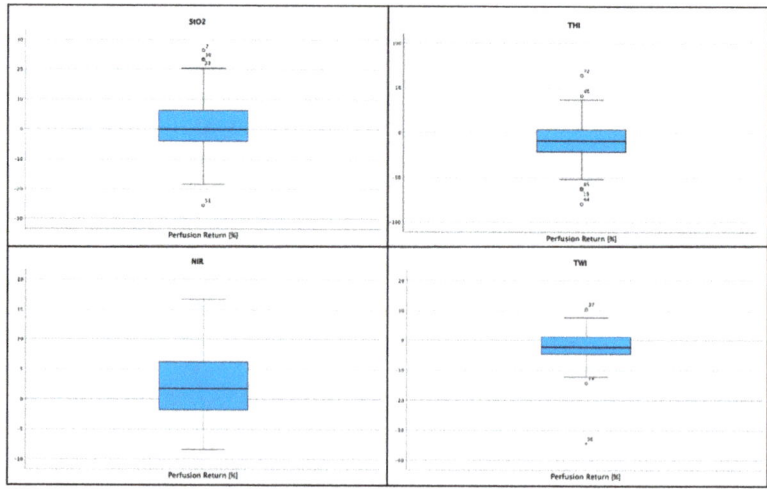

**Figure 4.** Boxplot diagrams for return-to-perfusion measurements for $StO_2$, NIR, THI and TWI values obtained from the population with a non-pathological modified Allen's Test.

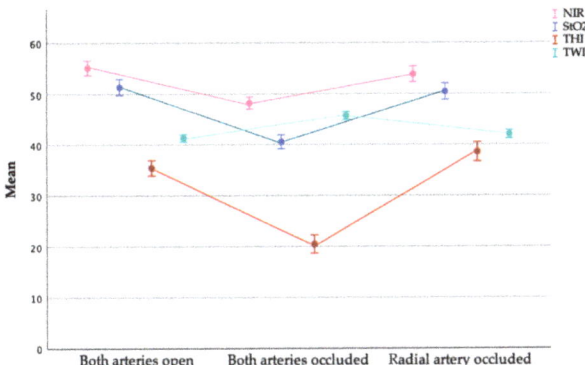

**Figure 5.** Measurements of the hyperspectral analysis over the time course of the experiment. The measured value at time point I symbolizes the baseline measurement, at time point II the values under occlusion of both vessels and at time point III the measured values after opening the ulnar artery. The NIR values (near infrared index/deep perfusion) are shown in pink, the $StO_2$ values (superficial perfusion) in blue, the THI (tissue hemoglobin index) in red and the TWI (tissue water index) in cyan.

### 3.2.2. Near Infrared Perfusion Index (NIR)

Once again, a Shapiro–Wilk test did not significantly contradict that measurements during occlusion and reperfusion were normally distributed ($p > 0.1$). The values measured at time point I (both arteries open), however, do not seem to follow a normal distribution ($p = 0.031$). At time point I, mean NIR was 55.11 (SD = 7.236; 95% CI: 53.67–56.55). After occlusion of both vessels, the perfusion decreased (Mean = 48.14 ± 5.946; 95% CI: 46.96–49.32) and increased up to 53.88 (SD = 7.876; 95% CI: 52.32–55.44) after release of the ulnar artery (Figures 4 and 5). Both, Pearson and Spearman correlation test showed statistically significant correlations between the different time points (each $p < 0.001$). Using Wilcoxon test, a significant difference between the distribution at the different time points could be demonstrated. Whereas for time points I and II as well as for II and III a strong effect ($r > 0.5$) was shown, between group I and III merely a weak effect was observed ($r = 0.241$).

### 3.2.3. Tissue Hemoglobin Index (THI)

Whereas a Shapiro–Wilk test could not reject that the measured values of both, perfusion and reperfusion were normally distributed ($p > 0.05$), the values obtained during occlusion do not seem to follow a normal distribution ($p = 0.005$). Mean THI was 35.39 ± 7.661 (95% CI: 33.87–36.91) while arterial blood flow was present, whereas THI decreased to 20.52 ± 8.973 (95% CI:18.74–22.20) after occlusion of the arteries. After release of the ulnar artery, mean THI increased up to 38.52 ± 9.517 (95% CI: 36.63–40.41) (Figures 4 and 5). Spearman and Pearson test showed statistically a significant correlation between all time points ($p < 0.001$). A significant difference between the mean ranks of the different time points could be shown by the Wilcoxon test. For time points I and II as well as for II and III a strong effect ($r > 0.6$) and between I and III a moderately strong effect could be shown.

### 3.2.4. Tissue Water Index (TWI)

Whereas the Shapiro–Wilk test indicated that for both, time points II (both arteries occluded) and III (only radial artery occluded), the normality assumption could not be rejected, this was not the case for the baseline measurement. Mean TWI was 41.28 (SD = 3.690; 95% CI: 40.55–42.01) at rest and increased to 45.68 ± 3.959 (95% CI: 44.89–46.47) when occluding both vessels. After release of the ulnar artery, TWI decreased to 42.01 (SD = 4.162; 95% CI: 41.18–42.84) (Figures 4 and 5). Both Spearman and Pearson correlation test showed statistically significant correlations between all time points ($p < 0.001$). Analyzing the difference in mean ranks, there were statistically significant differences between all groups corresponding to strong effects within the compared groups I and II as well as for II and III (r each > 0.5) and a weak effect for group comparison I with III (r = 0.231).

### 3.2.5. Return-to-Perfusion Measurement

The return-to-perfusion (RTP) value indicates the difference in percent between the measurements at time point III and time point I. Shapiro–Wilk and Kolmogorov–Smirnov could not reject a normal distribution for $StO_2$-RTP values. The mean difference for $StO_2$ was 1.46% (SD = 8.84%; 95% CI: −0.29–3.21%), for NIR 2.27% (SD = 5.74; 95% CI: 1.13–3.41%), for THI −10.21% (SD = 21.79%; 95% CI: −14.53– -5.88%) and for TWI −1.82% (SD = 5.63%; 95% CI: −2.93– -0.7%) (Figure 5). Correlation analysis between the MAT and RTP-measurements by Pearson and Spearman test showed no significant correlation between the MAT and RTP-values for $StO_2$ and NIR, whereas there was a statistically significant correlation between the MAT and THI values ($p < 0.05$) in the Spearmen test. On the other hand correlation analysis did not show a correlation between MAT and TWI.

### 3.3. Cases with Impaired Perfusion

#### 3.3.1. Allen's Test

A total of 14 patients had a MAT with a time to reperfusion of longer than 8 s. In three cases, time to reperfusion was 9 s, in four cases 10 s, in two cases 11 s, in one case 14 s and in four cases, there was no reperfusion detectable after more than 20 s, which is why the test was terminated in such cases (termed as AT max.).

#### 3.3.2. Tissue Oxygenation ($StO_2$)

A normal distribution of all time points analyzed within this study was detected. A statistically significant correlation between the different time points could be observed (each $p < 0.05$). Mean ranks differed significantly between the related samples time points I and II ($p < 0.001$) as well as between I and III ($p = 0.048$), whereas the values between time point II and III did not differ significantly ($p = 0.076$). This corresponded to a strong effect within the compared groups I and II (r = 0.6) and a moderately strong effect for group comparison I and III and II and III (r > 0.3).

#### 3.3.3. Near Infrared Perfusion Index (NIR)

A normal distribution for the measured values of all time points was seen. A statistically significant correlation between the different time points could be shown by Pearson and Spearman test with $p < 0.01$. There were significant differences in mean ranks between the related samples time points I and II as well as I and III ($p = 0.002$), whereas the values between time point II and III did not differ significantly ($p = 0.213$). This corresponded to a strong effect between the compred groups that showed significantly different mean ranks (r each > 0.5), whereas for group II and III only a weak effect could be shown (r = 0.235).

#### 3.3.4. Tissue Hemoglobin Index (THI)

The hypothesis of a normal distribution could not be rejected for time points I and III. Correlation analysis by Pearson and Spearman test could demonstrate a statistically significant correlation between the different time points with $p < 0.001$. Interestingly, statistically significant differences between mean ranks of time points I and II as well as II and III were shown, whereas time points I and III did not show such significant differences ($p = 0.133$). This corresponded to a strong effect between the compared groups that showed significantly different mean ranks (r each > 0.5), whereas for group I and III, a weak effect could be shown only (r = 0.284).

#### 3.3.5. Tissue Water Index (TWI)

For time points II and III, normally distributed values were observed. Both, Spearman and Pearson correlation test were able to show a statistically significant correlation between all time points. Mean ranks differed significantly between all groups, corresponding to a strong effect between time point I and II (r = 0.626) and a moderate effect between the other time points with r > 0.4.

### 3.3.6. Return-to-Perfusion Measurement

Shapiro–Wilk and Kolmogorov–Smirnov tests could not reject the hypothesis of normal distribution for $StO_2$, NIR, THI and TWI. There was a statistically significant correlation between the RTP-value and the MAT-measurements for $StO_2$ ($p < 0.001$), THI ($p = 0.004$) and TWI ($p = 0.011$), whereas no significant correlation could be shown for NIR-index ($p = 0.179$) (Figure 6).

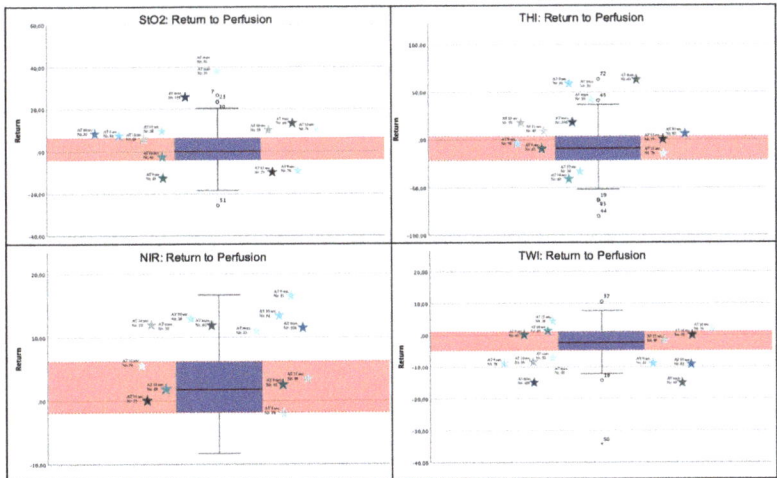

**Figure 6.** Boxplot diagram of the Return-to-Perfusion (RTP) measurements. The red box highlights the area between the 1st and 3rd quartile. The stars indicate the different subjects' measurements that had a MAT >8 s. As can be observed, some values lie between the 1st and the 3rd quartile, whereas others are located within the 4 inter quartiles range (IQR). Others lie due to their extreme values beyond these areas and are therefore considered outliers. With few exceptions, the measurements defined as outliers belong to the same patients. As can be seen, RTP-values for $StO_2$, THI and TWI of patients with a clear pathological MAT typically lie beyond the 4 IQR (Nr. 30, 35, 60, 108). Others, with a MAT of 9–15 s–depending on the definition–rated as pathologic or non-pathologic, typically fall within the 4 IQR. The allocation of the values on the X-axis has no meaning.

### 3.4. Patient Case

A 63-year-old patient presented with an oral mucosal lesion of the right floor of the mouth that had been present for a year. Clinically, there was an ulcerating lesion of about 2 cm. During staging, no further suspicions lesions could be detected; radiologically, neither lymphatic, nor osseus metastases were found. The interdisciplinary head and neck tumor board recommended resection of the tumor and bilateral neck dissection. To cover the defect, we planned to harvest a RFFF. However, the MAT showed a very poor perfusion of the right arm with a reperfusion time of over 20 s; the results could be confirmed by HSI. When the MAT was performed of the left arm, a time to reperfusion of 11 s was measured. However, the HSI measurement showed adequate perfusion with a satisfactory RTP-value for $StO_2$, NIR, THI, and TWI (Figure 7). Considering the measurable reperfusion, the decision was made to harvest a RFFF from the left arm. With constant monitoring of the oxygen saturation by means of pulse oximetry, the RFFF could be harvested without complications. In the postoperative follow-up, the graft was adequately perfused and healed well (Figure 8).

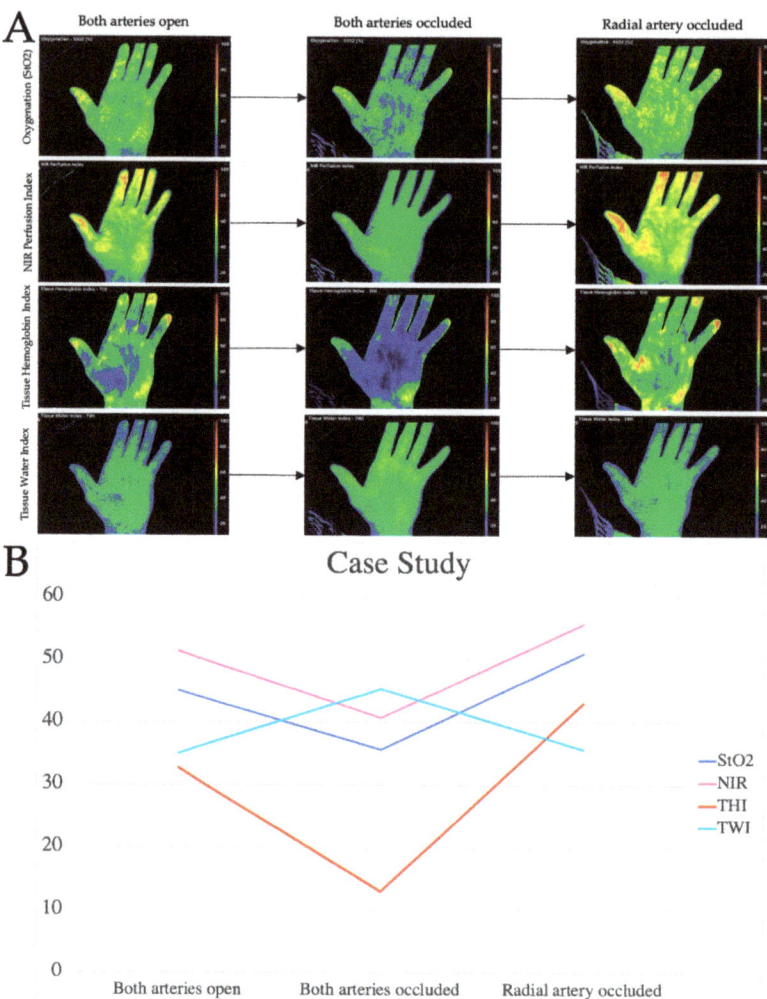

**Figure 7.** In (**A**) the measurements at the three different time points are shown. A baseline measurement was taken (time point I, both arteries open), then both, the radial and the ulnar artery were occluded (time point II) and at time point III, the ulnar artery was released. At time point I, tissue oxygenation (StO$_2$) was 45%. After occluding the arteries, the values decreased to 35.67% and increased again after release of the ulnar artery (51%) as can be seen in (**B**). This observation is consistent with the measurements of the NIR perfusion index (NIR) showing values of 51.33 at time point I, 40.67 at time point II and 55.67 at time point III (see B). The image shows very impressively the trend of the hemoglobin index (THI) during the course of the experiment. With both arteries open, the THI was 32.67; after occlusion of both arteries, the values decreased to 13 and increased again after release of the ulnar artery (43). As can be seen in the images in A, tissue water index (TWI) increased during artery occlusion showing values of 45.33 while both, the baseline measurement and the measurement after release of the ulnar artery showed values of 35. The Return-to-perfusion (RTP) value indicates the difference in percent between the measurements at time point III and time point I. Here, RTP-values for StO$_2$ were −13.33%, for NIR −8.46%, for THI −31.62% and for TWI −1.91%. Those values corresponded to a strong return to perfusion after release of the ulnar artery showing a save perfusion of the hand by the ulnar artery alone.

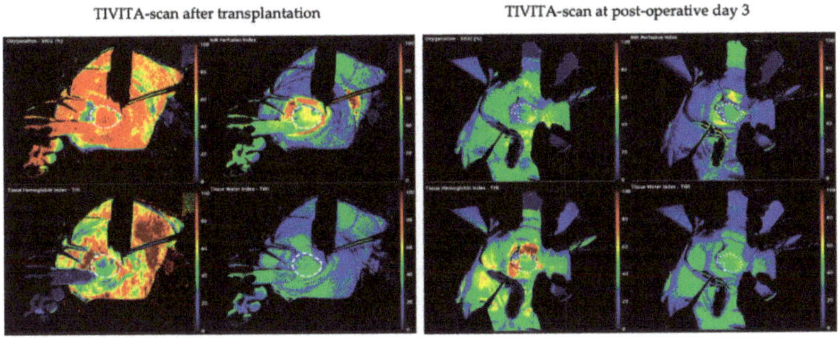

**Figure 8.** A TIVITA scan immediately after transplantation of the RFFF into the floor of the mouth is shown on the left. The circular mark (white dotted line) indicates the graft inside the patient's mouth. The measurement shows a (typical) initially very high oxygenation of the graft with correspondingly high NIR values and adequately low THI values. In the course of time, up to postoperative day 3 shown on the right, a reduction of the StO$_2$ and NIR values and a homogenization of the measured values over the area of the graft are visible. Based on previous studies [21], it could be determined that this process is typical for the proper healing and perfusion of the graft.

## 4. Discussion

The radial artery is located in the lateral intermuscular septum between the brachioradialis and flexor carpi radialis muscles [1]. Entering the hand, the radial artery gives rise to the princeps pollicis artery and radial indices artery. The deep palmar arch is formed by the dorsal radial artery and the deep branch of the ulnar artery. Four palmar metacarpal arteries arise from the deep palmar arch and converge with the common palmar digital arteries. The superficial palmar arch is formed by the ulnar artery and the superficial branch of the radial artery with four common palmar digital arteries arising from the arch. The common digital arteries then divide into two proper palmar digital arteries [22,27,28] (Figure 9).

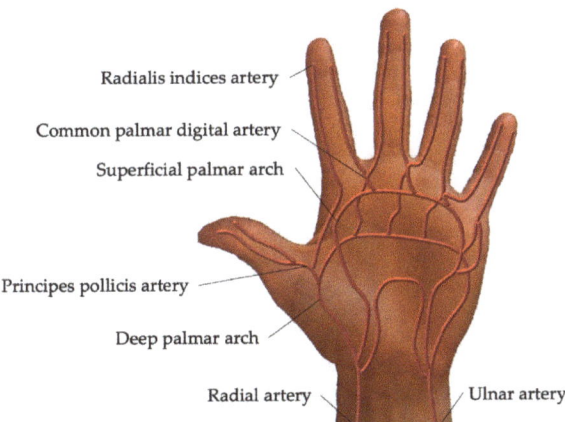

**Figure 9.** Palmar arch of the right hand. Entering the hand, the radial artery gives rise to the princeps pollicis artery and radial indices artery. The deep palmar arch is formed by the dorsal radial artery and the deep branch of the ulnar artery. The superficial palmar arch is formed by the ulnar artery and the superficial branch of the radial artery.

The vascular abnormality leading to impaired perfusion after raising the RFFF is a combined condition of an incomplete ulnar arterial supply to the hand and a missing communication between deep and superficial palmar arch. Coleman and Anson reported 12% of specimens to show a combination of the two abnormalities [29]. Strauch et al. reported the superficial arch and the deep arch to be incomplete in 21% and in 3% of cases, respectively. Other studies found the collateral circulation to be absent in 2% up to 20% of cases [28]. Complete superficial arches occur in 84% up to 90% of cases [4,27,30–32].

In this regard, a higher incidence of pathological results in Allen's test could be expected. In a large study with 1000 patients undergoing cardiac catheterization, 49% had a normal Allen's test (cut-off time <5 s). The authors classified 24% as borderline (5–9 s) and 27% as abnormal (>10 s) [22]. In 1990, Hosokawa et al. showed 5.8% of 1470 patients examined within the hospital to have an abnormal Allen's test (time until recover of color 5 s). Unilateral abnormality was observed in 4.4%, bilateral abnormality in 1.4% of cases [2]. The incidence of an abnormal test increased with age (incidence of abnormality >80 years 6.9%). Since the average age of developing oral cancer is 62 years [33], a more accurate and safer test method is needed to ensure adequate blood supply by the ulnar artery when harvesting RFFF.

Nuckols et al. reported a sensitivity of 65% and a specificity of 76% (positive predictive value (PPV) = 93%, negative predictive value (NPV) = 35%) for Allen's test with a cut-off time of 5 s [28]. This corresponds to the results of Husum et al. who indicated a NPV of 0.992, which yields a false-positive rate of to a 0.8% (1/100 hands with normal Allen's test and an inadequate collateral circulation) [28]. According to this study, a normal test result would incorrectly indicate inadequacy in about 50% of cases [28]. A systematic review by Romeu-Bordas et al. evaluated the reliability and validity of Allen's test in patients prior to radial artery puncture. They concluded Allen's test to show inadequate diagnostic validity for screening deficits in the collateral circulation. Because of this, Allen's test is termed to be no adequate predictor of hand ischemia: "Therefore, Allen's test should not be systematized prior to performing an arterial puncture as an isolated screening test for collateral arterial circulation deficits of the hand and should not be considered an absolute contraindication for performing a transradial puncture presenting an abnormal result in the Allen's test" [8]. False-negative Allen's test could result in hand ischemia and necrosis, whereas false-positive test results cause a change of primary treatment plan, possibly resulting in a suboptimal therapy situation [4]. Initially, ischemic hand complications (IHC) appear in the form of pallor and progressive darkening of the skin. Chronic complications include pain, cold intolerance, ulceration, tissue necrosis and gangrene of the digits [4].

Therefore, a secure method for vascular assessment is needed. In daily routine, some supplemental properties are necessary to make the test feasible: the test should be noninvasive, fast as well as easy to perform and the evaluation needs to be objective and reproducible. Furthermore, the method needs to have a good predictive ability with a high sensitivity, specificity and accuracy. In this study, HSI was shown to detect perfusion deficits during MAT. HSI provides both, topographical and spectral information in an objective, reproductive and measurable manner. Combinations of values allows drawing conclusions about tissue perfusion. High THI and low $StO_2$ indicates venous congestion, whereas low THI and low $StO_2$ points to an arterial occlusion. A high NIR and a low $StO_2$ indicated that deep tissue perfusion is given whereas superficial layers are undersupplied, whereas the contrary case points to a critical situation as superficial supply can clinically hide saturation problems in deeper tissue layers [21]. Moreover, if the reliability of Allen's test as a screening tool is shown by a high number of successful and complication-free radial forearm free flap transfers, the remaining percentage of hand ischemia in the presence of non-pathological test results suggests the need for a more secure measurement method to increase patients' safety.

The results of this study indicate that in patients with a non-pathological MAT (blood-refill time of less than nine seconds) all parameters collected during hyperspectral imaging significantly differ between both, the baseline measurement and the measurements taken during complete artery occlusion as well as between the measurement after release of the ulnar artery and during artery occlusion. Furthermore, THI-RTP values correlated with the MAT results. Hence, it can be concluded that the calculated ratio between the HSI-measurements at the beginning and the end of the test (RTP value) representing the ability to full reperfusion by only the ulnar artery reflects the time to reperfusion measured during MAT.

On the one hand, this indicates a reliable differentiation between perfusion and occlusion–as already shown by Grambow et al. in a rat in vivo model [26]–as well as the confirmation of non-pathological MAT. Therefore, the use of hyperspectral imaging for additional diagnostics in combination with MAT would be a useful tool to verify the correct performance of the test (differentiation of occlusion and perfusion) as well as to confirm the final diagnosis of a non-pathological MAT. With the aid of the RTP-value, a correlation between hyperspectral imaging and MAT could further be supported. We could not only show a safe differentiation between perfusion and occlusion status during a non-pathological MAT, but the system can also detect a pathological reperfusion based on the different parameters. This can be observed by the no longer significant differences between time points I and II as well as between II and III, but–due to the impaired reperfusion at time point III–significant differences between perfusion (time point I) and occlusion (time point II) as well as between perfusion (time point I) and reperfusion (time point III). Interestingly, we could show a statistically significant correlation between the RTP-value and the MAT results. This is in accordance with the observed outliers when comparing the hyperspectral data of patients with a non-pathological MAT and those with a pathological MAT. Here, it is clearly shown that the hyperspectral measurement values that are far beyond the norm correlate well with certainly pathological MAT values (AT max.).

Due to the overall group size and especially the rather small number of pathological MAT readings in our study, it was not possible to define safe cut-off values, rendering the fitting of neural-networks impossible. Nonetheless, the trends observed in this study indicate a potential use of hyperspectral imaging for reperfusion analysis thus offering an alternative or supplementary method to the gold standard.

Based on current data, an advantage of HSI over clinical assessment alone has already been observed for perfusion monitoring of microvascular anastomosed grafts, particularly by inexperienced personnel. Compared to visual assessment of the hand reperfusion during MAT, HSI offers some clear advantages as it provides an objective, reproducible method also feasible for non-medical personnel that has no interobserver error and–in contrast to the MAT–gives a visual and measurable feedback in case of insufficient artery occlusion or potential test error due to palmar hyperextension.

HSI is used both clinically and experimentally for numerous indications: In anesthesia and ICU, the technique is already used in critically ill patients to monitor micro- and macro-circulatory changes, tissue perfusion and oedema formation to reduce the negative effects of hemodynamic incoherence. Prior to HSI, skin mottling and capillary refill time were used to assess hemodynamic parameter, but, as in MAT, the inter-observer variability demonstrated contradictory findings and a variety of cut-off values were suggested [34]. In vascular surgery, HSI is used to provide objective decision criteria for determining the extent of amputation and to make predictions about the chance of healing of the amputation wound [35]. What is more, HSI has been frequently used in monitoring perfusion in microvascular anastomoses, both in experimental setups and in the clinical practice. Here, a clear advantage over the visual assessment of the grafts could be shown in numerous studies [21,26,36]. Similar results could also be shown in transplant medicine. Here Sucher et al. proved that by means of HSI it is possible to objectively assess whether an organ (the kidney) is suitable for transplantation even before the surgery. In addition, it is possible to check immediately after the transplantation whether the blood vessels have been sutured correctly and the organ is sufficiently supplied with blood. Until now, this was also decided by visual assessment, so the new HSI technique offers a clear advantage [37]. In visceral surgery, HSI is used for blood flow analysis, for example, to determine the extent of resection in the case of mesenteric ischemia, but also to assess anastomoses, as well as tubular gastric blood flow in esophageal resections [38,39]. At the current time, numerous other applications of the hyperspectral camera have already been developed. In addition to special products for the analysis of wounds and soft tissue, camera systems for the operating room and an endoscopic version have also been developed. For the resection of brain tumors, MRI scans are taken preoperatively in order to locate the tumor and subsequently plan the surgical intervention. Intraoperatively, there is currently a lack of tools to locate the tumor with certainty. Data to date indicate that it will most likely be possible to identify the tumor and resect it safely using this method [40]. This large number of potential application areas and the already established use in everyday clinical life point to a great benefit of hyperspectral technology in the future. In particular, subjective assessment criteria can be replaced by means of this technique and thus the therapy of patients can be improved.

As the ambient light conditions affect the parameter values, cautious interpretation is demanded. To the authors knowledge, this is the first study assessing the feasibility of HSI to collateral circulation prior to RFFF harvest. Regarding the number of cases within this study, the present results need to be classified as of descriptive nature. Further clinical studies must be conducted in order to set cut-off values indicating a save arterial refill during HSI assisted MAT. In general, perfusion markers should return to the level of the baseline measurement after releasing the ulnar artery. If the parameters stay low, an adequate perfusion is not guaranteed. What is more, in addition to the measurements performed during this study, further measurements at later time points could have been performed to assess the long-term which could have provided further insight. However, in this study, further measurements were deliberately omitted because we aimed to (1) to ensure the greatest comparability possible between the gold standard and the new method and (2) develop a new method for everyday clinical use. This method should be as simple, fast, and objective as possible, so further, time-consuming follow-up measurements were not necessary. With this study, we aimed to investigate the new method exactly as it should be applied in clinical practice. Despite the more limited assessability of long-term perfusion due to the reduction in the number of measurements, we were able to demonstrate that this method can clearly distinguish between appropriate, questionable, and non-appropriate donor sites. Nevertheless, especially in patients with impaired perfusion (questionable and non-appropriate), the assessment of tissue perfusion in later recordings would be of interest. A clear distinction could be made between delayed complete reperfusion and lack of reperfusion, thus identifying patients who would be expected to develop long-term tissue damage.

As the assessment of collateral perfusion by the ulnar artery is not just mandatory in the field of flap raising, but also for arterial puncture in anesthesia, coronary artery intervention and bypass, there is a high need for such a technique.

## 5. Conclusions

This study was able to show that, using HSI, a safe differentiation between perfusion and occlusion is possible and that this method has a good correlation to the present gold standard, the MAT. Therefore, HSI could serve as an additional method for the assessment of the collateral circulation of the hand prior to invasive interventions involving the damage or harvesting of radial artery. HSI provides some advantages over the single visual assessment, as it provides objective, reproducible results without interobserver error, can also be applied by non-medical personnel, and gives a visual and measurable feedback. Yet, limitations are imposed by the poor data situation and examination-related measurement errors.

**Author Contributions:** Conceptualization, P.W.K., D.H. and D.G.E.T.; methodology, P.W.K., D.H. and D.G.E.T.; software, P.W.K. and D.G.E.T.; validation, P.W.K., D.G.E.T., D.H., P.B., R.K. and S.K.; formal analysis, P.B., D.H. and R.K.; investigation, P.B. and D.H.; resources, P.W.K. and D.G.E.T.; data curation, P.B. and D.H.; writing—original draft preparation, D.H., P.B. and R.K.; writing—review and editing, D.H., P.B., D.G.E.T., R.K., S.K. and P.W.K.; visualization, D.H.; supervision, P.W.K. and D.H.;

project administration, P.W.K. and D.H. All authors have read and agreed to the published version of the manuscript.

**Funding:** This research received no external funding.

**Institutional Review Board Statement:** The study was conducted according to the guidelines of the Declaration of Helsinki, and approved by the Ethics Committee of Rhineland-Palatinate (registration number: 2020-15022_1, date of approval: 06/25/2020).

**Informed Consent Statement:** Informed consent was obtained from all subjects involved in the study.

**Data Availability Statement:** The data supporting the conclusions of the article is included within the article. The raw data analyzed during the current study is available from the corresponding author on reasonable request.

**Conflicts of Interest:** The authors declare no conflict of interest.

## References

1. Wolff, K.D.; Hölzle, F. *Raising of Microvascular Flaps—A Systematic Approach*; Springer: New York, NY, USA, 2011; Volume 2.
2. Hosokawa, K.; Hata, Y.; Yano, K.; Matsuka, K.; Ito, O.; Ogli, K. Results of the Allen test on 2,940 arms. *Ann. Plast. Surg.* **1990**, *24*, 149–151. [CrossRef] [PubMed]
3. Kerawala, C.J.; Martin, I.C. Palmar arch backflow following radial forearm free flap harvest. *Br. J. Oral. Maxillofac. Surg.* **2003**, *41*, 157–160. [CrossRef]
4. Wood, J.W.; Broussard, K.C.; Burkey, B. Preoperative testing for radial forearm free flaps to reduce donor site morbidity. *JAMA Otolaryngol. Head Neck Surg.* **2013**, *139*, 183–186. [CrossRef]
5. Rashid, M.; Kwok, C.S.; Pancholy, S.; Chugh, S.; Kedev, S.A.; Bernat, I.; Ratib, K.; Large, A.; Fraser, D.; Nolan, J.; et al. Radial artery occlusion after transradial interventions: A systematic review and meta-analysis. *J. Am. Heart Assoc.* **2016**, *5*. [CrossRef]
6. Ganesan, K.; Stead, L.; Smith, A.B.; Ong, T.K.; Mitchell, D.A.; Kanatas, A.N. Duplex in the assessment of the free radial forearm flaps: Is it time to change practice? *Br. J. Oral. Maxillofac. Surg.* **2010**, *48*, 423–426. [CrossRef]
7. Abdullakutty, A.; Bajwa, M.S.; Patel, S.; D'Souza, J. Clinical audit and national survey on the assessment of collateral circulation before radial forearm free flap harvest. *J. Cranio-Maxillofac. Surg.* **2017**, *45*, 108–112. [CrossRef] [PubMed]
8. Romeu-Bordas, O.; Ballesteros-Pena, S. Reliability and validity of the modified Allen test: A systematic review and metanalysis. *Emergencias* **2017**, *29*, 126–135.
9. Sachithanandan, A.; Ahmed, A.; Muir, A.; Graham, A. Simple method for monitoring hand perfusion following radial artery harvest for coronary artery bypass grafting. *Interact. Cardiovasc. Thorac. Surg.* **2002**, *1*, 50–51. [CrossRef]
10. Yudovsky, D.; Nouvong, A.; Pilon, L. Hyperspectral imaging in diabetic foot wound care. *J. Diabetes Sci. Technol.* **2010**, *4*, 1099–1113. [CrossRef]
11. Khaodhiar, L.; Dinh, T.; Schomacker, K.T.; Panasyuk, S.V.; Freeman, J.E.; Lew, R.; Vo, T.; Panasyuk, A.A.; Lima, C.; Giurini, J.M.; et al. The use of medical hyperspectral technology to evaluate microcirculatory changes in diabetic foot ulcers and to predict clinical outcomes. *Diabetes Care* **2007**, *30*, 903–910. [CrossRef]
12. Nouvong, A.; Hoogwerf, B.; Mohler, E.; Davis, B.; Tajaddini, A.; Medenilla, E. Evaluation of diabetic foot ulcer healing with hyperspectral imaging of oxyhemoglobin and deoxyhemoglobin. *Diabetes Care* **2009**, *32*, 2056–2061. [CrossRef] [PubMed]
13. Lu, G.; Fei, B. Medical hyperspectral imaging: A review. *J. Biomed. Opt.* **2014**, *19*, 10901. [CrossRef]
14. Calin, M.A.; Parasca, S.V.; Savastru, R.; Manea, D. Characterization of burns using hyperspectral imaging technique—A preliminary study. *Burns* **2015**, *41*, 118–124. [CrossRef]
15. Zuzak, K.J.; Schaeberle, M.D.; Lewis, E.N.; Levin, I.W. Visible reflectance hyperspectral imaging: Characterization of a noninvasive, in vivo system for determining tissue perfusion. *Anal. Chem.* **2002**, *74*, 2021–2028. [CrossRef]
16. Meier, J.K.; Prantl, L.; Muller, S.; Moralis, A.; Liebsch, G.; Gosau, M. Simple, fast and reliable perfusion monitoring of microvascular flaps. *Clin. Hemorheol. Microcirc.* **2012**, *50*, 13–24. [CrossRef] [PubMed]
17. Kulcke, A.; Holmer, A.; Wahl, P.; Siemers, F.; Wild, T.; Daeschlein, G. A compact hyperspectral camera for measurement of perfusion parameters in medicine. *Biomed. Tech.* **2018**, *63*, 519–527. [CrossRef]
18. Holmer, A.; Tetschke, F.; Marotz, J.; Malberg, H.; Markgraf, W.; Thiele, C.; Kulcke, A. Oxygenation and perfusion monitoring with a hyperspectral camera system for chemical based tissue analysis of skin and organs. *Physiol. Meas.* **2016**, *37*, 2064–2078. [CrossRef] [PubMed]
19. Marotz, J.; Siafliakis, A.; Holmer, A.; Kulcke, A.; Siemers, F. First results of a new hyperspectral camera system for chemical based wound analysis. *Wound Med.* **2015**, *10*, 17–22. [CrossRef]
20. Holmer, A.; Marotz, J.; Wahl, P.; Dau, M.; Kammerer, P.W. Hyperspectral imaging in perfusion and wound diagnostics—Methods and algorithms for the determination of tissue parameters. *Biomed. Tech.* **2018**, *63*, 547–556. [CrossRef] [PubMed]
21. Thiem, D.G.E.; Frick, R.W.; Goetze, E.; Gielisch, M.; Al-Nawas, B.; Kammerer, P.W. Hyperspectral analysis for perioperative perfusion monitoring-a clinical feasibility study on free and pedicled flaps. *Clin. Oral. Investig.* **2021**, *25*, 933–945. [CrossRef]

22. Habib, J.; Baetz, L.; Satiani, B. Assessment of collateral circulation to the hand prior to radial artery harvest. *Vasc. Med.* **2012**, *17*, 352–361. [CrossRef] [PubMed]
23. Abu-Omar, Y.; Mussa, S.; Anastasiadis, K.; Steel, S.; Hands, L.; Taggart, D.P. Duplex ultrasonography predicts safety of radial artery harvest in the presence of an abnormal Allen test. *Ann. Thorac. Surg.* **2004**, *77*, 116–119. [CrossRef]
24. Ruengsakulrach, P.; Brooks, M.; Hare, D.L.; Gordon, I.; Buxton, B.F. Preoperative assessment of hand circulation by means of Doppler ultrasonography and the modified Allen test. *J. Thorac. Cardiovasc. Surg.* **2001**, *121*, 526–531. [CrossRef]
25. Kranke, P.; Schuster, F.; Muellenbach, R.; Kranke, E.-M.; Roewer, N.; Smul, T. Grundlagen und Prinzipien klinischer Studien: Wie viele Patienten sollen (müssen) untersucht werden? Fallzahlschätzung in klinischen Studien. *Kardiotechnik* **2008**, *4*, 114–117.
26. Grambow, E.; Dau, M.; Holmer, A.; Lipp, V.; Frerich, B.; Klar, E.; Vollmar, B.; Kammerer, P.W. Hyperspectral imaging for monitoring of perfusion failure upon microvascular anastomosis in the rat hind limb. *MicroVasc. Res.* **2018**, *116*, 64–70. [CrossRef] [PubMed]
27. Baetz, L.; Satiani, B. Palmar arch identification during evaluation for radial artery harvest. *Vasc. Endovasc. Surg.* **2011**, *45*, 255–257. [CrossRef] [PubMed]
28. Nuckols, D.A.; Tsue, T.T.; Toby, E.B.; Girod, D.A. Preoperative evaluation of the radial forearm free flap patient with the objective Allen's test. *Otolaryngol. Head Neck Surg.* **2000**, *123*, 553–557. [CrossRef]
29. Coleman, S.; Anson, B. Arterial patterns in the hand based upon a study of 650 specimens. *Surg. Gynecol. Obstet.* **1961**, *113*, 409–424. [CrossRef] [PubMed]
30. Ruengsakulrach, P.; Eizenberg, N.; Fahrer, C.; Fahrer, M.; Buxton, B.F. Surgical implications of variations in hand collateral circulation: Anatomy revisited. *J. Thorac. Cardiovasc. Surg.* **2001**, *122*, 682–686. [CrossRef]
31. Loukas, M.; Holdman, D.; Holdman, S. Anatomical variations of the superficial and deep palmar arches. *Folia Morphol.* **2005**, *64*, 78–83.
32. Gellman, H.; Botte, M.J.; Shankwiler, J.; Gelberman, R.H. Arterial patterns of the deep and superficial palmar arches. *Clin. Orthop. Relat. Res.* **2001**, 41–46. [CrossRef]
33. American Cancer Society. Key Statistics for Oral Cavity and Oropharyngeal Cancers. Available online: https://www.cancer.org/cancer/oral-cavity-and-oropharyngeal-cancer/about/key-statistics.html (accessed on 8 June 2021).
34. Dietrich, M.; Marx, S.; Bruckner, T.; Nickel, F.; Muller-Stich, B.P.; Hackert, T.; Weigand, M.A.; Uhle, F.; Brenner, T.; Schmidt, K. Bedside hyperspectral imaging for the evaluation of microcirculatory alterations in perioperative intensive care medicine: A study protocol for an observational clinical pilot study (HySpI-ICU). *BMJ Open* **2020**, *10*, e035742. [CrossRef]
35. Grambow, E.; Dau, M.; Sandkuhler, N.A.; Leuchter, M.; Holmer, A.; Klar, E.; Weinrich, M. Evaluation of peripheral artery disease with the TIVITA(R) Tissue hyperspectral imaging camera system. *Clin. Hemorheol. Microcirc.* **2019**, *73*, 3–17. [CrossRef] [PubMed]
36. Schulz, T.; Marotz, J.; Stukenberg, A.; Reumuth, G.; Houschyar, K.S.; Siemers, F. Hyperspectral imaging for postoperative flap monitoring of pedicled flaps. *Handchir. Mikrochir. Plast. Chir.* **2020**, *52*, 316–324. [CrossRef] [PubMed]
37. Sucher, R.; Wagner, T.; Kohler, H.; Sucher, E.; Guice, H.; Recknagel, S.; Lederer, A.; Hau, H.M.; Rademacher, S.; Schneeberger, S.; et al. Hyperspectral imaging (HSI) of human kidney allografts. *Ann. Surg.* **2020**. [CrossRef] [PubMed]
38. Jansen-Winkeln, B.; Holfert, N.; Kohler, H.; Moulla, Y.; Takoh, J.P.; Rabe, S.M.; Mehdorn, M.; Barberio, M.; Chalopin, C.; Neumuth, T.; et al. Determination of the transection margin during colorectal resection with hyperspectral imaging (HSI). *Int. J. Colorectal Dis.* **2019**, *34*, 731–739. [CrossRef] [PubMed]
39. Mehdorn, M.; Kohler, H.; Rabe, S.M.; Niebisch, S.; Lyros, O.; Chalopin, C.; Gockel, I.; Jansen-Winkeln, B. Hyperspectral Imaging (HSI) in acute mesenteric ischemia to detect intestinal perfusion deficits. *J. Surg. Res.* **2020**, *254*, 7–15. [CrossRef]
40. Muhle, R.; Ernst, H.; Sobottka, S.B.; Morgenstern, U. Workflow and hardware for intraoperative hyperspectral data acquisition in neurosurgery. *Biomed. Tech.* **2020**. [CrossRef]

*Article*

# Free Myocutaneous Flap Assessment in a Rat Model: Verification of a Wireless Bioelectrical Impedance Assessment (BIA) System for Vascular Compromise Following Microsurgery

Yao-Kuang Huang [1], Min Yi Wong [1,2], Chi-Rung Wu [2], Yung-Ze Cheng [3] and Bor-Shyh Lin [2,3,*]

[1] Division of Thoracic and Cardiovascular Surgery, Chia Yi Chang Gung Memorial Hospital, College of Medicine, Chia-Yi and Chang Gung University, Taoyuan 33302, Taiwan; huang137@icloud.com (Y.-K.H.); mynyy001@gmail.com (M.Y.W.)
[2] Institute of Imaging and Biomedical Photonics, National Yang Ming Chiao Tung University, Tainan 71150, Taiwan; luck511286@gmail.com
[3] Department of Medical Research, Chi-Mei Medical Center, Tainan 71004, Taiwan; asaliea.cheng@gmail.com
* Correspondence: borshyhlin@gmail.com

**Abstract:** Background: Microvascular tissue transfer is a common reconstructive procedure. We designed a bioelectrical impedance assessment (BIA) system for quantitative analysis of tissue status. This study attempts to verify it through the animal model. Methods: The flaps of the rat model were monitored by the BIA system. Results: The BIA variation of the free flap in the rat after the vascular compromise was recorded. The non-vascular ligation limbs of the same rat served as a control group. The bio-impedance in the experimental group was larger than the control group. The bio-impedances of both the **thigh/feet** flaps in the experimental group were increased over time. In the **thigh**, the difference in bio-impedance from the control group was first detected at 10 kHz at the 3rd and last at 1 kHz at the 6th h, after vascular compromise. The same finding was observed in the **feet**. Compared with the control group, the bio-impedance ratio (1 kHz/20 kHz) of the experimental group decreased with time, while their variation tendencies in the thigh and feet were similar. Conclusions: The flap may be monitored by the BIA for vascular status.

**Keywords:** flap grafting; microsurgery; biosensor; bioelectrical impedance; rat

## 1. Introduction

Free tissue transfer by microsurgery is a commonly performed procedure within reconstructive surgery [1–3]. Using the autograft method, microvascular free tissue transfer can effectively rescue lethal surgical complications [3,4]. Monitoring of perfusion status, detection of thrombus formation within the capillaries after microsurgery and timely rescue of the flap are the crucial elements that contribute to a perfect free skin flap surgery. Physicians often observe variations in the flap edge, flap color and flap flexibility and use their previous experience to evaluate the state of the flap [5,6]. However, there are no objective parameters to help the physician make a correct judgement.

Measuring the surface temperature of grafted skin flaps is the simplest way of monitoring skin flap grafting. Physicians used skin temperature indicators to conduct free flap monitoring [7]. When the center location of the skin dropped by more than 3 °C from the baseline, it might have encountered arterial thrombosis. However, the sensitivity for monitoring the surface temperature of skin flap grafts is not high enough [8]. Several pieces of equipment, such as the Doppler ultrasound, a microdialysis system, a tissue pH monitoring system, laser Doppler flowmetry and color Duplex sonography, have been previously used to evaluate skin flaps [7–9]. The Doppler ultrasound device and the color Duplex sonograph can monitor blood flow within the transferred flaps to indirectly evaluate their condition. The microdialysis system is based on a perfusion sampling and dialysis technique that estimates free transverse rectus abdominis myocutaneous (TRAM) flaps [9].

Partial ischemia in free TRAM flaps could be indirectly estimated through variations in glucose, glycerol and lactate concentrations. The tissue pH monitoring system indirectly estimates the failure of free flaps and vascular complications using variations in pH that are caused by blockages in the artery. Laser Doppler flowmetry and tissue spectrophotometry use blood flow parameters and oxygen saturation to distinguish between blocked arteries and venous congestion [10]. Although the above methods could help the physician evaluate the condition of flaps, most of them are invasive and expensive and require the operator to be experienced.

Bioelectrical impedance analysis (BIA) has been developed to evaluate changes in human tissue composition and animal experiments [11]. The basic concept of BIA is to inject a current with different frequencies into the tissue to estimate the whole bio-impedance of the human tissue, which is contributed to by the bio-impedances of the different human tissue components [12,13]. It is a non-invasive measurement and can be used to monitor changes in human tissue composition in real-time.

The advantages of BIA are that it is non-invasive and provides real-time measurements, and it could have the potential as a helpful tool for evaluating the status of tissue flaps after microsurgery. In the current study, physiological parameters were monitored using the BIA technique to measure changes in bio-impedance and to verify the effectiveness of BIA in a rat model.

## 2. Materials and Methods

### 2.1. Bioelectrical Impedance Analysis

When an electrical current passes through different types of human cells or tissues (fluids, adipose, muscles, etc.), these tissues have different levels of conductivity due to the different numbers of electrolytes in them. In general, adipose tissue and bone have poorer conductivity, whereas fluids and muscles provide better conductivity. Lower frequency electrical currents have difficulty penetrating the cell membrane when they pass through a biological cell (i.e., most of the electrical current passes through the extracellular cell). Higher frequency bio-impedance may give more information on the intracellular and extracellular fluid [14]. Multiple-frequency BIA can be easily classified into several different frequency bands: the alpha domain (1~10 kHz), the beta domain (10~50 kHz) and the gamma domain (>100 kHz) [15]. Bio-impedance in the alpha domain may be associated with information on tissue interfaces, while the beta domain is associated with the polarization of cellular membranes, proteins and other organic macromolecules. Bio-impedance in the gamma domain may be associated with the polarization of water molecules [16]. Bio-impedance in the alpha and beta domains is most frequently used because the differences between normal and pathological tissues can be observed in their variations. Therefore, the change in the health of the flap may be effectively observed by the bio-impedance measurement in the alpha and beta domains.

Bio-impedance systems typically use a voltage-controlled current source, such as a Howland current source, to inject a known current into the tissue primarily for safety purposes but also to eliminate the need to measure the injected current into the tissue. In addition, safety limits according to international standards have been set with regards to currents into tissues: 100 µA from 0.1 Hz to 1 kHz, 100f µA from 1 to 100 kHz, and 10 mA for frequencies greater than 100 kHz, where f is the frequency in kHz. A 5 µA can be beneficial in terms of power consumption but maybe not that great for the signal-to-noise ratio. The self-assembled bio-impedance parameter monitoring device used in the current study is shown in Figure 1a. The bio-impedance parameter monitoring device was designed to measure tissue bio-impedance signals. The back-end host system was designed to analyze the raw data and to estimate, display and store the bio-impedance parameters. To ensure no damage or pain was caused, the current passing through the biological tissue was <5 µA. The excitation buffer can provide 2.5 Vp-p steady excitation voltage, and the reference resistance is set to about 5 M ohm. Therefore, the injected current will be limited below 5 uA. The block diagram for the bio-impedance parameter monitoring device is shown in Figure 1b. It mainly contains a microprocessor, a wireless transmission circuit, a steady voltage source circuit, a voltage divider circuit, a voltage acquisition circuit and a probe. The cost of this system is 200 USD.

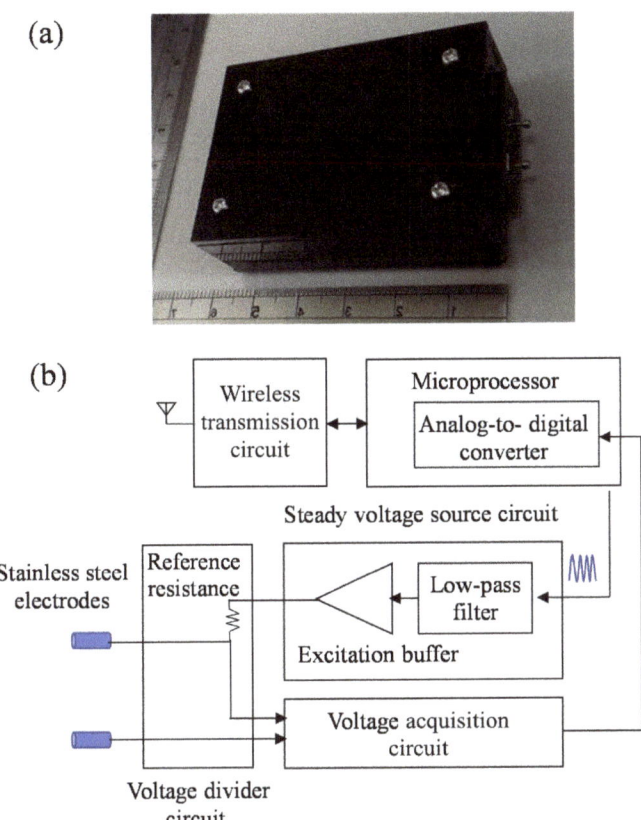

Figure 1. (a) Photograph and (b) block diagram of the self-assembled bio-impedance parameter monitoring device.

For functional bio-impedance analysis, the steady voltage source circuit was designed to provide a steady voltage with a specific frequency ranging from 1 to 20 kHz, which can be controlled by the microprocessor. The cut-off frequency of the low-pass filter in the steady voltage source circuit was set to 25 kHz. The generated steady voltage will then pass through the voltage divider circuit and the stainless-steel electrodes. The pair of stainless-steel electrodes will be placed on the region of tissue being measured. When generated, the steady voltage passes through the tissue via the electrodes and will then be attenuated due to tissue bio-impedance. The voltage acquisition circuit then receives the attenuated steady voltage signal and estimates the bio-impedance of the tissue. The gain of the voltage acquisition circuit is adjustable and can be set to 1, 2, 5 or 10. The sampling rate of the analog-to-digital converter in the microprocessor is set to 200 kHz. Under the consideration of simple operation and implementation of the designed device, bipolar measurement is used in this study. In bipolar measurement, the electrode interface impedance may cause the contributor in the measured impedance. Under the same measurement condition, the relative impedance change caused by the change in the health of the flap was monitored. Here, the distance between the two electrodes is set to 10 mm. Because the thickness of the flaps is about 1–3 mm, the measuring depth of the designed device should be sufficient.

Here, the shape of the used electrodes is a round tip needle, and it can reduce the risk of injuring the flaps. The used electrodes are made of stainless steel can improve the issue of metal oxidation.

## 2.2. Animal Experiment Design and Procedure

In the animal experiment, adult male Sprague Dawley albino rats with a weight of 325 ± 25 g were used. The experimental procedure was approved by the Animal Care and Use Committee of Chi-Mei Medical Center to minimize the discomfort to the animals during the study period. All rats were kept in a temperature-controlled air-conditioned room (23 ± 2 °C) for at least 7 days before this experiment began and were maintained in a 12-h light/dark cycle. After the experiment, all rats were sacrificed using urethane. During the experiment, all rats were first anesthetized by intraperitoneal injection with ketamine, and their hair was trimmed using a razor blade. Then, the right thigh of the animal was surgically dissected, and its muscles, nerves and skin tissue were all divided; their vascular pedicle was isolated but not transected. The left thigh of the animal that did not undergo surgery was still able to supply blood and nutrition from the femoral vessels and was used as the control group (Figure 2). Next, the skin on the right thighs was sutured, and probes from the BIA system were attached to both limbs. After the BIA system started to record, the right vascular pedicles were ligated. The BIA system probes were placed on the thighs of the animal to acquire the bio-impedance every hour using a self-assembling holder to stabilize the probe on the target surface. The total length of the experimental procedure was >8 h.

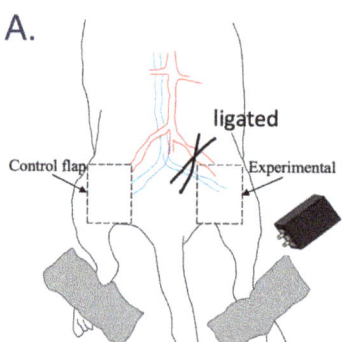
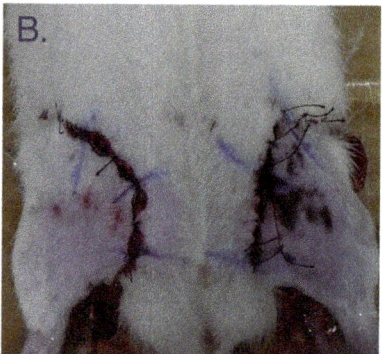

**Figure 2.** (**A**) A visualized experimental protocol. (**B**) Skin repair before measurement.

Six same reparative manipulations were done in rats. Power analysis is listed in Table 1. One-way analysis of variance (ANOVA) was used to analyze the experimental results, and $p < 0.05$ was considered to indicate a significant difference.

**Table 1.** Post hoc power analysis for comparing two group means.

| Group | Impact Region | 1 kHz | 5 kHz | 10 kHz | 20 kHz |
|---|---|---|---|---|---|
| Experimental group | Thigh | 28.60% | 50.90% | 81.40% | 45.40% |
|  | Feet | 31.40% | 40.50% | 91.60% | 3.30% |
| Control group |  |  |  |  |  |

Post hoc was estimated using the means and standard derivation and the sample size of each group ($n = 6$). The control group was defined as group 1, and the experimental group was defined as group 2. The significance level of alpha was defined as 0.05.

## 3. Results

The bio-impedance variation of the skin flap after surgery was investigated. The bio-impedances of both the thigh and feet skin flaps in the experimental group were clearly increased over time. Figures 3 and 4 show the time courses of the average bio-impedance in the thigh and feet skin flaps for the different frequencies. The average bio-impedances were obtained from six separate experimental trials. The standard deviation of the bio-impedance in the experimental group was significantly larger than the control group. In the thigh, the difference in bio-impedance from the control group was first detected at 10 kHz (Figure 3c) at the 3rd h and last detected at 1 kHz (Figure 3a) at the 6th h, after vascular compromise. The same finding was observed in the feet. (earliest in 10 Hz at the 3rd h and latest in 1 Hz at the 6th h). Moreover, with the increase in time, the difference between the bio-impedances of the thigh and feet flaps for the control and experimental groups also significantly increased. Figure 5 shows the average bio-impedance ratio (1/20 kHz). Compared with the control group, the bio-impedance ratio of the experimental group decreased with time, while their variation tendencies in the thigh and feet were similar.

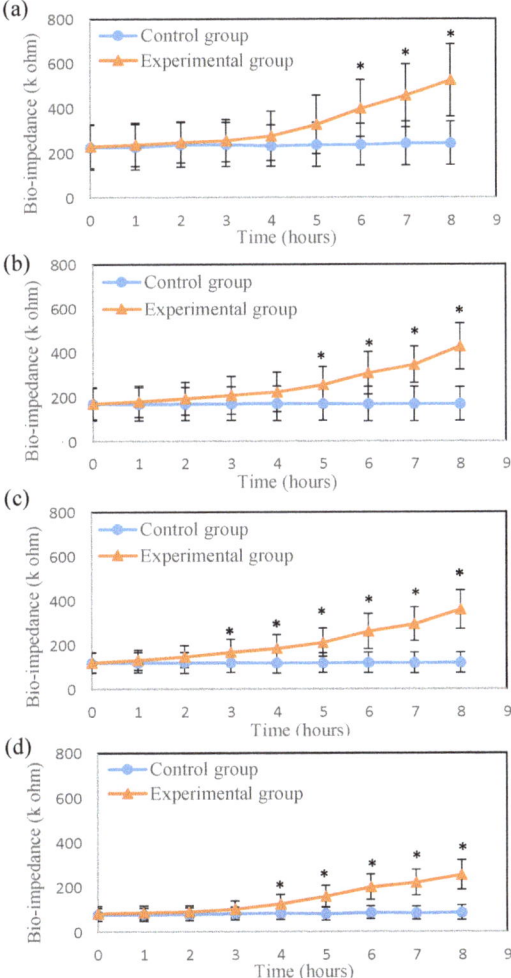

**Figure 3.** The time course of (**a**) 1 kHz, (**b**) 5 kHz, (**c**) 10 kHz and (**d**) 20 kHz average bio-impedance in the **thigh** flaps (* $p < 0.05$).

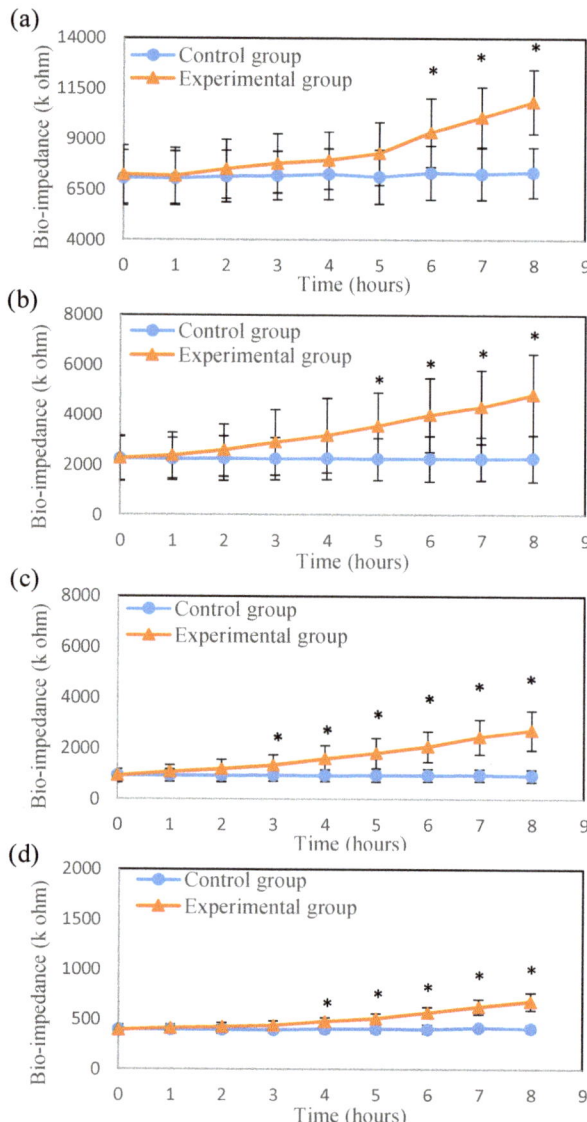

**Figure 4.** The time course of (**a**) 1 kHz, (**b**) 5 kHz, (**c**) 10 kHz and (**d**) 20 kHz average bio-impedance in the **feet** flaps (* $p < 0.05$).

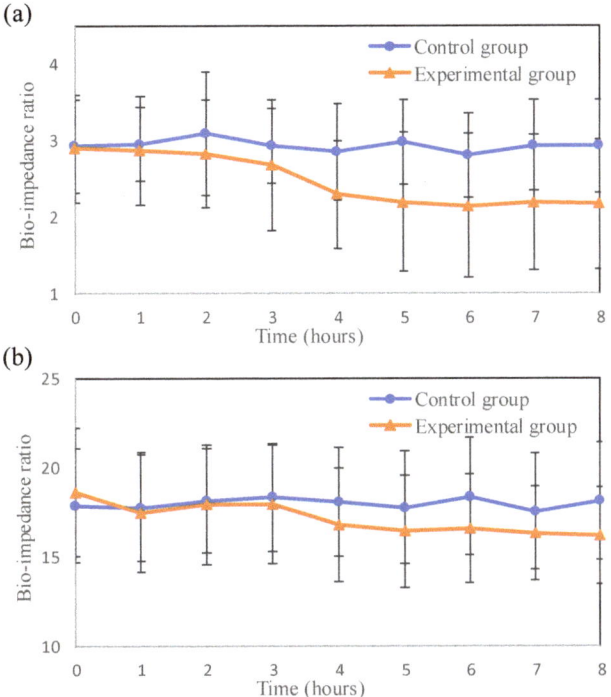

**Figure 5.** (**a**) Time course of the average bio-impedance ratio (1 kHz/20 kHz) in the **thigh**. (**b**) The time course of the average bio-impedance ratio (1 kHz/20 kHz) in the **feet**.

## 4. Discussion

Free tissue transfer by microsurgery is a meticulous procedure for reconstructive surgery following cancer or trauma. The first 48 h after surgery are critical for identifying and salvaging a failing flap. Most clinical teams can only provide routine spot checks on patients with the overwhelming workload. Therefore, continuous monitoring can reduce the flap failing rate. Some devices have been developed for continuous monitoring of tissue flaps after surgery, guts perfusion and myocardium by measuring microvascular parameters [11,13,17,18].

Our study demonstrated that after free flap ischemia after vascular compromise, the bio-impedances of the experimental group gradually increased over time. Metabolically active tissues can encounter a lack of oxygen and nutrition, which can cause severe ischemic injuries [19]. When ischemic injuries exceed the tolerance level of flap cells, the flaps will be destroyed [20,21]. Previous studies have indicated that hypoxia-ischemia directly affects the change in tissue bio-impedance and causes an increase in tissue bio-impedance [22–24].

The bio-impedance decreased as the frequency increased. This is because higher frequency currents have a better penetrating ability in tissue, as shown in Figures 3 and 4. When the frequency of the electrical current increases, it penetrates not only the extracellular fluid but also the cell membrane and intracellular fluid [25,26]. At 1 and 5 kHz bio-impedance, the experimental group was significantly different from the control group for 5 h after surgery. At 10 and 20 kHz bio-impedance, the bio-impedance of the experimental group was significantly different from the control group for 3 h after surgery. This also indicates that higher frequency bio-impedance (at about beta domain) may be more sensitive to tissue changes after perfusion compromise of skin flaps grafts. In Figure 5, the average bio-impedance ratio (1/20 kHz) decreased with time after surgical occlusion of the vessels. When ischemic injuries occur, extracellular fluid flowing into intracellular fluid results in an increase in capacitive reactance and resistance [13,18]. However, high-frequency currents have better penetration and can provide more sensitive results associated with skin flap necrosis in deeper tissue. Therefore, compared with the control group, the average bio-impedance ratio of the experimental group decreased with time, and the differences between the groups were higher in the thigh (proximal part of the flap near the vessel stalk) than in feet (Figure 5).

Several techniques, such as pH monitoring, microdialysis and laser Doppler flowmetry, might also be used to enhance survival following skin flap grafting. In 1996, WJ Issing et al. used a pH monitoring system to evaluate skin flap viability [27]. The pH monitoring system, which can be used to estimate the degree of ischemia, has to plant a pH microelectrode into the tissue, and then the pH value will change as the biological tissue becomes ischemic [28]. The pH monitoring system has low complexity, is not expensive and provides real-time data. However, the device is invasive (probe insertion into the flap). The microdialysis system can also be used to analyze the ratio of lactate to pyruvic acid in the cell substance to determine the degree of hypoxia-ischemia and is thus a useful tool for monitoring the viability of free flaps [29,30]. In 2016, L Liasis et al. also used the microdialysis system to evaluate the ischemic condition of limbs in patients with diabetes mellitus after amputation [31]. Although the microdialysis system is accurate, it is expensive and invasive and is not suitable for long-term free flap monitoring. Moreover, the microdialysis system requires an experienced operator to conduct the monitoring. Laser Doppler flowmetry is also used in the clinic to estimate the blood flow value. From the variation in blood flow rate, the physician can indirectly evaluate the state of the grafted skin flap [8]. This method is non-invasive but is highly dependent on the experience of the operator. Our BIA system is non-invasive and gives a fast response for detecting the state of the grafted flap; it was easy to use in this rat model. It is potentially useful in a clinical setting after microsurgery with free flaps. However, the change in this BIA after vascular complication is a minimum of 3 h; thus, the system has no sufficient clinical impact yet. Combination with the other bio-signals, for example, near-infrared spectrum, may increase its clinical usability further.

## 5. Conclusions

This BIA system was validated in this animal experiment for its usefulness in monitoring the vascularity and tissue status of grafted flaps. In the experimental group (transected femoral vessels in the groin to stop the blood supply to the flaps), the bio-impedance values of the flaps were significantly increased over time. Higher frequency electrical currents can better penetrate the tissue and are more stable. The 10 kHz detected the bio-impedance difference earliest (3rd h), and the 1 kHz detected the latest bio-impedance difference between the experimental group and the control group after vascular compromise.

**Author Contributions:** Conceptualization, Y.-K.H. and Y.-Z.C.; methodology, C.-R.W. and B.-S.L.; software, B.-S.L.; validation, Y.-K.H., M.Y.W. and B.-S.L.; formal analysis, B.-S.L.; investigation, B.-S.L.; resources, Y.-K.H.; writing—original draft preparation, Y.-Z.C. and B.-S.L.; writing—review and editing, B.-S.L.; visualization, B.-S.L.; supervision, B.-S.L.; funding acquisition, Y.-K.H., Y.-Z.C., C.-R.W. and B.-S.L. All authors have read and agreed to the published version of the manuscript.

**Funding:** This research was partly supported by Ministry of Science and Technology in Taiwan, under grants MOST 108-2221-E-009-054-MY2). This research was also partly supported by the Higher Education Sprout Project of the National Yang Ming Chiao Tung University and Ministry of Education (MOE), Taiwan, the Research Funding by Chi Mei Medical Center, Taiwan. The present study was also partly supported by the Chang Gung Medical Foundation of Taiwan (grant no. CORP G6E0111, CORP G6E0112 and CORP G6E0113).

**Institutional Review Board Statement:** All of the experimental procedures conformed to the guidelines of the National Institute of Health, Taiwan, and were approved by the Animal Care and Use Committee of Chi-Mei Medical Center (IACUC approval No 1040810001).

**Acknowledgments:** The authors thank the Chi-Mei Medical Center, Tainan, Taiwan for their instrumental support.

**Conflicts of Interest:** The authors declare no conflict of interest.

## References

1. el-Gammal, T.A.; Wei, F.C. Microvascular reconstruction of the distal digits by partial toe transfer. *Clin. Plast Surg.* **1997**, *24*, 49–55. [CrossRef]
2. Chen, H.C.; Tang, Y.B.; Chuang, D.; Wei, F.C.; Noordhoff, M.S. Microvascular free posterior interosseous flap and a comparison with the pedicled posterior interosseous flap. *Ann. Plast Surg.* **1996**, *36*, 542–550. [CrossRef] [PubMed]
3. Chen, H.C.; Mosely, L.H.; Tang, Y.B.; Wei, F.C.; Noordhoff, M.S. Difficult reconstruction of an extensive injury in the lower extremity with a large cross-leg microvascular composite-tissue flap containing fibula. *Plast Reconstr. Surg.* **1989**, *83*, 723–727. [CrossRef]
4. Tukiainen, E.; Popov, P.; Asko-Seljavaara, S. Microvascular reconstructions of full-thickness oncological chest wall defects. *Ann. Surg.* **2003**, *238*, 794–801. [CrossRef]
5. Lutz, B.S.; Ng, S.H.; Cabailo, R.; Lin, C.H.; Wei, F.C. Value of routine angiography before traumatic lower-limb reconstruction with microvascular free tissue transplantation. *J. Trauma* **1998**, *44*, 682–686. [CrossRef] [PubMed]
6. Kroll, S.S.; Schusterman, M.A.; Reece, G.P.; Miller, M.J.; Evans, G.R.; Robb, G.L.; Baldwin, B.J. Timing of pedicle thrombosis and flap loss after free-tissue transfer. *Plast. Reconstr. Surg.* **1996**, *98*, 1230–1233. [CrossRef]
7. Chiu, E.S.; Altman, A.; Allen, R.J., Jr.; Allen, R.J., Sr. Free flap monitoring using skin temperature strip indicators: Adjunct to clinical examination. *Plast. Reconstr. Surg.* **2008**, *122*, 144e–145e. [CrossRef]
8. Khouri, R.K.; Shaw, W.W. Monitoring of free flaps with surface-temperature recordings: Is it reliable? *Plast Reconstr. Surg.* **1992**, *89*, 495–499. [CrossRef]
9. Edsander-Nord, A.; Rojdmark, J.; Wickman, M. Metabolism in pedicled and free TRAM flaps: A comparison using the microdialysis technique. *Plast. Reconstr. Surg.* **2002**, *109*, 664–673. [CrossRef] [PubMed]
10. Mucke, T.; Rau, A.; Merezas, A.; Loeffelbein, D.J.; Wagenpfeil, S.; Mitchell, D.A.; Wolff, K.D.; Steiner, T. Identification of perioperative risk factor by laser-doppler spectroscopy after free flap perfusion in the head and neck: A prospective clinical study. *Microsurgery* **2014**, *34*, 345–351. [CrossRef] [PubMed]
11. Wtorek, J.; Jozefiak, L.; Polinski, A.; Siebert, J. An averaging two-electrode probe for monitoring changes in myocardial conductivity evoked by ischemia. *IEEE Trans. Biomed. Eng.* **2002**, *49*, 240–246. [CrossRef] [PubMed]
12. Kyle, U.G.; Bosaeus, I.; De Lorenzo, A.D.; Deurenberg, P.; Elia, M.; Gomez, J.M.; Heitmann, B.L.; Kent-Smith, L.; Melchior, J.C.; Pirlich, M.; et al. Bioelectrical impedance analysis—Part I: Review of principles and methods. *Clin. Nutr.* **2004**, *23*, 1226–1243. [CrossRef] [PubMed]
13. Berthelot, M.; Yang, G.Z.; Lo, B. A Self-Calibrated Tissue Viability Sensor for Free Flap Monitoring. *IEEE J. Biomed. Health Inform.* **2018**, *22*, 5–14. [CrossRef] [PubMed]
14. Steijaert, M.; Deurenberg, P.; Van Gaal, L.; De Leeuw, I. The use of multi-frequency impedance to determine total body water and extracellular water in obese and lean female individuals. *Int. J. Obes. Relat. Metab. Disord.* **1997**, *21*, 930–934. [CrossRef]
15. Schwan, H.P. Electrical properties of tissue and cell suspensions. *Adv. Biol. Med. Phys.* **1957**, *5*, 147–209. [CrossRef]
16. Dean, D.A.; Ramanathan, T.; Machado, D.; Sundararajan, R. Electrical Impedance Spectroscopy Study of Biological Tissues. *J Electrostat* **2008**, *66*, 165–177. [CrossRef]
17. Tahirbegi, I.B.; Mir, M.; Schostek, S.; Schurr, M.; Samitier, J. In vivo ischemia monitoring array for endoscopic surgery. *Biosens. Bioelectron.* **2014**, *61*, 124–130. [CrossRef]
18. Lingwood, B.E.; Dunster, K.R.; Colditz, P.B.; Ward, L.C. Noninvasive measurement of cerebral bioimpedance for detection of cerebral edema in the neonatal piglet. *Brain Res.* **2002**, *945*, 97–105. [CrossRef]
19. Briggs, S.E.; Banis, J.C., Jr.; Kaebnick, H.; Silverberg, B.; Acland, R.D. Distal revascularization and microvascular free tissue transfer: An alternative to amputation in ischemic lesions of the lower extremity. *J. Vasc. Surg.* **1985**, *2*, 806–811. [CrossRef]
20. Gurlek, A.; Kroll, S.S.; Schusterman, M.A. Ischemic time and free flap success. *Ann. Plast. Surg.* **1997**, *38*, 503–505. [CrossRef]
21. Keller, A. Noninvasive tissue oximetry for flap monitoring: An initial study. *J. Reconstr. Microsurg.* **2007**, *23*, 189–197. [CrossRef] [PubMed]
22. Ahn, H.; Shin, H.; Yun, S.; Kim, J.; Choi, J. Measurement of bioimpedance and cell viability during ischemia-reperfusion in the rat liver. *Conf. Proc. IEEE Eng. Med. Biol. Soc.* **2005**, *2005*, 1945–1947. [CrossRef] [PubMed]
23. Gomez, R.; Ivorra, A.; Villa, R.; Godignon, P.; Millan, J.; Erill, I.; Sola, A.; Hotter, G.; Palacios, L. A SiC microdevice for the minimally invasive monitoring of ischemia in living tissues. *Biomed. Microdevices.* **2006**, *8*, 43–49. [CrossRef] [PubMed]
24. Ivorra, A.; Gomez, R.; Noguera, N.; Villa, R.; Sola, A.; Palacios, L.; Hotter, G.; Aguilo, J. Minimally invasive silicon probe for electrical impedance measurements in small animals. *Biosens. Bioelectron.* **2003**, *19*, 391–399. [CrossRef]
25. Kun, S.; Ristic, B.; Peura, R.A.; Dunn, R.M. Algorithm for tissue ischemia estimation based on electrical impedance spectroscopy. *IEEE Trans. Biomed. Eng.* **2003**, *50*, 1352–1359. [CrossRef]
26. Gabriel, S.; Lau, R.W.; Gabriel, C. The dielectric properties of biological tissues: II. Measurements in the frequency range 10 Hz to 20 GHz. *Phys. Med. Biol.* **1996**, *41*, 2251–2269. [CrossRef]
27. Issing, W.J.; Naumann, C. Evaluation of pedicled skin flap viability by pH, temperature and fluorescein: An experimental study. *J. Craniomaxillofac. Surg.* **1996**, *24*, 305–309. [CrossRef]

28. Schepel, S.J.; Koning, G.; Oeseburg, B.; Langbroek, A.J.; Zijlstra, W.G. Performance of a pH monitoring system in vivo. *Med. Biol. Eng. Comput.* **1987**, *25*, 63–67. [CrossRef]
29. Rojdmark, J.; Heden, P.; Ungerstedt, U. Prediction of border necrosis in skin flaps of pigs with microdialysis. *J. Reconstr. Microsurg.* **2000**, *16*, 129–134. [CrossRef]
30. Rojdmark, J.; Blomqvist, L.; Malm, M.; Adams-Ray, B.; Ungerstedt, U. Metabolism in myocutaneous flaps studied by in situ microdialysis. *Scand J. Plast. Reconstr. Surg. Hand. Surg.* **1998**, *32*, 27–34. [CrossRef]
31. Liasis, L.; Malietzis, G.; Galyfos, G.; Athanasiou, T.; Papaconstantinou, H.T.; Sigala, F.; Zografos, G.; Filis, K. The emerging role of microdialysis in diabetic patients undergoing amputation for limb ischemia. *Wound Repair Regen.* **2016**, *24*, 1073–1080. [CrossRef] [PubMed]

MDPI
St. Alban-Anlage 66
4052 Basel
Switzerland
Tel. +41 61 683 77 34
Fax +41 61 302 89 18
www.mdpi.com

*Journal of Personalized Medicine* Editorial Office
E-mail: jpm@mdpi.com
www.mdpi.com/journal/jpm

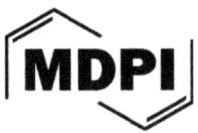